I0885431

Chatbots and Mental Healthcare in Psychology and Psychiatry

Kadir Uludag
Shanghai Jiao Tong University, China

Nafees Ahmad
Central South University, China

IGI Global
Scientific Publishing
Publishing Tomorrow's Research Today

Published in the United States of America by
IGI Global Scientific Publishing
701 East Chocolate Avenue
Hershey, PA, 17033, USA
Tel: 717-533-8845
Fax: 717-533-8661
Website: https://www.igi-global.com E-mail: cust@igi-global.com

Library of Congress Cataloging-in-Publication Data

Names: Uludağ, Kadir, 1994- editor. | Ahmad, Nafees, 1987- editor.
Title: Chatbots and mental healthcare in psychology and psychiatry / edited by: Kadir Uludag, Nafees Ahmad.
Description: Hershey PA : IGI Global Scientific Publishing, [2025] | Includes bibliographical references. | Summary: "The objective of this book is to examine the transformative impact of chatbots in the field of mental health"-- Provided by publisher.
Identifiers: LCCN 2024047673 (print) | LCCN 2024047674 (ebook) | ISBN 9798369331125 (hardcover) | ISBN 9798337300924 (paperback) | ISBN 9798369331132 (ebook)
Subjects: LCSH: Mental health services--Technological innovations. | Artificial intelligence--Medical applications. | Chatbots.
Classification: LCC RA790.5 .C538 2025 (print) | LCC RA790.5 (ebook) | DDC 362.20285--dc23/eng/20250207
LC record available at https://lccn.loc.gov/2024047673
LC ebook record available at https://lccn.loc.gov/2024047674

British Cataloguing in Publication Data
A Cataloguing in Publication record for this book is available from the British Library.

Table of Contents

Detailed Table of Contents

Artificial intelligence has allowed programmers to create human-like meaningful texts. As a result, chatbots have recently gained great attention. Many people have praised how novel chat applications can create original and human-like essays. However, few studies discuss the use of AI chatbots in psychology. The authors aimed to discuss the use of AI chatbots in the field of Psychology. Also, they summarize previous studies on ChatGPT. This chapter discusses how AI can be used in this process. They used ChatGPT to create a brief literature review to show the progress of the OpenAI ChatGPT AI application. Studies on Pubmed were searched. Overall, the authors found eight studies using the keyword of "ChatGPT." Most studies claim that ChatGPT can write original essays, and it is hard to distinguish ChatGPT from human-like writing. They found no study discussing the impact of ChatGPT on psychology. ChatGPT can allow writing essays on various topics and be used in many fields, including psychology, medicine, engineering, philosophy, medical education, literature, and computer sciences.

Artificial intelligence (AI) offers significant potential for enhancing mental healthcare. Its ability to detect patterns in vast datasets can reveal insights into risk factors and symptoms, aiding the creation of tailored treatment plans. As an emerging research field, AI faces numerous challenges, particularly in its practical application. AI tools provide additional support for therapy and patient interaction. However, they cannot substitute the expertise of mental health professionals. AI's role in crisis intervention is promising but requires extensive validation to confirm its reliability and effectiveness. The ethical considerations of AI in mental health are complex, demanding careful scrutiny of its impact. This chapter examines AI's intersection with mental health, evaluating AI's practical efficacy and the ethical concerns it raises. The discussion presents a comprehensive perspective on mental healthcare's

As chatbots gain prominence across diverse fields, including education, their static knowledge base poses limitations. This study investigates the utilization of an internet wizard to enhance the knowledge base of an open-domain question-answering chatbot. The proposed approach leverages search engines, particularly Google, and their features, such as feature snippets, knowledge graph, and organic search, by integrating data science and natural language models. This enables the chatbot to access real-time and up-to-date answers from web documents, providing dynamic responses to user queries. A pilot study in higher education assessed the chatbot's mechanism and features, demonstrating its ability to generate responses across a wide range of educational and non-educational topics, supported by positive feedback and user satisfaction. The chatbot's dynamic feature of retrieving related or follow-up questions from search engines significantly enhances student engagement and facilitates exploration of additional information beyond the curriculum.

ChatGPT is a large language model trained on a vast amount of text and can generate human-like responses to natural language queries. However, the extent to which ChatGPT can be considered a creative system is still unclear. There is a need to develop methods to test the creativity of ChatGPT and assess its potential for generating novel and valuable responses. In this study, the authors have only focused on the creativity of ChatGPT in the field of psychology. In this study, they asked questions for testing the creativity of ChatGPT. They used a combination of quantitative and qualitative methods to evaluate the creative potential of ChatGPT. They assessed the novelty and usefulness of ChatGPT-generated responses. However, it is not clear how to assess the novelty of ChatGPT. The results suggest that ChatGPT has the potential to generate creative responses. Additionally, the responses generated by ChatGPT were found to be similar in quality to those developed by human experts in certain domains. ChatGPT could produce texts by logic without directly citing previous texts.

AI's integration into mental healthcare has opened new frontiers in the diagnosis, treatment, and management of mental disorders. This leap brings with it a host of ethical considerations. This chapter provides an analysis of the ethical dimensions of AI interventions in mental healthcare, examining the implications for patient autonomy, privacy, and the integrity of the therapeutic relationship. It discusses the challenges of ensuring informed consent in the context of complex AI systems, the risks of algorithmic bias, its impact on equitable care, and the importance of maintaining confidentiality in the face of expansive data requirements. The chapter also explores the need for transparent AI algorithms that can be scrutinized and understood by both practitioners and patients. Furthermore, it addresses the ethical responsibility of AI developers and healthcare providers to prevent harm and ensure the beneficence of AI applications. By highlighting these ethical issues, the chapter aims to foster a responsible approach to the development and deployment of AI interventions.

The ethical considerations surrounding chatbots extend well beyond simple functionality, touching on nuanced areas of trust, societal impact, and moral responsibility. Chatbots frequently handle sensitive user data, such as personal information, financial details, or health records. This raises significant privacy and data security concerns. Developers must ensure that data collection adheres to stringent standards, such as those outlined in the General Data Protection Regulation (GDPR) or other privacy regulations. Any misuse, such as sharing data with third parties without consent, undermines user trust and poses legal and ethical dilemmas. The importance of encryption, secure servers, and transparent data handling policies cannot be overstated in mitigating these risks. Here the authors discuss some ethical aspects such as bias in chatbot algorithms, transparency, accountability, and emotional impact.

Preface

In an era where digital technology is seamlessly woven into the fabric of daily life, the intersection of chatbots and mental healthcare stands at the forefront of innovation in psychology and psychiatry. Once limited to basic customer service functions, chatbots have evolved into sophisticated digital entities capable of engaging in meaningful human interactions. With the rapid advancements in artificial intelligence (AI) and natural language processing (NLP), these digital agents are increasingly being designed to support mental health initiatives, enhance therapeutic interventions, and facilitate behavioral change.

This book delves into the complex and evolving relationship between chatbots and psychological practice, shedding light on their expanding role in mental healthcare. We explore how chatbots are being developed to provide psychological support, assist in therapy, and serve as educational and behavioral tools. By analyzing the principles that underpin effective chatbot design—such as empathy, rapport-building, and conversational adaptability—we uncover the ways in which these technologies can be optimized to create more engaging and impactful interactions.

CHAPTER OVERVIEWS

Chapter 1: The Use of AI-Supported Chatbots in Psychology

This chapter explores the growing role of AI chatbots in psychology, assessing their ability to generate human-like text and their potential applications in psychological research and practice. It reviews existing literature on AI-based chatbots, particularly ChatGPT, and highlights the gap in research on their psychological impact. The chapter also discusses how AI tools can assist in writing, education, and therapy while emphasizing the need for further studies to understand their full potential in psychological settings.

Chapter 2: Revolutionizing Mental Healthcare Through Artificial Intelligence

This chapter examines how AI is transforming mental healthcare by enhancing diagnostic accuracy, identifying risk factors, and supporting therapy. While AI-driven tools offer promising applications, they cannot replace human expertise. The chapter evaluates the practical effectiveness of AI in crisis intervention, its role in improving patient outcomes, and the ethical concerns surrounding its use. It provides an insightful discussion on the future of AI in mental health, emphasizing the need to balance technological advancements with ethical considerations.

Chapter 3: Chatbots as Tools for Psychoeducation and Self-Help in Mental Health

This chapter investigates the role of mental health chatbots in addressing global challenges in mental healthcare. By offering accessible, affordable, and anonymous support, chatbots enhance psychoeducation and self-help interventions. The authors explore their effectiveness in improving treatment outcomes, screening for mental health conditions, and disseminating knowledge. They also emphasize the importance of collaboration between psychologists, physicians, and engineers to develop more responsive AI-driven tools tailored to user needs.

Chapter 4: AI in Mental Healthcare: Exploring Technology Acceptance, Emotional and Cognitive Innovation, and Cultural Influences

This chapter presents a comprehensive study on the acceptance of AI in mental healthcare among college students in Karnataka, India. Using a mixed-methods approach, the research evaluates factors such as cognitive and sensory innovativeness, emotional responses, and cultural influences on AI adoption. The findings offer insights into how technology acceptance models can inform AI integration in mental health services, highlighting the importance of emotional and cognitive factors in user adoption.

Chapter 5: Tracing the Development and Influence of Chatbots in Contemporary Healthcare Systems

This chapter explores the evolution of chatbot technology in healthcare, from simple automated scripts to advanced AI-powered systems. It examines how chatbots improve healthcare accessibility, efficiency, and patient-provider interactions, particularly in crisis situations such as the COVID-19 pandemic. The chapter also addresses key concerns regarding data privacy, security, and ethical challenges, offering recommendations for the responsible integration of AI-driven chatbots into modern healthcare systems.

Chapter 6: A Conversation With ChatGPT on Its Role in Teaching and Learning Real-World Problem Solving in School Mathematics

Through a detailed dialogue with ChatGPT, this chapter explores its capabilities in teaching and solving real-world mathematical problems. It evaluates the AI's ability to generate meaningful problem-solving strategies, contextualize mathematical concepts, and support educators in the learning process. The chapter also examines ChatGPT's effectiveness in mathematical problem-solving based on the author's expertise, assessing both its strengths and limitations as an educational tool.

Chapter 7: Internet Wizard for Enhancing Open-Domain Question Answering Chatbot Knowledge-Base in Information Seeking

This chapter investigates how integrating internet-based resources can enhance chatbots' knowledge base, making them more dynamic and responsive to user queries. By leveraging search engines and data science techniques, AI chatbots can generate real-time, up-to-date answers across diverse topics. The chapter presents a pilot study in higher education, demonstrating how chatbots enriched with internet-based knowledge retrieval can significantly improve student engagement and information exploration.

Chapter 8: Testing Creativity of ChatGPT in Psychology: Interview With ChatGPT

This chapter explores the creative capabilities of ChatGPT within the field of psychology. Through a structured interview and analysis, the study assesses ChatGPT's ability to generate novel and valuable responses. It examines the AI's potential for creativity, comparing its responses to human expert-generated content. The discussion highlights the challenges in defining and evaluating AI creativity and underscores the need for further research to refine assessment methodologies.

Chapter 9: Ethical Considerations Surrounding the Use of AI Interventions in Mental Healthcare

This chapter provides an in-depth exploration of the ethical challenges associated with AI-driven mental health interventions. Topics include patient autonomy, informed consent, data privacy, algorithmic bias, and the integrity of the therapeutic relationship. The chapter emphasizes the necessity of transparent AI algorithms and the ethical responsibility of developers and mental health practitioners in ensuring safe and equitable AI applications in mental healthcare.

Chapter 10: The Ethical Aspects of Chatbots and Beyond

Expanding on broader ethical concerns, this chapter addresses issues such as trust, bias, accountability, and the societal impact of chatbot technology. It explores privacy risks associated with chatbot data collection and storage, emphasizing the importance of compliance with data protection regulations like GDPR. Additionally, the chapter discusses how biases in chatbot algorithms can impact decision-making and user trust, calling for greater transparency and ethical oversight in AI development.

Chapter 11: Data Security and Privacy Considerations in Mental Health Settings

Focusing on the critical issue of data security in mental health services, this chapter examines the risks and vulnerabilities associated with chatbot integration in psychology and psychiatry. It highlights legal and ethical frameworks, such as HIPAA and GDPR, that guide data protection practices. The chapter also presents strategies for enhancing cybersecurity, including encryption, secure communication protocols, and periodic audits, ensuring that chatbot applications in mental health maintain patient confidentiality and trust.

Beyond their use in therapy, chatbots are also playing a significant role in promoting mental well-being through early intervention, psychoeducation, and self-help applications. Whether they are used to screen for psychological conditions, provide cognitive-behavioral techniques, or offer crisis support, these digital tools are reshaping the way mental health resources are accessed and delivered. At the same time, ethical considerations, challenges related to trust and privacy, and the limitations of AI in replicating human emotions remain critical areas of discussion.

By bringing together perspectives from psychology, psychiatry, AI research, and human-computer interaction, this volume offers an in-depth examination of how chatbot technology is being leveraged to enhance mental healthcare. We aim to provide insights for researchers, clinicians, developers, and policymakers seeking to navigate this rapidly evolving landscape.

As we stand at the cusp of a new era in mental healthcare, it is crucial to examine both the opportunities and challenges presented by chatbot-assisted interventions. We hope this book serves as a valuable resource for understanding the transformative potential of AI-driven chatbots in psychology and psychiatry—offering a glimpse into the future of digital mental health and human-machine collaboration.

Chapter 1
The Use of AI-Supported Chatbot in Psychology

Kadir Uludag
https://orcid.org/0000-0003-3713-4670
Shanghai Jiao Tong University, China

ABSTRACT

Artificial intelligence has allowed programmers to create human-like meaningful texts. As a result, chatbots have recently gained great attention. Many people have praised how novel chat applications can create original and human-like essays. However, few studies discuss the use of AI chatbots in psychology. The authors aimed to discuss the use of AI chatbots in the field of Psychology. Also, they summarize previous studies on ChatGPT. This chapter discusses how AI can be used in this process. They used ChatGPT to create a brief literature review to show the progress of the OpenAI ChatGPT AI application. Studies on Pubmed were searched. Overall, the authors found eight studies using the keyword of "ChatGPT." Most studies claim that ChatGPT can write original essays, and it is hard to distinguish ChatGPT from human-like writing. They found no study discussing the impact of ChatGPT on psychology. ChatGPT can allow writing essays on various topics and be used in many fields, including psychology, medicine, engineering, philosophy, medical education, literature, and computer sciences.

1. INTRODUCTION

Artificial intelligence (AI) has allowed programmers to create original human-like texts (Uludag, 2023b). As a result, AI Chatbots have recently gained great attention (C.-C. Lin, Huang, & Yang, 2023). Chatbots have become essential aids for writing and conducting research, serving as indispensable assistants for a range

DOI: 10.4018/979-8-3693-3112-5.ch001

of tasks. From a psychological standpoint, the integration of AI chatbots into writing and research represents a profound shift in how we understand creativity, writing, intellectual labor, and ethical responsibility.

To begin, we can explain what a chatbot is: To understand what ChatGPT is, we should ask him. In his own words, ChatGPT defines himself as follows:

''I am ChatGPT. I am a state-of-the-art natural language processing (NLP) and machine learning system, designed to assist with a wide range of language-based tasks'' (Michael R. King, 2022).

Recent studies have investigated the use of Chatbots in academy (Bin-Nashwan, Sadallah, & Bouteraa, 2023; Else, 2023; Kim & Wong, 2023; Yu, 2023), academic libraries (Adetayo, 2023; Ehrenpreis & DeLooper, 2022; Hussain & Ahmad, 2024; Kaushal & Yadav, 2022; Mckie & Narayan, 2019), fashion (Chung, Ko, Joung, & Kim, 2020; Landim et al., 2022; Sawada, Tanabe, & Nakada, 2022; Seo, 2022; Zeng, Vignali, & Ryding, 2023), tourism (Melián-González, Gutiérrez-Taño, & Bulchand-Gidumal, 2021; Pillai & Sivathanu, 2020; Ukpabi, Aslam, & Karjaluoto, 2019), education (Jauhiainen & Guerra, 2023; Mhlanga, 2023; Okonkwo & Ade-Ibijola, 2021; Pérez, Daradoumis, & Puig, 2020), economy (Korinek, 2023; Rotman, 2023), mathematics (D. Lee & Yeo, 2022; Moral-Sánchez, Rey, & Cebrián-de-la-Serna, 2023; Wardat, Tashtoush, AlAli, & Jarrah, 2023; Wijaya, Su, Cao, Weinhandl, & Houghton, 2024), programming (Bucaioni, Ekedahl, Helander, & Nguyen, 2024; Castelvecchi, 2022; Hörnemalm, 2023; Kashefi & Mukerji, 2023), and essay writing (Graham, 2022; M. P.-C. Lin & Chang, 2020; M Pitychoutis, 2024). However, ChatGPT could potentially pose a threat to one's creative writing skills (Niloy, Akter, Sultana, Sultana, & Rahman, 2024). Moreover, another research suggested that ChatGPT could potentially exhibit greater creativity compared to humans (Cropley, 2023). The connection between creativity in writing and psychology is deep and multifaceted, involving various psychological theories, processes, and research findings that explore how creativity emerges, develops, and functions within the human mind.

Overall, previous studies collectively contribute to the growing understanding of ChatGPT's versatility and effectiveness in diverse fields such as academy, tourism, literature, and economy. More and more studies are expected to investigate its impact on various fields, such as psychology (Uludag, 2023c, 2023d). For example, chatbots can be used to help individuals to socialize. Although, the current version of the chatbot program cannot speak (2023 version). It can give comprehensive feedback about certain situations. In addition, it is unclear if Chatbots can process emotional inputs. Therefore, future studies are needed to explore the use of AI chatbots in psychology. We have compiled information from various sources on the intersection of AI and psychology.

Taken together, our chapter aimed to discuss the use of AI chatbots in psychology.

2. METHODS

This manuscript discusses how chat programs supported by Artificial Intelligence (AI) can be used in various fields such as tourism and fashion. Notably, we have investigated studies on the practical use of ChatGPT. We used ChatGPT to create a literature review article to show the process of the OpenAI ChatGPT artificial intelligence application. Studies on Pubmed were searched. Overall, using the ChatGPT, we found eight studies. We have searched all studies published before 19 January 2023 (Table 1). We have listed the main goals of the studies as well. Listing previous literature related to ChatGPT is crucial.

3. RESULTS

Table 1. Studies related to ChatGPT found on PubMed

Title of Study	Author of Study	Goal of Study
Abstracts written by ChatGPT fool scientists	(Else, 2023)	The study discusses whether abstracts written by ChatGPT are distinct from human writing.
Are ChatGPT and AlphaCode going to replace programmers	(Castelvecchi, 2022)	The study discusses whether ChatGPT can be used to program.
Daily briefing: Will ChatGPT kill the essay assignment?	(Graham, 2022)	The study discusses the function of ChatGPT on essay assignments.
AI bot ChatGPT writes smart essays - should professors worry?	(Stokel-Walker, 2022)	The study discusses the function of ChatGPT on academic assignments.
Are ChatGPT's knowledge and interpretation ability comparable to those of medical students in Korea for taking a parasitology examination?: a descriptive study	(Huh, 2023)	The study discusses whether or not ChatGPT's knowledge and interpretation skills are comparable to medical students.
A conversation with ChatGPT on the role of computational systems biology in stem cell research	(Cahan & Treutlein, 2023)	The study discusses the function of computational systems biology in stem cell research.
Open artificial intelligence platforms in nursing education: Tools for academic progress or abuse?	(O'Connor & ChatGpt, 2023)	The study discusses the function of AI platforms in nursing education.
Rapamycin in the context of Pascal's Wager: generative pre-trained transformer perspective	(Zhavoronkov, 2022)	The study discusses the potential of ChatGPT to provide philosophical arguments

4. DISCUSSION

Chatbots are used in academy (Else, 2023; Gammoh, 2024), programming (Biswas, 2023; Bucaioni et al., 2024; Castelvecchi, 2022; Kashefi & Mukerji, 2023), philosophy (Adewumi, Liwicki, & Liwicki, 2019; Hanna; Peters et al., 2024; Zhavoronkov, 2022), medical education (H. Lee, 2024; O'Connor & ChatGpt, 2023), biology (Agathokleous, Saitanis, Fang, & Yu, 2023; Cahan & Treutlein, 2023; Chuang, Lo, & Wu, 2023; Uludag, 2023a; J. Wang et al., 2024), and essay writing (Graham, 2022). To our knowledge, this is the first academic work discussing the impact of ChatGPT in Psychology. While chatbots are a familiar concept, the emergence of ChatGPT has instilled a sense of great promise within the field.

It is crucial to keep in mind that AI-supported chatbot can make mistakes. For example, in the following example, the chatbot thinks that the next article is the first time it has written a scientific article.

''This is the first time an AI-enabled chatbot has written a scientific article for publication'' (Michael R. King, 2022). Therefore, AI chatbots can mislead or misguide individuals needing personal psychological feedback.

ChatGPT could inadvertently result in plagiarism and alter the perception of plagiarism among individuals (Uludag, 2023e). Numerous other publications have explored the association between chatbots and plagiarism (Anders, 2023; Baron, 2024; Hassanipour et al., 2024; Jarrah, Wardat, & Fidalgo, 2023; Michael R King & ChatGPT, 2023). Additionally, chatbots have the potential to alter perceptions of plagiarism. This shift in perception brought about by the influence of chatbots could potentially impact academic integrity by influencing individuals' attitudes towards originality, proper citation practices, and the boundaries of intellectual property rights within academic settings. It may lead to a reevaluation of what constitutes ethically sound research practices and the importance of upholding academic integrity standards in scholarly work.

The way plagiarism is perceived in relation to chatbots and AI is shaped by a mix of cognitive biases, ethical factors, and changing social norms. While traditional views of plagiarism emphasize human agency, creativity, and intent, the advent of AI disrupts these ideas, complicating ethical standards. As AI increasingly influences creative and professional domains, it is essential to understand these perceptions and develop new frameworks to navigate the challenges surrounding originality, authorship, and intellectual property in the era of artificial intelligence.

4.1. Use of Artificial intelligence Chatbots in Psychology

A few studies have discussed the role of AI chatbots in psychology. For example, the chatbot format can provide positive psychology skills to individuals with cancer and reduce their anxiety (Greer et al., 2019).

More and more studies are expected to investigate ChatGPTs impact on psychology. Chatbots can be used to help individuals to socialize since ChatGPTs can create meaningful human-like essays. Although, the current version of the AI-supported chat program cannot speak. It can give comprehensive feedback about certain situations. A previous study found that the impacts of emotional disclosure were equal whether participants thought they were talking to a bot or a human (Ho, Hancock, & Miner, 2018).

However, it is unclear if chatGPT can process emotional inputs. Moreover, a previous study claimed that psychotherapy chatbots could not easily replace psychological experts (Xu & Zhuang, 2022). Therefore, future studies are needed to explore the use of AI chatbots in psychology.

4.2. Adding Chatbots as an Author

Several research projects employed ChatGPT to draft a paper, subsequently attributing authorship to Chatbot. Nevertheless, the appropriateness of including Chatbot as an author remains debatable. Moreover, defining the chatbot's affiliation poses an additional challenge.

Morever, whether we have to include statistical analysis tools as an author is doubtful. However, if additional programs supported the authors, they should mention it in their articles. In the future, if chatbots gain the ability to independently compose articles, they could be considered authors. Similar to advancements in chess engine development where they might surpass human capacities in terms of creativity and reliability.

Transparency regarding the tools and software utilized in the research process is essential, and if these programs significantly contributed to the study, it is advisable for authors to disclose their involvement in the publication. This not only enhances the clarity of the research process but also gives due credit to the tools that facilitated the study's execution. Multiple written works debated whether a chatbot should be included as an author (Baveye, 2024; Coghlan et al., 2023; de Vasconcellos, 2023; Goto & Katanoda, 2023; Ide, Hawke, & Nakayama, 2023; J. Y. Lee, 2023; Scerbo, 2023; Thorp, 2023). Nowadays, journals inquire about the use of chatbots but do not require authors to include chatbots as co-authors. It also aids reviewers in analyzing the scientific paper. Chatbots are capable of producing scientifically sound papers, but they may not effectively convey the intended meaning to the audience.

Nevertheless, there is a possibility that in the future, chatbots could reach the same level of scientific accuracy as humans. However, humans should still review the content to make the final decision. Furthermore, it is crucial to establish guidelines for reporting the utilization of chatbots.

In conclusion, while journals now consider the use of chatbots without mandating their inclusion as co-authors, their potential for generating scientifically accurate content poses challenges in effectively communicating intended meanings, which underscores the importance of human oversight in reviewing and setting standardized reporting guidelines for chatbot applications in scientific research.

It is also worth mentioning that some publishers utilize automated systems, such as chatbots, to provide authors with information by extracting specific details from the manuscript and displaying them for readers.

4.2.1. Recognition for Chatbots

As artificial intelligence continues to develop, one question looms large in the literary and creative spheres: *Will chatbots ever receive literary awards or recognition for their work?* This question touches on the intersections of technology, creativity, and tradition in the world of literature. It raises fundamental issues about authorship, creativity, and how we define literary merit in a world where AI can generate written content with increasing sophistication.

4.3. Chatbot Personality

Consistency is key in maintaining a chatbot's personality. The tone and language used by the chatbot should remain consistent across interactions to build trust and familiarity with users. Incorporating elements of humor, empathy, and understanding can make a chatbot more relatable and engaging. However, it's important to strike a balance and ensure that the chatbot's personality enhances the user experience without overshadowing the primary goal of the interaction. Another research discovered that personality plays a crucial role in influencing the user experience of chatbot interfaces, yet this influence varies depending on the context, the tasks it undertakes, and the demographics of its users (Ruane, Birhane, & Ventresque, 2019). Furthermore, a chatbot that frequently switches between different tones and styles, causing confusion among users. Inconsistencies in language and behavior can make the chatbot appear unreliable and untrustworthy.

Additionally, the memory of chatbots is crucial as it can influence their personality. In simpler terms, having access to past conversations enables them to learn more about other individuals.

4.3.1. Challenges in Designing Chatbot Personalities

Creating a chatbot personality goes beyond simply programming a bot to reply to user input; it demands thoughtful attention to psychological, cultural, and functional elements.

4.4. Ethical Considerations in AI-Powered Therapy Chatbots:

Numerous recent research projects have focused on the ethical considerations surrounding chatbots (Chauncey & McKenna, 2023; Kretzschmar et al., 2019; Ng, Haller, & Murray, 2022; Parviainen & Rantala, 2022; Rivas & Zhao, 2023; Ruane et al., 2019; Sebastian & Sebastian, 2024; Vilaza & McCashin, 2021; Williams, 2024; Zarifhonarvar, 2024). The conversations with a chatbot might become accessible to third parties, potentially leading to additional complications. Moreover, the inadvertent disclosure of chatbot conversations could have repercussions on individuals' mental well-being, relationships, and overall sense of security. It underscores the importance of robust data protection measures, encryption protocols, and stringent access controls to safeguard the confidentiality and integrity of chatbot interactions, ensuring that users feel secure and protected while engaging with AI-driven conversational agents. Moreover, it is crucial to understand that it is uncertain who should be held accountable if issues arise from chatbot inquiries. Another manuscript has identified and explored four significant ethical concerns using a established ethical framework consisting of five fundamental principles. The article provides suggestions to assist chatbot creators, providers, researchers, and mental health professionals in ethically developing and implementing mental health chatbots (Coghlan et al., 2023).

4.5. Creating Psychology studies with Chatbot

Creating psychology studies with a chatbot like ChatGPT can be an innovative approach to understanding human behavior, cognition, and interaction. Chatbots can be used for various types of studies, including surveys, experiments, and therapeutic interventions. Creating original psychology studies with chatbots requires blending psychological theories, innovative applications, and the chatbot's interactive capabilities.

4.5.1. Creative Possibilities

This blending of theory, technology, and interactivity enables psychologists to:

- Explore novel questions (e.g., Can AI influence emotional resilience?).
- Test traditional theories in digital contexts (e.g., Does emotional contagion occur with chatbots?).
- Develop interventions that scale efficiently and adapt to individual needs (e.g., mental health chatbots).

It is uncertain whether chatbots have the capability to develop entirely original studies. It remains uncertain and unlikely that chatbots, in their current form, can independently develop entirely original studies. Their value lies in supporting and enhancing human-led research rather than replacing it. True originality in research still requires the depth of understanding, intuition, and creativity that are uniquely human traits. Additionally, it's challenging to assess the originality and impact of research endeavors.

4.5.2. AI-Generated Content vs. Human Creativity: The Perception of Originality and Authorship

In terms of psychology, the perception of originality and authorship plays a crucial role in how individuals value creative work, with AI-generated content often being viewed as less authentic or innovative compared to human-created works. This bias may stem from cognitive heuristics that associate creativity with human emotion, intention, and experience, leading to a diminished sense of ownership and value when the creator is an artificial intelligence, even if the output is equally novel.

Future studies can explore certain textual parameters such as sentence length (Uludag, 2024) and how, in terms of psychology, the perception of originality and authorship influences the value individuals place on creative work, with AI-generated content often seen as less authentic or innovative due to cognitive heuristics linking creativity with human emotion, intention, and experience, thus diminishing the sense of ownership and value despite equally novel outputs.

4.5.3. Chatbots for Brainstorming: Enhancing Creativity and Idea Generation

AI-powered chatbots have become increasingly valuable tools in creative processes like brainstorming, assisting individuals and teams in generating a diverse array of ideas quickly and efficiently. Through simulated conversation, chatbots provide a unique form of support that challenges conventional thought patterns, encourages innovative solutions, and promotes divergent thinking. The literature on the use of chatbots for brainstorming is limited (Cheddak, Ait Baha, Es-Saady, El Hajji, &

Baslam, 2024; Lavrič & Škraba, 2023; Memmert, 2024; Wang, Claudy, & Yan, 2024; Wieland, de Wit, & de Rooij, 2022).

In conclusion, while AI-powered chatbots offer promising potential for enhancing creativity and idea generation, further research is needed to explore their full capabilities and impact on brainstorming processes.

4.5.3.1. Comparison of Chatbots in the field of psychology

In the field of psychology, chatbots have emerged as promising tools for providing mental health support, counseling, and therapy services. These AI-powered conversational agents offer a range of advantages, such as accessibility, affordability, anonymity, and scalability.

The success of psychology-therapy chatbots can be influenced by the algorithms they employ.

Therefore, understanding the version of the chatbot is crucial.

4.5.3.2. Possible detrimental effects of chatbots on human communication

As chatbots become increasingly integrated into daily life and various sectors, their impact on human communication is a topic of growing concern. While chatbots offer convenience, especially in areas like customer serviceand education, there are potential detrimental effects on human communication that should not be overlooked.

Sexting, the act of sending sexually explicit messages, images, or videos via digital platforms, has become a prevalent form of communication in the digital age. While sexting is often viewed as a normal part of adult relationships, it can sometimes evolve into problematic behavior, leading to what is increasingly referred to as "sexting addiction." The intersection between sexting addiction and emerging technologies, such as chatbots, introduces new concerns about the development, perpetuation, and management of this issue as mentioned in the previous work (Uludag, 2023f).

4.6. Conclusion

In conclusion, ChatGPT can produce human-like texts and be a useful tool, especially in psychology. Human-like texts can mirror clients' responses and act like a psychotherapist. This feature can be particularly beneficial in therapeutic settings, where the generation of empathetic and understanding responses can aid in mirroring a supportive and responsive environment for clients. By emulating human-like conversations, ChatGPT has the potential to enhance psychological interventions and support individuals seeking mental health assistance.

4.7. Limitations

We did not include preprint studies in this review. Although ChatGPT can create human-like texts. It does not have consciousness and memory like humans. Furthermore, ChatGPT cannot store personalized information to give different answers to different people. One limitation is that we only considered initial studies concerning ChatGPT. Moreover, there are currently a multitude of chatbots like Gemini available. Additionally, it is not a systematic review.

4.8. Suggestions for Further Studies

Further studies should investigate the use of Chatbots in psychology with empirical design. Furthermore, inducing vibrant visualization of the products approved by the chatbots is an essential factor (Jin & Youn, 2022). Future studies can evaluate how AI chatbots perform in relation to traditional in-person therapy and other digital mental health interventions. Explore the distinctive strengths and weaknesses associated with incorporating chatbots into psychological treatment. Further studies can investigate how the integration of textual analysis methods can augment and enrich conventional psychological research approaches to achieve a deeper insight into human behavior, as demonstrated in the preceding manuscript (Uludag, 2024). Moreover, upcoming research could concentrate on the psychology of chatbots and how they influence user experience. Additionally, future research endeavors can explore collaborations with ChatGPT as a co-author. The quality and features of abstracts authored by chatbots can be compared with those created by humans.

Further studies can create a longitudinal study with adolescents using ChatGPT to engage in emotional conversations or role-play scenarios, with pre- and post-assessments of empathy and emotional intelligence.

CONFLICT OF INTEREST STATEMENT

There is no conflict of interest to state.

AUTHOR STATEMENT

K.U. wrote the book chapter and is the only author.

FUNDING

There is no funding information to state.

ACKNOWLEDGMENT

Thanks to the authors who made this literature review possible. It was previously disseminated as a preprint at the following link: https://papers.ssrn.com/sol3/papers.cfm?abstract_id=4331367.

DATA AVAILABILITY STATEMENT

None. There is no available data.

REFERENCES

Adetayo, A. J. (2023). Artificial intelligence chatbots in academic libraries: The rise of ChatGPT. *Library Hi Tech News*, 40(3), 18–21. DOI: 10.1108/LHTN-01-2023-0007

Adewumi, T. P., Liwicki, F., & Liwicki, M. (2019). Conversational systems in machine learning from the point of view of the philosophy of science—Using alime chat and related studies. *Philosophies*, 4(3), 41. DOI: 10.3390/philosophies4030041

Agathokleous, E., Saitanis, C. J., Fang, C., & Yu, Z. (2023). Use of ChatGPT: What does it mean for biology and environmental science? *The Science of the Total Environment*, 888, 164154. DOI: 10.1016/j.scitotenv.2023.164154 PMID: 37201835

Anders, B. A. (2023). Is using ChatGPT cheating, plagiarism, both, neither, or forward thinking? *Patterns (New York, N.Y.)*, 4(3), 100694. DOI: 10.1016/j.patter.2023.100694 PMID: 36960444

Baron, P. (2024). Are AI detection and plagiarism similarity scores worthwhile in the age of ChatGPT and other Generative AI? *Scholarship of Teaching and Learning in the South*, 8(2), 151–179. DOI: 10.36615/sotls.v8i2.411

Baveye, P. C. (2024). Authorship for chatbots on scholarly publications: The time has not yet come. *European Science Editing*, 50, e139657. DOI: 10.3897/ese.2024.e139657

Bin-Nashwan, S. A., Sadallah, M., & Bouteraa, M. (2023). Use of ChatGPT in academia: Academic integrity hangs in the balance. *Technology in Society*, 75, 102370. DOI: 10.1016/j.techsoc.2023.102370

Biswas, S. (2023). Role of ChatGPT in Computer Programming. *Mesopotamian Journal of Computer Science*, 2023, 9–15. DOI: 10.58496/MJCSC/2023/002

Bucaioni, A., Ekedahl, H., Helander, V., & Nguyen, P. T. (2024). Programming with ChatGPT: How far can we go? *Machine Learning with Applications*, 15, 100526. DOI: 10.1016/j.mlwa.2024.100526

Cahan, P., & Treutlein, B. (2023). A conversation with ChatGPT on the role of computational systems biology in stem cell research. *Stem Cell Reports*, 18(1), 1–2. DOI: 10.1016/j.stemcr.2022.12.009 PMID: 36630899

Castelvecchi, D. (2022). Are ChatGPT and AlphaCode going to replace programmers? *Nature*. Advance online publication. DOI: 10.1038/d41586-022-04383-z PMID: 36481949

Chauncey, S. A., & McKenna, H. P. (2023). A framework and exemplars for ethical and responsible use of AI Chatbot technology to support teaching and learning. *Computers and Education: Artificial Intelligence*, 5, 100182. DOI: 10.1016/j.caeai.2023.100182

Cheddak, A., Ait Baha, T., Es-Saady, Y., El Hajji, M., & Baslam, M. (2024). BERTopic for Enhanced Idea Management and Topic Generation in Brainstorming Sessions. *Information (Basel)*, 15(6), 365. DOI: 10.3390/info15060365

Chuang, C.-H., Lo, J.-H., & Wu, Y.-K. (2023). Integrating chatbot and augmented reality technology into biology learning during COVID-19. *Electronics (Basel)*, 12(1), 222. DOI: 10.3390/electronics12010222

Chung, M., Ko, E., Joung, H., & Kim, S. J. (2020). Chatbot e-service and customer satisfaction regarding luxury brands. *Journal of Business Research*, 117, 587–595. DOI: 10.1016/j.jbusres.2018.10.004

Coghlan, S., Leins, K., Sheldrick, S., Cheong, M., Gooding, P., & D'Alfonso, S. (2023). To chat or bot to chat: Ethical issues with using chatbots in mental health. *Digital Health*, 9, 20552076231183542. DOI: 10.1177/20552076231183542 PMID: 37377565

Cropley, D. (2023). Is artificial intelligence more creative than humans?: ChatGPT and the divergent association task. *Learning Letters*, 2, 13–13. DOI: 10.59453/ll.v2.13

de Vasconcellos, V. G. (2023). *Artificial Intelligence and Co-Authorship of Scientific Manuscripts: Discussions about Using ChatGPT in Scientific Research and Writing* (Vol. 9). HeinOnline.

Ehrenpreis, M., & DeLooper, J. (2022). Implementing a chatbot on a library website. *Journal of Web Librarianship*, 16(2), 120–142. DOI: 10.1080/19322909.2022.2060893

Else, H. (2023). Abstracts written by ChatGPT fool scientists. *Nature*, 613(7944), 423. DOI: 10.1038/d41586-023-00056-7 PMID: 36635510

Gammoh, L. A. (2024). ChatGPT in academia: Exploring university students' risks, misuses, and challenges in Jordan. *Journal of Further and Higher Education*, 48(6), 608–624. DOI: 10.1080/0309877X.2024.2378298

Goto, A., & Katanoda, K. (2023). Should we acknowledge ChatGPT as an author? *Journal of Epidemiology*, 33(7), 333–334. DOI: 10.2188/jea.JE20230078 PMID: 37032108

Graham, F. (2022). Daily briefing: Will ChatGPT kill the essay assignment? *Nature*. Advance online publication. DOI: 10.1038/d41586-022-04437-2 PMID: 36517680

Greer, S., Ramo, D., Chang, Y.-J., Fu, M., Moskowitz, J., & Haritatos, J. (2019). Use of the chatbot "vivibot" to deliver positive psychology skills and promote well-being among young people after cancer treatment: Randomized controlled feasibility trial. *JMIR mHealth and uHealth*, 7(10), e15018. DOI: 10.2196/15018 PMID: 31674920

Hanna, R. (2023). *Philosophy That Can't Be Done By Chatbots: Rational Anthropology*. Unpublished MS. https://www. academia. edu/74562370/Philosophy_That_Can_t_Be_Done_By_Chatbots_ Rational_Anthropology_April_2023_version_

Hassanipour, S., Nayak, S., Bozorgi, A., Keivanlou, M.-H., Dave, T., Alotaibi, A., & Kuriyakose, D. (2024). The ability of ChatGPT in paraphrasing texts and reducing plagiarism: A descriptive analysis. *JMIR Medical Education*, 10(1), e53308. DOI: 10.2196/53308 PMID: 38989841

Ho, A., Hancock, J., & Miner, A. S. (2018). Psychological, Relational, and Emotional Effects of Self-Disclosure After Conversations With a Chatbot. *Journal of Communication*, 68(4), 712–733. DOI: 10.1093/joc/jqy026 PMID: 30100620

Hörnemalm, A. (2023). Chatgpt as a software development tool: The future of development.

Huh, S. (2023). Are ChatGPT's knowledge and interpretation ability comparable to those of medical students in Korea for taking a parasitology examination?: A descriptive study. *Journal of Educational Evaluation for Health Professions*, 20, 1. DOI: 10.3352/jeehp.2023.20.01 PMID: 36627845

Hussain, A., & Ahmad, S. (2024). Mapping the literature on artificial intelligence in academic libraries: A bibliometrics approach. *Science & Technology Libraries*, 43(2), 131–146. DOI: 10.1080/0194262X.2023.2238198

Ide, K., Hawke, P., & Nakayama, T. (2023). Can ChatGPT be considered an author of a medical article? *Journal of Epidemiology*, 33(7), 381–382. DOI: 10.2188/jea.JE20230030 PMID: 37032109

Jarrah, A. M., Wardat, Y., & Fidalgo, P. (2023). Using ChatGPT in academic writing is (not) a form of plagiarism: What does the literature say. *Online Journal of Communication and Media Technologies*, 13(4), e202346. DOI: 10.30935/ojcmt/13572

Jauhiainen, J. S., & Guerra, A. G. (2023). Generative AI and ChatGPT in school children's education: Evidence from a school lesson. *Sustainability (Basel)*, 15(18), 14025. DOI: 10.3390/su151814025

Jin, S. V., & Youn, S. (2022). Social Presence and Imagery Processing as Predictors of Chatbot Continuance Intention in Human-AI-Interaction. *International Journal of Human-Computer Interaction*, 1–13. DOI: 10.1080/10447318.2022.2129277

Kashefi, A., & Mukerji, T. (2023). ChatGPT for programming numerical methods. *Journal of Machine Learning for Modeling and Computing*, 4(2), 1–74. DOI: 10.1615/JMachLearnModelComput.2023048492

Kaushal, V., & Yadav, R. (2022). The role of chatbots in academic libraries: An experience-based perspective. *Journal of the Australian Library and Information Association*, 71(3), 215–232. DOI: 10.1080/24750158.2022.2106403

Kim, S.-K. A., & Wong, U.-H. (2023). *ChatGPT impacts on academia.* Paper presented at the 2023 International Conference on System Science and Engineering (ICSSE). DOI: 10.1109/ICSSE58758.2023.10227188

King, M. R. (2022). The Future of AI in Medicine: A Perspective from a Chatbot. *Annals of Biomedical Engineering*. Advance online publication. DOI: 10.1007/s10439-022-03121-w PMID: 36572824

King, M. R., & Chat, G. P. T. (2023). A conversation on artificial intelligence, chatbots, and plagiarism in higher education. *Cellular and Molecular Bioengineering*, 16(1), 1–2. DOI: 10.1007/s12195-022-00754-8 PMID: 36660590

Korinek, A. (2023). Generative AI for economic research: Use cases and implications for economists. *Journal of Economic Literature*, 61(4), 1281–1317. DOI: 10.1257/jel.20231736

Kretzschmar, K., Tyroll, H., Pavarini, G., Manzini, A., & Singh, I. (2019). Can your phone be your therapist? Young people's ethical perspectives on the use of fully automated conversational agents (chatbots) in mental health support. *Biomedical Informatics Insights*, 11, 1178222619829083. DOI: 10.1177/1178222619829083 PMID: 30858710

Landim, A., Pereira, A., & Vieira, T., de B. Costa, E., Moura, J., Wanick, V., & Bazaki, E. (. (2022). Chatbot design approaches for fashion E-commerce: An interdisciplinary review. *International Journal of Fashion Design, Technology and Education*, 15(2), 200–210. DOI: 10.1080/17543266.2021.1990417

Lavrič, F., & Škraba, A. (2023). *Group Brainstorming Support by ChatGPT & Ayoa at the Design of Regional Development Plan.* Paper presented at the 42th International Conference on Organizational Science Development, Portorož, Slovenia. DOI: 10.18690/um.fov.3.2023.43

Lee, D., & Yeo, S. (2022). Developing an AI-based chatbot for practicing responsive teaching in mathematics. *Computers & Education*, 191, 104646. DOI: 10.1016/j.compedu.2022.104646

Lee, H. (2024). The rise of ChatGPT: Exploring its potential in medical education. *Anatomical Sciences Education*, 17(5), 926–931. DOI: 10.1002/ase.2270 PMID: 36916887

Lee, J. Y. (2023). Can an artificial intelligence chatbot be the author of a scholarly article? *Journal of Educational Evaluation for Health Professions*, 20. PMID: 36842449

Lin, C.-C., Huang, A. Y., & Yang, S. J. (2023). A review of ai-driven conversational chatbots implementation methodologies and challenges (1999–2022). *Sustainability (Basel)*, 15(5), 4012. DOI: 10.3390/su15054012

Lin, M. P.-C., & Chang, D. (2020). Enhancing post-secondary writers' writing skills with a chatbot. *Journal of Educational Technology & Society*, 23(1), 78–92.

Mckie, I. A. S., & Narayan, B. (2019). Enhancing the academic library experience with chatbots: An exploration of research and implications for practice. *Journal of the Australian Library and Information Association*, 68(3), 268–277. DOI: 10.1080/24750158.2019.1611694

Melián-González, S., Gutiérrez-Taño, D., & Bulchand-Gidumal, J. (2021). Predicting the intentions to use chatbots for travel and tourism. *Current Issues in Tourism*, 24(2), 192–210. DOI: 10.1080/13683500.2019.1706457

Memmert, L. (2024). Brainstorming with a Generative Language Model: Understanding Performance Through Brainstorming Group Effects.

Mhlanga, D. (2023). ChatGPT in education: Exploring opportunities for emerging economies to improve education with ChatGPT. *Available atSSRN* 4355758. DOI: 10.2139/ssrn.4355758

Moral-Sánchez, S. N., Rey, F. J. R., & Cebrián-de-la-Serna, M. (2023). Analysis of artificial intelligence chatbots and satisfaction for learning in mathematics education. *IJERI: International Journal of Educational Research and Innovation*, (20), 1–14. DOI: 10.46661/ijeri.8196

Ng, J., Haller, E., & Murray, A. (2022). The ethical chatbot: A viable solution to socio-legal issues. *Alternative Law Journal*, 47(4), 308–313. DOI: 10.1177/1037969X221113598

Niloy, A. C., Akter, S., Sultana, N., Sultana, J., & Rahman, S. I. U. (2024). Is Chatgpt a menace for creative writing ability? An experiment. *Journal of Computer Assisted Learning*, 40(2), 919–930. DOI: 10.1111/jcal.12929

O'Connor, S. (2023). Open artificial intelligence platforms in nursing education: Tools for academic progress or abuse? *Nurse Education in Practice*, 66, 103537. DOI: 10.1016/j.nepr.2022.103537 PMID: 36549229

Okonkwo, C. W., & Ade-Ibijola, A. (2021). Chatbots applications in education: A systematic review. *Computers and Education: Artificial Intelligence*, 2, 100033. DOI: 10.1016/j.caeai.2021.100033

Parviainen, J., & Rantala, J. (2022). Chatbot breakthrough in the 2020s? An ethical reflection on the trend of automated consultations in health care. *Medicine, Health Care, and Philosophy*, 25(1), 61–71. DOI: 10.1007/s11019-021-10049-w PMID: 34480711

Pérez, J. Q., Daradoumis, T., & Puig, J. M. M. (2020). Rediscovering the use of chatbots in education: A systematic literature review. *Computer Applications in Engineering Education*, 28(6), 1549–1565. DOI: 10.1002/cae.22326

Peters, M. A., Jackson, L., Papastephanou, M., Jandrić, P., Lazaroiu, G., Evers, C. W., & Tesar, M. (2024). AI and the future of humanity: ChatGPT-4, philosophy and education–Critical responses. *Educational Philosophy and Theory*, 56(9), 828–862. DOI: 10.1080/00131857.2023.2213437

Pillai, R., & Sivathanu, B. (2020). Adoption of AI-based chatbots for hospitality and tourism. *International Journal of Contemporary Hospitality Management*, 32(10), 3199–3226. DOI: 10.1108/IJCHM-04-2020-0259

Pitychoutis, K. (2024). Harnessing AI Chatbots for EFL Essay Writing: A Paradigm Shift in Language Pedagogy. *Arab World English Journal.*

Rivas, P., & Zhao, L. (2023). Marketing with chatgpt: Navigating the ethical terrain of gpt-based chatbot technology. *AI*, 4(2), 375–384. DOI: 10.3390/ai4020019

Rotman, D. (2023). ChatGPT is about to revolutionize the economy. We need to decide what that looks like. *MIT Technology Review*.

Ruane, E., Birhane, A., & Ventresque, A. (2019). Conversational AI: Social and Ethical Considerations. *AICS*, 2563, 104–115.

Sawada, Y., Tanabe, A., & Nakada, Y. (2022). *A chatbot to search for similar fashion photos and reference fashion coordinators via body part and fashion item segmentations.* Paper presented at the 2022 IEEE Symposium Series on Computational Intelligence (SSCI). DOI: 10.1109/SSCI51031.2022.10022245

Scerbo, M. W. (2023). *Can Artificial Intelligence Be My Coauthor?* (Vol. 18). LWW.

Sebastian, G., & Sebastian, S. R. (2024). Exploring ethical implications of ChatGPT and other AI chatbots and regulation of disinformation propagation. *Annals of Engineering Mathematics and Computational Intelligence*, 1(1), 1–12.

Seo, M. J. (2022). Consumers' Negative Responses to the Communication Failure of Chatbots in Online Fashion Shopping Malls. *Fashion & Textile Research Journal*, 24(2), 183–194. DOI: 10.5805/SFTI.2022.24.2.183

Stokel-Walker, C. (2022). AI bot ChatGPT writes smart essays - should professors worry? *Nature*. Advance online publication. DOI: 10.1038/d41586-022-04397-7 PMID: 36494443

Thorp, H. H. (2023). *ChatGPT is fun, but not an author* (Vol. 379). American Association for the Advancement of Science.

Ukpabi, D. C., Aslam, B., & Karjaluoto, H. (2019). Chatbot adoption in tourism services: A conceptual exploration. In *Robots, artificial intelligence, and service automation in travel, tourism and hospitality* (pp. 105–121). Emerald Publishing Limited. DOI: 10.1108/978-1-78756-687-320191006

Uludag, K. (2023a). Brain Imaging Analysis with ChatGPT and Python's Powerful NumPy Package. *Available atSSRN* 4449615. DOI: 10.2139/ssrn.4449615

Uludag, K. (2023b). Chatbots Can Be Trained to Represent Humans after Death: Interview with ChatGPT. *Available atSSRN* 4399732. DOI: 10.2139/ssrn.4399732

Uludag, K. (2023c). ChatGPT Can Distinguish Paranoid Thoughts in Patients with Schizophrenia. *Available atSSRN* 4391941. DOI: 10.2139/ssrn.4391941

Uludag, K. (2023d). ChatGPT Can Help to Distinguish Delusional Jealousy. *Available atSSRN* 4406212. DOI: 10.2139/ssrn.4406212

Uludag, K. (2023e). Revealing the hidden aspects of ChatGPT: An inquiry into concerns surrounding plagiarism rates.

Uludag, K. (2023f). Understanding Sexting Addiction: Exploring the Role of Chatbots in Its Development and Definition. *Available atSSRN* 4398059. DOI: 10.2139/ssrn.4398059

Uludag, K. (2024). Exploring the Association Between Textual Parameters and Psychological and Cognitive Factors. *Psychology Research and Behavior Management*, 17, 1139–1150. DOI: 10.2147/PRBM.S460503 PMID: 38505355

Vilaza, G. N., & McCashin, D. (2021). Is the automation of digital mental health ethical? Applying an ethical framework to chatbots for cognitive behaviour therapy. *Frontiers in Digital Health*, 3, 689736. DOI: 10.3389/fdgth.2021.689736 PMID: 34713163

Wang, J., Cheng, Z., Yao, Q., Liu, L., Xu, D., & Hu, G. (2024). Bioinformatics and biomedical informatics with ChatGPT: Year one review. *Quantitative Biology*, 12(4), 345–359. DOI: 10.1002/qub2.67 PMID: 39364207

Wang, S., Claudy, M., & Yan, Q. (2024). Collaborating with AI in Brainstorming: How Gender Cues of Virtual Agents Affect User Idea Generation and Selection.

Wardat, Y., Tashtoush, M. A., AlAli, R., & Jarrah, A. M. (2023). ChatGPT: A revolutionary tool for teaching and learning mathematics. *Eurasia Journal of Mathematics, Science and Technology Education*, 19(7), em2286. DOI: 10.29333/ejmste/13272

Wieland, B., de Wit, J., & de Rooij, A. (2022). Electronic brainstorming with a chatbot partner: A good idea due to increased productivity and idea diversity. *Frontiers in Artificial Intelligence*, 5, 880673. DOI: 10.3389/frai.2022.880673 PMID: 36213166

Wijaya, T. T., Su, M., Cao, Y., Weinhandl, R., & Houghton, T. (2024). Examining Chinese preservice mathematics teachers' adoption of AI chatbots for learning: Unpacking perspectives through the UTAUT2 model. *Education and Information Technologies*, 1–29.

Williams, R. T. (2024). *The ethical implications of using generative chatbots in higher education.* Paper presented at the Frontiers in Education. DOI: 10.3389/feduc.2023.1331607

Xu, B., & Zhuang, Z. (2022). Survey on psychotherapy chatbots. *Concurrency and Computation*, 34(7), e6170. DOI: 10.1002/cpe.6170

Yu, H. (2023). Reflection on whether Chat GPT should be banned by academia from the perspective of education and teaching. *Frontiers in Psychology*, 14, 1181712. DOI: 10.3389/fpsyg.2023.1181712 PMID: 37325766

Zarifhonarvar, A. (2024). Economics of chatgpt: A labor market view on the occupational impact of artificial intelligence. *Journal of Electronic Business & Digital Economics*, 3(2), 100–116. DOI: 10.1108/JEBDE-10-2023-0021

Zeng, N., Vignali, G., & Ryding, D. (2023). Understanding the Application of AI-enabled Chatbots in Luxury Fashion Retailing. In *The Garment Economy: Understanding History, Developing Business Models, and Leveraging Digital Technologies* (pp. 369-388): Springer. DOI: 10.1007/978-3-031-33302-6_19

Zhavoronkov, A. (2022). Rapamycin in the context of Pascal's Wager: Generative pre-trained transformer perspective. *Oncoscience*, 9, 82–84. DOI: 10.18632/oncoscience.571 PMID: 36589923

Chapter 2

Revolutionizing Mental Healthcare Through Artificial Intelligence

Mirza Jahanzeb K. Beg
https://orcid.org/0000-0002-6308-2678
Lovely Professional University, India

Manish Kumar Verma
Lovely Professional University, India

ABSTRACT

Artificial intelligence (AI) offers significant potential for enhancing mental healthcare. Its ability to detect patterns in vast datasets can reveal insights into risk factors and symptoms, aiding the creation of tailored treatment plans. As an emerging research field, AI faces numerous challenges, particularly in its practical application. AI tools provide additional support for therapy and patient interaction. However, they cannot substitute the expertise of mental health professionals. AI's role in crisis intervention is promising but requires extensive validation to confirm its reliability and effectiveness. The ethical considerations of AI in mental health are complex, demanding careful scrutiny of its impact. This chapter examines AI's intersection with mental health, evaluating AI's practical efficacy and the ethical concerns it raises. The discussion presents a comprehensive perspective on mental healthcare's future, highlighting AI's potential benefits and the critical need to navigate its intricate challenges and limitations for psychological health.

DOI: 10.4018/979-8-3693-3112-5.ch002

INTRODUCTION

Artificial Intelligence (AI) has been explored in several fields such as administration, security, environmental management, research, education, healthcare, and commerce, because to its ability to improve efficiency and results (Karimian et al., 2022). Advancements in digital data and computational capabilities in healthcare are enabling the use of artificial intelligence (AI) to assist with many activities, including disease detection, decision-making, personalised therapy, research, drugs development, administrative streamlining, and reducing health inequities (Bak et al., 2022; Lee & Yoon, 2021).

In 2019, the World Health Organisation (WHO) said that around one in eight people worldwide had a mental disorder, with anxiety and depression being the prevailing conditions. The COVID-19 pandemic worsened these circumstances, with forecasts indicating a 26% surge in anxiety and a 28% escalation in severe depressive disorders over a span of one year (World Mental Health Report, 2022). The pandemic has underscored the pressing need for inventive remedies to tackle growing disparity in mental healthcare (World Health Organization, 2022b). Researchers propose the incorporation of digital technologies into mental health services, arguing that combining evidence-based policies and decision-support systems with conventional treatment might create a powerful hybrid model. This technique is corroborated by other research (Adiukwu et al., 2020; Gavin et al., 2020; Halms et al., 2022; Li, 2023; Peng et al., 2020; Prescott et al., 2022; SAMHSA, 2022).

Psychotherapy is a fundamental approach to addressing mental health problems. It utilises several methods, such as cognitive-behavioral therapy or psychodynamic therapy, which may be administered in person or online. Nevertheless, the extent of its influence is often constrained by variables such as social disapproval, expenses, and availability. Artificial intelligence (AI) offers novel approaches to tackle these difficulties by offering customised, flexible, and adjustable remedies (Panesar & Panesar, 2021). Chatbots, digital phenotyping, and precision medicine are capable of customising treatments to suit individual requirements.

Global concerns arise from mental health illnesses, including issues such as insufficient resources and stigma. Digital health technologies provide supportive, preventative, and therapeutic solutions that may help reduce the medical and social effects of mental health conditions (Wies et al., 2021). This chapter investigates the impact of artificial intelligence (AI) on the transformation of mental health treatment. It examines the present uses of AI, assesses their usefulness and practicality, and discusses the ethical considerations associated with their implementation.

FUNDAMENTALS OF ARTIFICIAL INTELLIGENCE

John McCarthy, a renowned computer scientist, coined the term "artificial intelligence" to include the scientific and technological concepts related to the creation of intelligent machines (McCarthy, 1989). Alan Turing, renowned as a trailblazer in the field of artificial intelligence, authored a seminal article in 1950 entitled "Computing Machinery and Intelligence." The article provided an overview of the standards used to assess machine intelligence, as proposed by Turing in 1950. The field of artificial intelligence has had periods of progress and lack of progress throughout time (McCorduck & Cfe, 2004). In contemporary society, it serves as a mechanism to expedite the process of diagnosing diseases and effectively controlling them. This technology also enables the development of novel therapy approaches for both physical and mental ailments.

Artificial Intelligence (AI) is not a one, cohesive entity, but rather a collection of several unique subsets. Each of these subcategories, or types of AI has unique characteristics and applications. The range of systems include rule-based systems, machine learning models, natural language processing, and robotics. Each category plays a crucial role in shaping the AI landscape and contributes to its vast potential in transforming many aspects of society. The constituents of artificial intelligence include the following elements:

- **Machine learning**: Machine learning is a discipline that uses algorithms trained on datasets to construct models capable of making predictions and classifying data without human intervention. This methodology uses data-driven algorithms to extract valuable insights from existing information and provide forecasts for forthcoming data or future occurrences. The emphasis is placed on formulating hypotheses rather than being influenced by preconceived notions (Graham et al., 2019).
- **Deep learning:** Deep learning is a kind of machine learning method that use many layers to extract complex features from raw input data. Each layer gains the capacity to transform the information into a little more abstract representation. Image recognition often begins with a pixel matrix as the first input. Following layers of the model subsequently examine the matrix in order to identify edges and combinations of edges. Ultimately, the model becomes capable of identifying intricate formations such as face features or objects. Deep learning algorithms autonomously choose the most beneficial features to extract at each layer of the network (Schmidhuber, 2015). Deep learning is very effective in tasks like as detecting depression, providing diagnoses, and predicting the response to treatment (Squires et al., 2023).

- **Transfer learning**: Transfer learning is the practice of applying knowledge gained from addressing one problem to another similar one. This aspect of machine learning enables the preservation and use of information that has been acquired in the past (Tajbakhsh et al., 2016).

Additional significant terms in the realm of artificial intelligence encompass:

- **Expert knowledge**: Expert knowledge systems are computer programmes that use artificial intelligence techniques to solve complex issues and provide decision-making capabilities. They do this by gathering data from their knowledge base via the application of logical reasoning and inference rules, which are developed from user queries (Leondes, 2001).
- **Neural networks (NN)**: Neural networks are interconnected collections of artificial neurons that use a mathematical or computational framework to handle and manipulate information. They draw inspiration from a connectionist approach and are often used in the field of artificial intelligence. Neural networks are adaptive systems that alter their configuration in reaction to external or internal stimuli. They are used to depict complex relationships between inputs and outputs, as well as to identify patterns in data (Hopfield, 1982).
- **Predictive analytics**: Predictive analytics is the use of historical data, statistical algorithms, and machine learning methods to assess the likelihood of future occurrences. The aim is to go beyond mere understanding of past events and instead provide the best accurate prediction of future occurrences possible (Hahn et al., 2017).
- **Natural Language Processing (NLP)**: Natural Language Processing (NLP) is the discipline that concentrates on the computer examination and comprehension of human language in its unorganised state. It includes activities such as translating languages, extracting information, and understanding meaning (Singh et al., 2024). It explores how computers can analyse and modify natural language text or voice for different objectives.

Machine learning and natural language processing (NLP) are becoming more relevant in mental health research due to their capacity to analyse extensive datasets and identify significant trends. These strategies often strengthen current clinical concepts by offering a data-driven basis to substantiate beliefs. Utilising social media data in natural language processing (NLP) may enhance forecast accuracy by including linguistic subtleties, while it may not provide a comprehensive representation of the complete population. Prior to incorporating these technologies into clinical practice, it is essential to tackle ethical issues such as data protection, informed permission, and possible biases. These factors are vital for maintaining confidence and integrity in mental health treatment. The combination of machine learning and natural language processing (NLP) has the potential to improve clinical treatment, as emphasised by Le Glaz et al. (2021). However, it is important to approach this integration with caution and responsibility.

AUTOMATED PROCESSES IN AI SYSTEMS

The integration of artificial intelligence (AI) into psychotherapy is a developing phenomenon, presenting possible advantages but also raising significant ethical concerns. Artificial intelligence (AI) chatbots have the potential to enhance the accessibility and affordability of treatment, while also streamlining administrative procedures. AI-augmented virtual and robotic treatments have the potential to assist in addressing the emotional, cognitive, and social dimensions of therapy (Holohan & Fiske, 2021). Nevertheless, it is essential to carefully examine the ethical, social, and therapeutic consequences of using AI in psychotherapy (Manríquez Roa et al., 2019). With the increasing use of AI in psychotherapy, it is essential to comprehend the intricate dynamics of AI-human relationships. This requires going beyond a simplified perspective of information exchange (Walsh, 2023).

Artificial intelligence (AI) may potentially contribute to the reduction of mental health stigma and the resolution of the scarcity of mental health providers. In India, the psychiatrist-to-population ratio is below the recommended level, with just 0.75 psychiatrists per 100,000 persons (Garg et al., 2019). Artificial Intelligence (AI) has the capacity to assist in closing this divide. The extensive proliferation of smartphones and internet connectivity, particularly in India, offers prospects for the integration of artificial intelligence (AI) and chatbots into mental health treatments. With the widespread use of smartphones worldwide and the expected increase in smartphone ownership and internet use, there is a significant potential for implementing AI interventions via applications and chatbots. These technologies have the potential to enhance the cost and accessibility of mental health treatment while also reducing the strain on mental health professionals. This might lead to improved efficiency and well-being for the professionals (Søvold et al., 2021).

AI IN RISK ASSESSMENT AND PREDICTIVE MODELLING

Predictive biomarkers are quantifiable biological characteristics that categorise individuals based on their likelihood of responding to certain treatments (De Grutolla et al., 2021; US Food and Drug Administration, 2020). For biomarkers to be considered reliable and useful in clinical decision-making, they need to demonstrate high levels of reliability, sensitivity, and specificity. Additionally, their validity should be proven by replication and verification in separate samples. Furthermore, it is crucial that they allow personalised predictions for each patient, with quantifiable levels of precision. After obtaining biomarkers that have been shown to be valid and reliable, it is important to consider variables related to safety and efficiency (Lueken & Hahn, 2020).

In order to effectively use these biomarkers and prediction models in precision medicine, a comprehensive evaluation of the risk factors linked to mental health disorders is required. This comprehensive method forms the foundation for assessing and controlling risks in psychiatry, eventually guiding therapy and decision-making procedures. Using digital technology allows for the measurement of clinical data and the use of decision models, making it easier to evaluate and create biomarkers based on empirical evidence. Using digital technology may improve patient care in psychiatry by measuring data, evaluating decision models, incorporating phenotypic data, and guiding treatment interventions (Barron et al., 2020).

Personalised predictive modelling has been crucial in advancing precision medicine as a field grounded in empirical evidence. Predictive models strive to improve their ability to reliably distinguish between individuals who do and do not achieve the anticipated outcome, a concept known as discrimination. Furthermore, their objective is to improve the correspondence between the frequencies of expected and actual outcomes, a concept known as calibration (Meehan et al., 2022). Recent research suggests that certain models have the potential to be useful in practical decision-making processes, particularly in the assessment of the risk of psychosis (Oliver et al., 2021).

Precisely identifying non-responsive people streamlines the process of developing and assessing novel medications and therapies. This allows for tailoring to certain subcategories of individuals. In the present group-statistical technique, an intervention is considered effective if it has a significant impact on the majority of participants and has a meaningful influence on the minority. Identifying individuals who do not respond to first treatment may aid in the creation of therapies that are customised for this subgroup, allowing for the early recognition of prospective benefits (Lueken & Hahn, 2020).

DIGITAL PHENOTYPING IN MENTAL HEALTH

Digital phenotyping, often referred to as personal sensing, is a data-driven approach that employs personal digital devices, namely smartphones, to predict psychological and psychometric outcomes, as well as mental health disorders (D'Alfonso, 2020).

This approach enhances the conventional methodology in psychiatry, leading to increased patient compliance and less adverse effects (Lueken & Hahn, 2020). Significant advancements have been achieved in addiction research via the use of digital phenotyping (Ferreri et al., 2018; Skinner et al., 2017). This technique shows potential for assisting in the clinical diagnosis and screening of Autism Spectrum Disorders (ASDs), a method that entails the analysis of tweets (Hswen et al., 2019). Precision medicine is a medical strategy that customises treatments based on the particular characteristics of individual patients, often using genetic data.

Clinical investigations are using digital phenotyping to detect first indications of depression, schizophrenia, and PTSD. The goal is to use data collected from mobile phones or wearable devices to improve or replace conventional clinical assessments (Huckvale et al., 2019; Jacobson et al., 2019; Kuhn et al., 2020; Lane et al., 2023; Waring et al., 2020). Ongoing research is being performed to evaluate smartphone data with the aim of identifying cognitive or behavioural characteristics that might possibly predict the probability of treatment success. In addition, digital phenotyping is used to monitor persons with serious mental illnesses, notifying healthcare practitioners of early indications of relapse for efficient care administration (Hirschtritt & Insel, 2018).

The association between digital phenotyping and precision medicine is essential as it reveals the potential benefits and constraints of precision medicine, resulting in enhanced healthcare outcomes and a transition towards proactive therapy. This combination has the capacity to generate substantial changes in the generation of medical knowledge, resulting in the creation of healthcare solutions that are more customised and effective (Baumgartner, 2021).

Machine Learning (ML) is suggested in psychiatry due to its ability to efficiently analyse extensive and complex datasets without requiring explicit instructions. This allows for the detection of underlying patterns within the data. The promise of machine learning's predictive models lies in its ability to improve clinical management by aiding in the prompt detection of illnesses, determining suitable therapies, and forecasting the probable prognosis for individual patients (Bzdok & Mayor-Lindenberg, 2018; Gillan & Whelan, 2017; Perna et al., 2018; Rutledge at al., 2019).

These technological advancements also generate ethical concerns. Ensuring data privacy and gaining consent are crucial, since these technologies often include the collection and analysis of sensitive personal data. The misuse of such data is a substantial concern, since it may lead to negative outcomes, such as employment or insurance prejudice. Stringent procedures should be enforced to guarantee the prevention of misuse. It is essential to prioritise accessibility and justice in order to prevent health disparities from worsening, since these technologies may not be equally available to those with less financial resources. Reliability and validity are essential ethical considerations because inaccurate positive or negative outcomes might lead to unnecessary therapy or missed diagnosis. In essence, digital phenotyping and precision medicine are cutting-edge approaches that give utmost importance to data and have the potential to revolutionise the healthcare industry.

BIAFFECT: AI-DRIVEN MOOD ANALYSIS

BiAffect is an advanced technology created by the University of Illinois Chicago. The system utilises an iPhone application to monitor users' typing patterns and evaluate their emotional and cognitive states. Mobile Typing Kinematics offers a non-intrusive and rapid method to detect and forecast mental health conditions. This has the capacity to augment patient autonomy, boost the availability of treatment, and optimise the cost-effectiveness of medical care (Cao et al., 2017; Jiang et al., 2020; Johnson, 2024; Sage Bionetworks, 2024).

DIGITAL TRANSFORMATION IN MENTAL HEALTHCARE

Data-based medicine, pioneered by David Sackett, is an approach that integrates the most dependable research and clinical data with practical clinical expertise and patient values to tackle clinical matters (Sackett, 1997). Decision-making is dependent on current and reliable scientific information, and data from real-world circumstances is undermining outdated hierarchies. The integration of Information and Communication Technologies (ICT) in the field of Psychology has been a rapidly growing topic of interest since the mid-20th century. Cybertherapy, coined by Isaac Marks (Marks et al., 2007), refers to the use of Information and Communication Technologies (ICTs) for therapeutic aims, such as e-therapy, virtual therapy, and Virtual Reality (VR) treatments. Computer-assisted therapy use computers to facilitate, enhance, or aid in treatment sessions, functioning as means for distant communication and as devices for creating virtual worlds.

TELEPSYCHIATRY: REMOTE TREATMENT VIA AI

Telepsychiatry is the progressive method of providing psychiatric care via various forms of communication (Ibrahim et al., 2020). The progress in healthcare is influencing patient behaviour, resulting in an increased need for online support from both professionals and peers. Telepsychiatry has evolved from simple consultations to complex models that include AI-driven evaluations using machine learning and deep learning methodologies. The use of smartphones, social media, digital communities, health applications, nutrition monitoring, wearables, and health IoT devices enables the conversion of human experiences into data, empowering patients to depend on their own gathered evidence. This has had a profound influence on the field of healthcare academics and our understanding of healthcare.

There has been a significant increase in the incorporation of Artificial Intelligence (AI) in the medical field, particularly in regard to physical well-being. However, the mental health sector has been rather hesitant to use AI (Jiang et al., 2017; Miller & Brown, 2018). The field of mental health has the potential to dramatically improve as a result of advancements in AI technology (Iniesta et al., 2016; Janssen et al., 2018; Luxton 2014; Mohr et al., 2017; Shatte et al., 2019). The potential of artificial intelligence (AI) to revolutionise the techniques used for diagnosing and comprehending mental disorders is immense. Utilising AI methods has the potential to enhance the development of enhanced pre-diagnostic screening tools and the creation of risk models for assessing an individual's susceptibility or likelihood of developing mental illnesses.

AI-assisted therapy is a novel method in the field of mental health treatment that makes use of machine learning and language processing technologies to provide therapeutic services. AI systems enhance the work of human therapists by analysing patient data, identifying patterns, and proposing treatment approaches. One significant benefit of AI therapy is its round-the-clock availability, ensuring immediate support during crises and addressing the shortage of mental health professionals in certain areas. An important characteristic of AI is its ability to independently evaluate clinical indications using various approaches, such as web-based interactions and gamified medicines.

The partnership between psychiatrists and technical professionals is crucial for the continuous progress in this field. In a study undertaken by Pham et al. (2022), the use of artificial intelligence (AI) in the field of psychiatry was investigated, with a special focus on patients exhibiting symptoms associated with Covid-19. The researchers used several artificial intelligence technologies, including chatbots like Woebot and Tess, to provide cognitive behavioural therapy and offer emotional support.

APPLICATIONS OF AI IN MENTAL HEALTH CONTEXTS

The use of Artificial Intelligence (AI) into digital healthcare is becoming widespread, offering significant potential to enhance patient outcomes, reduce costs, and optimise efficiency. Artificial intelligence (AI) is used in several fields such as mental health, medical diagnostics, therapeutic interventions, nursing, and hospital management. It enables the early diagnosis of illnesses, analyses medical imaging, and supervises administrative tasks. The objective of AI is not to replace human physicians, but rather to aid them in attaining more accurate diagnosis and treatments for patients. Integrating artificial intelligence (AI) into digital healthcare has the potential to revolutionise mental health services by offering personalised treatment plans, increased accuracy in diagnosis, and greater patient engagement (Thieme et al., 2020). The progression of artificial intelligence is expected to play a pivotal role in shaping the future of mental health care (Pandey & Misra, 2023).

AI-ENHANCED DIAGNOSTIC TECHNIQUES

Artificial intelligence (AI) can revolutionise the understanding and diagnosis of mental health disorders. An individual's mental well-being is shaped by their own bio-psycho-social characteristics, however our understanding of the interplay between biological, psychological, and social systems remains limited. The identification of biomarkers has the potential to lead to more precise and impartial categorizations of mental diseases. AI technology may provide advanced pre-diagnostic screening tools and develop risk models that can predict an individual's susceptibility to mental illness (Shatte et al., 2019).

Recent research has evaluated the effectiveness of artificial intelligence (AI) technologies in detecting affective diseases such as depression and anxiety disorders. Deep Learning (DL) databases are used to extract relevant data for people exhibiting common symptoms, such as sadness, emptiness, apathy, and sleep disturbances. Deep learning algorithms can examine extensive and varied datasets, such as health records and social media data, to identify particular factors that may contribute to an increased risk of depression. Deep learning techniques used to neuroimaging data, such as functional magnetic resonance imaging (fMRI) scans, facilitate the identification of alterations in brain structures and potential mental disorders. Deep learning has the potential to extract information directly from raw data, resulting in a more unbiased process with less bias. Online assessments and machine learning (ML) techniques enable the concurrent and iterative analysis of interrelated variables, resulting in the creation of predictive models utilising data. Machine learning has the ability to analyse complex non-linear correlations and combine diverse types of data from several sources (Andersson et al., 2021).

PERSONALIZATION OF TREATMENT THROUGH AI

Personalised Medicine, commonly referred to as precision medicine, is a cutting-edge strategy for customising illness prevention and treatment by considering variations in individuals' genes, surroundings, and lifestyles. It provides doctors with resources to get a deeper understanding of the intricate systems that contribute to a patient's well-being, illness, or condition, and to more accurately anticipate which therapies will provide the best results (National Research Council, 2011). The merging of clinical research with molecular biology, genetics, and computer science is driving advancements in personalised medicine. The process of integrating several factors is resulting in the discovery of specific molecules that cause diseases and the creation of treatments that specifically target these molecules (Jameson & Longo, 2015). Personalised medicine has the capacity to revolutionise healthcare by allowing the choice of therapies that have the highest probability of being beneficial for each unique patient, therefore enhancing health outcomes and perhaps decreasing healthcare expenses (Hamburg & Collins, 2010). Artificial Intelligence (AI) is widely acknowledged as a transformative force in the realm of personalised medicine. Artificial intelligence (AI), with its capacity to analyse and comprehend intricate information, is on the verge of transforming healthcare by facilitating data-driven decision-making, precise risk evaluation, accurate diagnoses, optimum therapy selection, and enhanced patient management. Artificial intelligence (AI) is used in personalised medicine in several important areas, such as genomic medicine, illness diagnosis, risk prediction, patient stratification, and clinical trials. The incorporation of artificial intelligence (AI) into digital health data is essential due to the growing trend in healthcare to customise treatments based on individual characteristics (Allen, 2024).

AI IN MANAGING MENTAL HEALTH EMERGENCIES

Artificial Intelligence (AI) has played a vital role in enhancing mental health care, especially in critical cases that need prompt intervention. AI chatbots, available 24/7, have played a crucial role in connecting mental health experts with those who want assistance (Khawaja & Bélisle-Pipon, 2023). They provide a cost-efficient and effective alternative to conventional therapy. These chatbots are capable of overcoming financial and logistical obstacles, offering assistance at the most crucial times and locations.

Nevertheless, the implementation of AI in this delicate domain is not devoid of its difficulties. Important problems that must be addressed include the potential risks of giving inadequate or damaging help, the exploitation of disadvantaged populations, and the development of biassed suggestions resulting from algorithmic prejudice. AI-generated replies, however efficient, can lack the authenticity, knowledge, and usefulness of human interactions, which are crucial in mental health crises (Lopes et al., 2023).

Research undertaken by Cheng & Jiang (2020) has investigated the factors that drive users to connect with healthcare chatbots. Their findings indicate that pro-active communication on the internet may impact users' behaviours in both online and offline mental health situations. This understanding is crucial for improving AI chatbots' ability to handle mental health emergencies and encourage user involvement and successful issue resolution. However, studies also suggest that AI companions sometimes have difficulties in accurately identifying or reacting suitably to indicators of distress, with only a limited number of discussions displaying signs of mental health crises. Freitas et al. (2022) have observed that users often respond unfavourably when chatbots provide useless or perhaps harmful replies. This constraint is exacerbated by the proprietary nature of the data and the cryptic nature of AI algorithms, which might disguise the efficacy of the interventions.

In order to address any ethical concerns, Mörch et al. (2021) have created a dedicated ethical checklist for the use of artificial intelligence in suicide prevention and mental health. This checklist recognises the inherent subjectivity of expert judgements and emphasises the need of doing more research including a more diverse collection of experts in order to guarantee the responsible use of AI.

To summarise, while AI has shown significant potential in the field of mental health care, especially in delivering instant assistance during critical situations, it is crucial to approach the ethical and technical obstacles with caution. To achieve success in this essential sector, it is crucial to guarantee the proper use of AI while constantly enhancing its capabilities.

AI CHATBOTS IN MENTAL HEALTH SUPPORT

Chatbots, which are software programmes that use artificial intelligence (AI) to imitate conversations in natural language, have becoming more popular in mental health environments due to their ability to provide companionship, support, and treatment. They provide benefits compared to conventional in-person or online treatments, including accessibility, cost, anonymity, and scalability. Nevertheless, chatbots present difficulties in terms of ethical, legal, and technological issues, as well as the need for human supervision and assessment.

The efficacy and adherence of a smartphone app called Shim, which utilises tactics from positive psychology and cognitive-behavioral therapy (CBT) via an automated chatbot, were evaluated in a research conducted by Ly et al. (2017) among a non-clinical population. The results revealed substantial interaction effects between the groups and time on psychological well-being and felt stress, in comparison to the control group. During the 2-week intervention period, participants showed a significant level of involvement, with an average of 17.71 instances of accessing the app.

A comprehensive evaluation was carried out by Aggarwal et al. (2023) to assess the features, effectiveness, and practicability of chatbots powered by artificial intelligence in encouraging healthy lifestyle modifications. The analysis examined 15 empirical publications published between 1980 and 2022. These articles specifically investigated treatments that used AI chatbots to address different health behaviours, including smoking cessation, medication adherence, and drug usage reduction. The findings shown a strong capacity to encourage the adoption of healthy habits and behavioural modifications. However, it is important to acknowledge several limitations such as the lack of internal validity, inadequate explanations of AI techniques, and difficulties in generalising the results.

Mobile mental health (MH) chatbots were the subject of Haque and Rubya's (2023) research, which aimed to discover user preferences and experiences by analysing reviews. Chatbots in mental health care function as digital aides, providing assistance, direction, and access to information via interactive dialogues. Nevertheless, there were constraints associated with depending on evaluations from certain platforms and the possibility of biases in user contributions.

The need for more comprehensive research and standardised result reporting to adequately evaluate the usefulness of conversational bots in psychiatric usage was highlighted by Vaidyam et al. (2019), who examined their potential. The main conclusions of the review are that conversational agents have great potential, especially in the fields of psychoeducation and self-adherence support. There is initial data that supports their usage in psychiatric settings. Nevertheless, the report emphasises the need for more research and a careful approach to incorporating conversational robots into mental therapy.

AI CHATBOTS FOR DEPRESSION AND ANXIETY MANAGEMENT

Researchers have made substantial progress in understanding and improving digital therapies by conducting a series of studies that investigate the use of AI chatbots in the treatment of depression and anxiety disorders. Fitzpatrick et al. (2017) started their investigation by conducting a research on 70 college students who exhibited signs of sadness and anxiety. They used Woebot, a conversational chatbot based on Cognitive Behavioural Therapy (CBT). During a span of two weeks, those who interacted with Woebot had a significant decrease in symptoms of depression.

However, their levels of anxiety did not show any improvement, indicating that the chatbot was specifically helpful in addressing depressed symptoms.

In addition to this, Fulmer et al. (2018) evaluated Tess, a different programme powered by artificial intelligence, across a wider range of college students from 15 universities in the United States. Their research, which allowed participants to freely use Tess, demonstrated a significant reduction in depression symptoms, especially in the group that interacted with Tess for two weeks. Both experimental groups had a drop in anxiety levels compared to the control group. Additionally, there was an improvement in positive affect ratings, suggesting that Tess has the potential to be a versatile tool for mental health.

Ip et al. (2016) used a culturally sensitive method by modifying a Western-designed online intervention to suit Chinese teenagers. Their randomised controlled experiment, including 257 teens, demonstrated the modest efficacy of "Grasping the Opportunity" in decreasing depressed symptoms over a 12-month duration. This highlights the significance of adapting digital mental health treatments to different cultures.

Leo et al. (2022) demonstrated the practicality of incorporating digital mental health care into conventional medical environments by introducing Wysa, a digital intervention, to adult orthopaedic patients. The significant levels of user retention and engagement, together with the enhanced anxiety ratings seen in regular users, highlight the feasibility and advantages of including such connections.

Liu et al. (2022) confirmed the effectiveness of therapeutic chatbots delivered via mobile devices in a university environment. The intervention resulted in significant decreases in symptoms of sadness and anxiety. Surprisingly, users found the therapeutic connection and process characteristics to be more significant than the material itself in digital therapy. This emphasises the significance of the user experience in the effectiveness of treatment.

Finally, Danieli et al. (2022) investigated the stress management capacities of "TEO," a conversational AI agent integrated with Cognitive Behavioural Therapy (CBT), for those impacted by the COVID-19 crisis in Italy. Although the study's findings are still pending, the project demonstrates the increasing use of AI chatbots as effective resources for mental health assistance, especially during times of global emergencies.

These studies demonstrate the potential of AI chatbots in mental health care, providing convenient, affordable, and tailored assistance for persons with depression and anxiety disorders. Additionally, they emphasise the need of continuous study to improve these digital tools, guaranteeing that they fulfil the various requirements of users and comply with ethical norms in mental health treatment.

AI IN FOR ADHD AND SUBSTANCE USE DISORDERS

The integration of artificial intelligence (AI) in the form of chatbots into mental health care has been the subject of various studies, each exploring the practicality and effectiveness of these digital tools in addressing different psychological conditions. In the domain of ADHD, Kaur et al. (2019) sought to categorise EEG data in order to distinguish between persons with ADHD and a control group. They achieved high levels of accuracy in differentiating between the two groups under varied scenarios. Tachmazidis et al. (2020) proposed a hybrid AI approach that integrated machine learning with medical knowledge to aid in the clinical diagnosis of adult ADHD, achieving a 95% accuracy rate.

In 2023, Chen et al. conducted a clinical experiment in the UK to demonstrate the diagnosis potential of AI for ADHD. They used a hybrid system named NeuroIntel, which achieved an accuracy rate of 93.61%. This research had an equitable sample of both positive and negative cases, demonstrating the capacity of artificial intelligence to improve diagnostic accuracy. Jang et al. (2021) delved into this by examining Todaki, a mobile application chatbot designed to provide cognitive behavioral therapy and psychoeducation for individuals with attention deficit symptoms. Their study, which included a diverse age group, demonstrated a significant reduction in attention-related symptoms among chatbot users, suggesting the potential of app-based chatbots as a viable method for mental health support. However, the study also highlighted the need for further validation through more extensive trials.

In a similar vein, Prochaska et al. (2021a) assessed Woebot-SUDs (W-SUDs), a digital intervention aimed at reducing substance abuse during the COVID-19 pandemic. The study, involving American individuals who reported drug abuse, found notable improvements in substance use and mental health outcomes for those engaging with W-SUDs. Despite these promising results, the research faced limitations due to its reliance on self-reported data and a high dropout rate.

Elmasri & Maeder (2016) focused on the use of chatbots for evaluating alcohol consumption patterns among young adults in Australia, a demographic known for high per capita alcohol use. They developed a chatbot program to conduct standardized assessments of drinking patterns, discovering that chatbots with varied behaviors and advanced conversational abilities significantly enhanced user satisfaction and perceived utility.

Further research by Prochaska et al. (2021b) looked into the feasibility and initial efficacy of Woebot for Substance Use Disorders (W-SUDs). Participants showed a high willingness to use the app and recommended it to others, although less than half felt that their needs were fully met by the intervention, indicating room for improvement in meeting user expectations.

Moghadasi et al. (2020) explored the use of a chatbot named Robo, designed to provide immediate information to individuals seeking help for opioid addiction on social media platforms. While the chatbot utilized deep learning to generate responses, the study acknowledged limitations in the dataset's scope and the chatbot's inability to offer medical advice.

Lastly, Barnett et al. (2021) raised concerns about the potential of chatbots to replace human therapists in online care for alcohol and drug-related issues. The study suggested that chatbots might lack the empathy and emotional intelligence necessary for providing empathetic care, though these findings were based on a small sample size and subjective participant feedback.

Collectively, these studies underscore the growing interest in AI chatbots as adjunct tools for mental health interventions. They reveal the nuanced benefits and challenges of implementing such technology, emphasizing the importance of continued research to enhance their effectiveness and address ethical considerations in their application. The exploration of chatbots in mental health care reflects a broader shift towards digital solutions that can complement traditional therapeutic approaches, offering accessible and personalized support for individuals with various psychological needs.

LANGUAGE ANALYSIS AND INTERVENTION OPTIMIZATION VIA AI

The subject of mental health has been greatly influenced by artificial intelligence (AI), which provides tools for language analysis and optimisation of interventions in psychotherapy. The use of AI in this field has been diverse, including the examination of therapists' language, which is naturally versatile, adaptive, and logical, as well as the creation of personalised digital treatments that address the specific requirements of each patient. State-of-the-art machine learning methods have been used to detect language patterns that are associated with positive results, therefore improving the effectiveness of therapeutic interventions.

Miner et al. (2022) devised a novel method where treatment sessions were transformed into a barcode structure, allowing for a detailed examination of therapist language at the level of individual words. This approach provides new opportunities for comprehending the intricacies of therapeutic communication. In a similar vein, Ryu et al. (2023) showcased the proficiency of natural language processing in identifying certain linguistic attributes that promote a robust therapeutic alliance, hence enhancing the connection between therapists and patients.

AI systems have played a crucial role in evaluating the accuracy and effectiveness of cognitive behavioural therapy (CBT) sessions. They automate the quality control process and assist in the training and supervision of therapists. However, there are problems associated with the use of AI into psychotherapy, notwithstanding the progress made in this field. Significant obstacles persist in the form of ethical and sociological issues, including the possibility of biases, the dissemination of false information, and the safeguarding of privacy.

However, AI represents a promising opportunity for the advancement of psychotherapy, namely in the management of anxiety disorders. It provides the potential for more individualised care, guaranteeing that mental health therapies are not only efficient but also readily available to a large number of people. With the ongoing advancement of technology, it is expected that AI will have a growing importance in improving mental health treatments and extending the availability of therapeutic services.

ADDRESSING AFFECTIVE DISORDERS WITH AI

Recent progress in artificial intelligence (AI) has shown encouraging uses in the management of affective disorders. Multiple researches have showcased the promise of machine learning and data analysis in this domain. In their study, Sau and Bhakta (2017) used machine learning techniques to create a prognostic model that accurately predicts anxiety and depression in older adults. The primary objective of this model is to aid general practitioners in identifying and intervening early in these mental health conditions. Nevertheless, they acknowledged the need of doing bigger, multi-centric research in order to improve the model's relevance to other communities.

Ay et al. (2019) developed a hybrid model that utilises EEG data to accurately diagnose depression, obtaining significant classification accuracy. This method signifies a notable advancement in the automated detection of depressed conditions. A study conducted by Mahato et al. (2020) examined electroencephalogram (EEG) data from 24 male patients diagnosed with depression and 20 control participants. The researchers specifically investigated both linear and non-linear features. Their research emphasised the specific influence of depression on the temporal area of the brain and its varying effects on each hemisphere, especially in relation to higher frequency bands.

Andersson et al. (2021) conducted research on a substantial group of 4313 women from the BASIC study in Uppsala, Sweden. They used random forest algorithms to detect individuals with a high likelihood of experiencing postpartum depression. The research emphasised the significance of variables such as unhappiness and anxiety experienced during pregnancy, resilience, and personality qualities in forecasting postpartum depression. The study indicates that the use of machine learning has the potential to enhance postpartum care by specifically focusing on those at a higher risk, thereby leading to an improvement in cost-effectiveness. Nevertheless, the research also recognised constraints, such as the need for enhanced screening techniques and the difficulty of precisely forecasting favourable results owing to the widespread occurrence of postpartum depression.

These research demonstrate how AI is continuously improving our comprehension and treatment of emotional diseases. The authors emphasise the potential of the technology to contribute to personalised treatment, while also stressing the need for more study to overcome existing limits and ethical concerns.

AI INNOVATIONS: SCHIZOPHRENIA TO ALZHEIMER'S CARE

The emergence of artificial intelligence (AI) is transforming the field of mental health diagnosis and treatment, as shown by several research showcasing its capacity to effectively handle intricate conditions like schizophrenia, Alzheimer's and ADHD. Appaji et al. (2019) conducted pioneering research in Bangalore, which included 300 participants. The participants included both healthy volunteers and patients who had been diagnosed with schizophrenia and bipolar illness. The researchers used a fundus camera to record retinal pictures and examine the vascular trajectory, revealing noteworthy disparities that indicate the potential use of retinal patterns as biomarkers for various mental health disorders. Although the study yielded encouraging results, it recognised several limitations, such as not including ocular factors and the potential impact of medicine on patients. This underscores the need for doing larger-scale research to confirm and verify these findings.

In a study done by Tikka et al. (2020), the researchers used high-density electroencephalographic data and a Support Vector Machine to differentiate between 38 male schizophrenia patients and 20 male healthy controls, therefore further investigating the potential of AI. The research obtained a classification accuracy of 78.95% in distinguishing individuals with schizophrenia from those without the condition, and 89.29% in identifying subgroups with positive and negative symptoms. Nevertheless, the study was limited to a particular subgroup of individuals, and its conclusions cannot be applied to a wider population.

Prabhakar et al. (2020) expanded the use of artificial intelligence (AI) in the field of mental health. They employed swarm intelligence computing to classify electroencephalogram (EEG) waves in persons diagnosed with schizophrenia. The research demonstrated a remarkable accuracy rate of 92.17% for individuals diagnosed with schizophrenia. However, it encountered difficulties with the limited size of the sample and possible biases in the selection of features. In a study conducted by Farooq et al. (2017), the connection between Alzheimer's disease and Mild Cognitive Impairment was examined using MRI scans. The researchers used a deep learning framework and reached a testing accuracy of 98.88% for multi-class classification. In their study, Lahmiri and Shmuel (2018) used artificial intelligence methods to examine MRI pictures and cognitive scores in order to detect Alzheimer's Disease. They discovered that a Support Vector Machine, trained using certain indices and test scores, was very successful in differentiating between healthy persons and those with Alzheimer's Disease. Farid et al. (2020) conducted a study on the use of artificial intelligence (AI) in the diagnosis of Alzheimer's Disease. They used a clinical dataset and proposed a composite hybrid feature selection approach that performed better than previous methodologies. The proposed method achieved an accuracy rate of 96.50%.

These findings highlight the significant potential of AI to revolutionise mental health care by providing individualised treatment plans, increasing the accuracy of diagnoses, and promoting patient involvement. Nevertheless, they also stress the need of resolving methodological limitations, guaranteeing ethical implementation, and broadening research to fully achieve the advantages of AI in therapeutic environments. The continuous advancement of AI has the potential to transform mental health services by offering tailored treatment and promoting more patient engagement.

ETHICAL CONSIDERATIONS IN AI DEPLOYMENT

The use of artificial intelligence (AI) into mental health care has been a revolutionary advancement, providing several advantages such as higher accuracy in diagnosis, customised treatment strategies, better results, increased efficiency, reduced costs, and expanded accessibility. Nevertheless, this integration is not without of its difficulties and gives rise to significant ethical deliberations.

An important concern is the occurrence of automation bias, which refers to the tendency of doctors to excessively depend on AI technology, possibly impacting the accuracy and effectiveness of clinical decision-making. Although AI models are very capable, they are not flawless and may include heuristics that decrease their accuracy when applied to certain patient populations. This may result in areas of limited visibility in AI performance, where the technology does not achieve its maximum potential. The generalizability of AI models and the efficacy of their explanations are also concerns that might affect their usefulness in therapeutic contexts.

Clinicians may demonstrate automation bias by relying on AI forecasts without considering their accuracy or relevance, highlighting the need for enhanced tools to assist physicians in comprehending and incorporating AI outputs into their practice. Gaining insight into the intricacies of human-AI cooperation is crucial for maximising the effectiveness of decision-making results.

It is essential to address the public's perception and knowledge gaps in order to establish trust and foster understanding between healthcare professionals and patients. AI systems should be designed and deployed with a primary focus on ethical issues to guarantee the safety, privacy, independence, and provision of excellent healthcare. Given the increasing integration of AI in mental health therapy, it is crucial to prioritise these ethical considerations in order to uphold patient safety, tackle privacy concerns, establish responsibility for AI choices, and promote ethical therapeutic partnerships.

CONCLUDING REMARKS ON AI IN MENTAL HEALTH

The use of Artificial Intelligence (AI) into mental health care has been a revolutionary influence, signalling a new period of accuracy in diagnosis, risk anticipation, and crisis handling. The underlying ideas and automation capabilities of AI have greatly enhanced the efficiency and efficacy of mental health therapies. Advanced predictive technologies have been created to detect possible hazards and provide prompt solutions, therefore improving patient outcomes. The efficient utilisation of digital technology, enabled by AI, has resulted in the automation and predictive abilities that enhance the effectiveness of treatments and interventions.

The influence of AI on mental health care is especially apparent in the areas of diagnosis and tailored treatment. Algorithms have been developed to carefully examine patient data, resulting in precise diagnoses that are essential for designing successful treatments. Moreover, AI has played a crucial role in developing personalised therapeutic approaches, specifically designed to address the individual requirements of patients, leading to enhanced treatment results. AI-powered chatbots have become indispensable tools in the field of mental health treatment, offering uninterrupted assistance to patients. These chatbots have shown to be effective in promptly connecting with patients, giving quick replies, and providing support during crises. Their ability to give instant aid in crucial circumstances has the potential to save lives.

Utilising artificial intelligence (AI) for language analysis and intervention optimisation has shown significant potential in improving patient outcomes. AI can identify indications of mental discomfort and provide early therapies by examining language patterns shown by patients. Moreover, AI may enhance the efficacy of mental health treatments by optimising therapy according to patient input.

Nevertheless, the use of artificial intelligence in mental health treatment also presents several ethical problems. Ensuring data protection and obtaining permission are of utmost importance. Given that AI systems are responsible for managing sensitive healthcare data, it is crucial to prioritise appropriate data management and safeguard patient privacy. Furthermore, it is essential that patients be provided with comprehensive information on the use of artificial intelligence in their medical care and provide their express consent.

The occurrence of automation bias, in which physicians may excessively depend on AI predictions, is a worrisome issue that might have an influence on clinical decision-making. AI models may use heuristics that reduce their accuracy for some patients, which might result in less than optimum clinical judgements. The presence of blind spots in AI models, resulting in suboptimal performance, and the limited ability of AI models to generalise, as well as the quality of their explanations, raise questions about their usefulness. Clinicians exhibiting automation bias may rely on AI predictions regardless of their precision or pertinence, underscoring the need for improved explanatory tools to assist physicians in comprehending AI model outputs and smoothly incorporating them into healthcare procedures.

Gaining insight into the intricacies of collaboration between humans and AI is essential for maximising the effectiveness of decision-making results. To cultivate trust and comprehension between practitioners and patients, it is crucial to tackle public perception and knowledge deficiencies. When developing AI systems, it is crucial to prioritise ethical issues to guarantee the safety, privacy, autonomy, and delivery of excellent healthcare to patients.

To put it briefly, AI has the capacity to greatly improve mental health treatment. Nevertheless, the incorporation of this technology requires careful and meticulous consideration in order to adequately tackle ethical issues. As artificial intelligence (AI) progresses, it will undeniably influence the future of mental health care by providing more tailored and efficient treatment approaches. However, it is essential to address these ethical concerns and guarantee the responsible use of AI in order to revolutionise mental health treatment. The potential advantages of using AI in mental health treatment are substantial, but, they must be counterbalanced with the need to safeguard patient confidentiality and maintain ethical principles. Continuing research on the potential applications of artificial intelligence in mental health treatment is crucial, since it also tackles the ethical implications that emerge.

REFERENCES

Adiukwu, F., de Filippis, R., Orsolini, L., Gashi Bytyçi, D., Shoib, S., Ransing, R., Slaih, M., Jaguga, F., Handuleh, J. I. M., Ojeahere, M. I., Ullah, I., Karaliuniene, R., Nagendrappa, S., Vahdani, B., Ashrafi, A., Ori, D., Noël, C., Abbass, Z., Jatchavala, C., & Shalbafan, M. (2022). Scaling up global mental health services during the COVID-19 pandemic and beyond. *Psychiatric Services (Washington, D.C.)*, 73(2), 231–234. DOI: 10.1176/appi.ps.202000774 PMID: 34235945

Aggarwal, A., Tam, C. C., Wu, D., Li, X., & Qiao, S. (2023). Artificial intelligence–based chatbots for promoting health behavioral changes: Systematic review. *Journal of Medical Internet Research*, 25, e40789. DOI: 10.2196/40789 PMID: 36826990

Allen, B. (2024). The Promise of Explainable AI in Digital Health for Precision Medicine: A Systematic Review. *Journal of Personalized Medicine*, 14(3), 277. DOI: 10.3390/jpm14030277 PMID: 38541019

Andersson, S., Bathula, D. R., Iliadis, S. I., Walter, M., & Skalkidou, A. (2021). Predicting women with depressive symptoms postpartum with machine learning methods. *Scientific Reports*, 11(1), 7877. DOI: 10.1038/s41598-021-86368-y PMID: 33846362

Appaji, A., Nagendra, B., Chako, D. M., Padmanabha, A., Jacob, A., Hiremath, C. V., Varambally, S., Kesavan, M., Venkatasubramanian, G., Rao, S. V., Webers, C. A. B., Berendschot, T. T. J. M., & Rao, N. P. (2019). Examination of retinal vascular trajectory in schizophrenia and bipolar disorder. *Psychiatry and Clinical Neurosciences*, 73(12), 738–744. DOI: 10.1111/pcn.12921 PMID: 31400288

Ay, B., Yildirim, O., Talo, M., Baloglu, U. B., Aydin, G., Puthankattil, S. D., & Acharya, U. R. (2019). Automated depression detection using deep representation and sequence learning with EEG signals. *Journal of Medical Systems*, 43(7), 1–12. DOI: 10.1007/s10916-019-1345-y PMID: 31139932

Bak, M., Madai, V. I., Fritzsche, M. C., Mayrhofer, M. T., & McLennan, S. (2022). You can't have ai both ways: Balancing health data privacy and access fairly. *Frontiers in Genetics*, 13, 929453. DOI: 10.3389/fgene.2022.929453 PMID: 35769991

Bansal, D., Chhikara, R., Khanna, K., & Gupta, P. (2018). Comparative analysis of various machine learning algorithms for detecting dementia. *Procedia Computer Science*, 132, 1497–1502. DOI: 10.1016/j.procs.2018.05.102

Barnett, A., Savic, M., Pienaar, K., Carter, A., Warren, N., Sandral, E., Manning, V., & Lubman, D. I. (2021). Enacting 'more-than-human' care: Clients' and counsellors' views on the multiple affordances of chatbots in alcohol and other drug counselling. *The International Journal on Drug Policy*, 94, 102910. DOI: 10.1016/j.drugpo.2020.102910 PMID: 33059955

Barron, D. S., Baker, J. T., Budde, K. S., Eickhoff, S. B., Friston, K. J., Fox, P. T., & Krystal, J. H. (2021). Decision models and technology can help psychiatry develop biomarkers. *Frontiers in Psychiatry*, 12, 706655. DOI: 10.3389/fpsyt.2021.706655 PMID: 34566711

Baumgartner, R. (2021). Precision medicine and digital phenotyping: Digital medicine's way from more data to better health. *Big Data & Society*, 8(2). DOI: 10.1177/20539517211066452

Bhagyashree, S. I. R., Nagaraj, K., Prince, M., Fall, C. H., & Krishna, M. (2018). Diagnosis of Dementia by Machine learning methods in Epidemiological studies: A pilot exploratory study from south India. *Social Psychiatry and Psychiatric Epidemiology*, 53(1), 77–86. DOI: 10.1007/s00127-017-1410-0 PMID: 28698926

Blackwell, S. E., Heisig, S., & Kuckertz, J. M. (2021). Optimizing delivery of recovery-oriented online self-help for depression: A randomized controlled trial. *Psychotherapy and Psychosomatics*, 90, 25–37.

Blackwell, S. E., Woud, M. L., & Margraf, J. (2020). A meta-analysis of cognitive-behavioural interventions for anxiety and depression in children and adolescents. *Child and Adolescent Mental Health*, 25, 37–46.

Botella, C., Díaz-García, A., Baños, R. M., & Quero, S. (2009). Cybertherapy: Advantages, limitations, and ethical issues.

Bzdok, D., & Meyer-Lindenberg, A. (2018). Machine learning for precision psychiatry: Opportunities and challenges. *Biological Psychiatry: Cognitive Neuroscience and Neuroimaging*, 3(3), 223–230. DOI: 10.1016/j.bpsc.2017.11.007 PMID: 29486863

Cao, B., Zheng, L., Zhang, C., Yu, P. S., Piscitello, A., Zulueta, J., & Leow, A. D. (2017, August). Deepmood: modeling mobile phone typing dynamics for mood detection. In *Proceedings of the 23rd ACM SIGKDD international conference on knowledge discovery and data mining* (pp. 747-755). DOI: 10.1145/3097983.3098086

Chen, T., Tachmazidis, I., Batsakis, S., Adamou, M., Papadakis, E., & Antoniou, G. (2023). Diagnosing attention-deficit hyperactivity disorder (ADHD) using artificial intelligence: A clinical study in the UK. *Frontiers in Psychiatry*, 14, 1164433. DOI: 10.3389/fpsyt.2023.1164433 PMID: 37363182

Cheng, Y., & Jiang, H. (2020). AI-Powered mental health chatbots: Examining users' motivations, active communicative action and engagement after mass-shooting disasters. *Journal of Contingencies and Crisis Management*, 28(3), 339–354. DOI: 10.1111/1468-5973.12319

D'Alfonso, S. (2020). AI in mental health. *Current Opinion in Psychology*, 36, 112–117. DOI: 10.1016/j.copsyc.2020.04.005 PMID: 32604065

Danieli, M., Ciulli, T., Mousavi, S. M., Silvestri, G., Barbato, S., Di Natale, L., & Riccardi, G. (2022). Assessing the impact of conversational artificial intelligence in the treatment of stress and anxiety in aging adults: Randomized controlled trial. *JMIR Mental Health*, 9(9), e38067. DOI: 10.2196/38067 PMID: 36149730

De Freitas, J., Uğuralp, A. K., Oğuz-Uğuralp, Z., & Puntoni, S. (2022). Chatbots and mental health: Insights into the safety of generative AI. *Journal of Consumer Psychology*.

De Gruttola, V. G., Clax, P., DeMets, D. L., Downing, G. J., Ellenberg, S. S., Friedman, L., Gail, M. H., Prentice, R., Wittes, J., & Zeger, S. L. (2001). Considerations in the evaluation of surrogate endpoints in clinical trials: Summary of a National Institutes of Health workshop. *Controlled Clinical Trials*, 22(5), 485–502. DOI: 10.1016/S0197-2456(01)00153-2 PMID: 11578783

Elmasri, D., & Maeder, A. (2016). A conversational agent for an online mental health intervention. In *Brain Informatics and Health:International Conference, BIH 2016,Omaha, NE, USA,October 13-16, 2016Proceedings* (pp. 243-251). Springer International Publishing. DOI: 10.1007/978-3-319-47103-7_24

Farid, A. A., Selim, G. I., & Khater, H. A. A. (2020). Applying artificial intelligence techniques to improve clinical diagnosis of Alzheimer's disease. *European Journal of Engineering Science and Technology*, 3(2), 58–79. DOI: 10.33422/ejest.v3i2.487

Farooq, A., Anwar, S., Awais, M., & Alnowami, M. (2017, September). Artificial intelligence based smart diagnosis of Alzheimer's disease and mild cognitive impairment. In *2017 International Smart cities conference (ISC2)* (pp. 1-4). IEEE. DOI: 10.1109/ISC2.2017.8090871

Ferreri, F., Bourla, A., Mouchabac, S., & Karila, L. (2018). e-Addictology: An overview of new technologies for assessing and intervening in addictive behaviors. *Frontiers in Psychiatry*, 9, 348832. DOI: 10.3389/fpsyt.2018.00051 PMID: 29545756

Fitzpatrick, K. K., Darcy, A., & Vierhile, M. (2017). Delivering cognitive behavior therapy to young adults with symptoms of depression and anxiety using a fully automated conversational agent (Woebot): A randomized controlled trial. *JMIR Mental Health*, 4(2), e7785. DOI: 10.2196/mental.7785 PMID: 28588005

Fleming, T. M., de Beurs, D., Khazaal, Y., Gaggioli, A., Riva, G., Botella, C., Baños, R. M., Aschieri, F., Bavin, L. M., Kleiboer, A., Merry, S., Lau, H. M., & Riper, H. (2016). Maximizing the impact of e-therapy and serious gaming: Time for a paradigm shift. *Frontiers in Psychiatry*, 7, 65. DOI: 10.3389/fpsyt.2016.00065 PMID: 27148094

Fulmer, R., Joerin, A., Gentile, B., Lakerink, L., & Rauws, M. (2018). Using psychological artificial intelligence (Tess) to relieve symptoms of depression and anxiety: Randomized controlled trial. *JMIR Mental Health*, 5(4), e9782. DOI: 10.2196/mental.9782 PMID: 30545815

Garg, K., Kumar, C. N., & Chandra, P. S. (2019). Number of psychiatrists in India: Baby steps forward, but a long way to go. *Indian Journal of Psychiatry*, 61(1), 104–105. PMID: 30745666

Gavin, B., Lyne, J., & McNicholas, F. (2020). Mental health and the COVID-19 pandemic: Looking back and moving forward. *Irish Journal of Psychological Medicine*, 37(4), 247–249. DOI: 10.1017/ipm.2020.128 PMID: 33323135

Gillan, C. M., & Whelan, R. (2017). What big data can do for treatment in psychiatry. *Current Opinion in Behavioral Sciences*, 18, 34–42. DOI: 10.1016/j.cobeha.2017.07.003

Graham, S., Depp, C., Lee, E. E., Nebeker, C., Tu, X., Kim, H. C., & Jeste, D. V. (2019). Artificial intelligence for mental health and mental illnesses: An overview. *Current Psychiatry Reports*, 21(11), 1–18. DOI: 10.1007/s11920-019-1094-0 PMID: 31701320

Hahn, T., Nierenberg, A. A., & Whitfield-Gabrieli, S. (2017). Predictive analytics in mental health: Applications, guidelines, challenges and perspectives. *Molecular Psychiatry*, 22(1), 37–43. DOI: 10.1038/mp.2016.201 PMID: 27843153

Halms, T., Strasser, M., Kunz, M., & Hasan, A. (2022). How to reduce mental health burden in health care workers during COVID-19?–a scoping review of guideline recommendations. *Frontiers in Psychiatry*, 12, 770193. DOI: 10.3389/fpsyt.2021.770193 PMID: 35126194

Hamburg, M. A., & Collins, F. S. (2010). The path to personalized medicine. *The New England Journal of Medicine*, 363(4), 301–304. DOI: 10.1056/NEJMp1006304 PMID: 20551152

Haque, M. R., & Rubya, S. (2023). An overview of chatbot-based mobile mental health apps: Insights from app description and user reviews. *JMIR mHealth and uHealth*, 11(1), e44838. DOI: 10.2196/44838 PMID: 37213181

Hirschtritt, M. E., & Insel, T. R. (2018). Digital technologies in psychiatry: Present and future. *Focus (San Francisco, Calif.)*, 16(3), 251–258. DOI: 10.1176/appi.focus.20180001 PMID: 31975919

Holohan, M., & Fiske, A. (2021). "Like I'm talking to a real person": Exploring the meaning of transference for the use and design of AI-based applications in psychotherapy. *Frontiers in Psychology*, 12, 720476. DOI: 10.3389/fpsyg.2021.720476 PMID: 34646209

Hopfield, J. J. (1982). Neural networks and physical systems with emergent collective computational abilities. *Proceedings of the National Academy of Sciences of the United States of America*, 79(8), 2554–2558. DOI: 10.1073/pnas.79.8.2554 PMID: 6953413

Hswen, Y., Gopaluni, A., Brownstein, J. S., & Hawkins, J. B. (2019). Using Twitter to detect psychological characteristics of self-identified persons with autism spectrum disorder: A feasibility study. *JMIR mHealth and uHealth*, 7(2), e12264. DOI: 10.2196/12264 PMID: 30747718

Huckvale, K., Venkatesh, S., & Christensen, H. (2019). Toward clinical digital phenotyping: A timely opportunity to consider purpose, quality, and safety. *NPJ Digital Medicine*, 2(1), 1–11. DOI: 10.1038/s41746-019-0166-1 PMID: 31508498

Ibrahim, F. A., Pahuja, E., Dinakaran, D., Manjunatha, N., Kumar, C. N., & Math, S. B. (2020). The future of telepsychiatry in India. *Indian Journal of Psychological Medicine*, 42(5, suppl), 112S–117S. DOI: 10.1177/0253717620959255 PMID: 33354056

Iniesta, R., Stahl, D., & McGuffin, P. (2016). Machine learning, statistical learning and the future of biological research in psychiatry. *Psychological Medicine*, 46(12), 2455–2465. DOI: 10.1017/S0033291716001367 PMID: 27406289

Ip, P., Chim, D., Chan, K. L., Li, T. M., Ho, F. K. W., Van Voorhees, B. W., Tiwari, A., Tsang, A., Chan, C. W. L., Ho, M., Tso, W., & Wong, W. H. S. (2016). Effectiveness of a culturally attuned Internet-based depression prevention program for Chinese adolescents: A randomized controlled trial. *Depression and Anxiety*, 33(12), 1123–1131. DOI: 10.1002/da.22554 PMID: 27618799

Jacobson, N. C., Weingarden, H., & Wilhelm, S. (2019). Using digital phenotyping to accurately detect depression severity. *The Journal of Nervous and Mental Disease*, 207(10), 893–896. DOI: 10.1097/NMD.0000000000001042 PMID: 31596769

Jameson, J. L., & Longo, D. L. (2015). Precision medicine—Personalized, problematic, and promising. *Obstetrical & Gynecological Survey*, 70(10), 612–614. DOI: 10.1097/01.ogx.0000472121.21647.38 PMID: 26014593

Jang, S., Kim, J. J., Kim, S. J., Hong, J., Kim, S., & Kim, E. (2021). Mobile app-based chatbot to deliver cognitive behavioral therapy and psychoeducation for adults with attention deficit: A development and feasibility/usability study. *International Journal of Medical Informatics*, 150, 104440. DOI: 10.1016/j.ijmedinf.2021.104440 PMID: 33799055

Janssen, R. J., Mourão-Miranda, J., & Schnack, H. G. (2018). Making individual prognoses in psychiatry using neuroimaging and machine learning. *Biological Psychiatry: Cognitive Neuroscience and Neuroimaging*, 3(9), 798–808. DOI: 10.1016/j.bpsc.2018.04.004 PMID: 29789268

Jiang, F., Jiang, Y., Zhi, H., Dong, Y., Li, H., Ma, S., Wang, Y., Dong, Q., Shen, H., & Wang, Y. (2017). Artificial intelligence in healthcare: Past, present and future. *Stroke and Vascular Neurology*, 2(4), 230–243. DOI: 10.1136/svn-2017-000101 PMID: 29507784

Jiang, X., Li, Y., Jokinen, J. P., Hirvola, V. B., Oulasvirta, A., & Ren, X. (2020, April). How we type: Eye and finger movement strategies in mobile typing. In *Proceedings of the 2020 CHI conference on human factors in computing systems* (pp. 1-14). DOI: 10.1145/3313831.3376711

Johnson, N. (2024, January 3). *Mental Illness Could Now be Detected Through an App*. YR Media. https://yr.media/health/mental-health/brain-mental-illness-biaffect-depression-bipolar-alex-leow/

Karimian, G., Petelos, E., & Evers, S. M. (2022). The ethical issues of the application of artificial intelligence in healthcare: A systematic scoping review. *AI and Ethics*, 2(4), 539–551. DOI: 10.1007/s43681-021-00131-7

Kaur, S., Singh, S., Arun, P., Kaur, D., & Bajaj, M. (2020). Phase space reconstruction of EEG signals for classification of ADHD and control adults. *Clinical EEG and Neuroscience*, 51(2), 102–113. DOI: 10.1177/1550059419876525 PMID: 31533446

Khawaja, Z., & Bélisle-Pipon, J. C. (2023). Your robot therapist is not your therapist: Understanding the role of AI-powered mental health chatbots. *Frontiers in Digital Health*, 5, 1278186. DOI: 10.3389/fdgth.2023.1278186 PMID: 38026836

Kuhn, E., & Owen, J. E. (2020). Advances in PTSD treatment delivery: The role of digital technology in PTSD treatment. *Current Treatment Options in Psychiatry*, 7(2), 88–102. DOI: 10.1007/s40501-020-00207-x

Lahmiri, S., & Shmuel, A. (2019). Performance of machine learning methods applied to structural MRI and ADAS cognitive scores in diagnosing Alzheimer's disease. *Biomedical Signal Processing and Control*, 52, 414–419. DOI: 10.1016/j.bspc.2018.08.009

Lane, E., D'Arcey, J., Kidd, S., Onyeaka, H., Alon, N., Joshi, D., & Torous, J. (2023). Digital Phenotyping in Adults with Schizophrenia: A Narrative Review. *Current Psychiatry Reports*, 25(11), 699–706. DOI: 10.1007/s11920-023-01467-z PMID: 37861979

Le Glaz, A., Haralambous, Y., Kim-Dufor, D. H., Lenca, P., Billot, R., Ryan, T. C., Marsh, J., DeVylder, J., Walter, M., Berrouiguet, S., & Lemey, C. (2021). Machine learning and natural language processing in mental health: Systematic review. *Journal of Medical Internet Research*, 23(5), e15708. DOI: 10.2196/15708 PMID: 33944788

Lee, D., & Yoon, S. N. (2021). Application of artificial intelligence-based technologies in the healthcare industry: Opportunities and challenges. *International Journal of Environmental Research and Public Health*, 18(1), 271. DOI: 10.3390/ijerph18010271 PMID: 33401373

Leo, A. J., Schuelke, M. J., Hunt, D. M., Metzler, J. P., Miller, J. P., Areán, P. A., Armbrecht, M. A., & Cheng, A. L. (2022). A digital mental health intervention in an orthopedic setting for patients with symptoms of depression and/or anxiety: Feasibility prospective cohort study. *JMIR Formative Research*, 6(2), e34889. DOI: 10.2196/34889 PMID: 35039278

Leondes, C. T. (Ed.). (2001). *Expert systems: the technology of knowledge management and decision making for the 21st century*. Elsevier.

Li, J. (2023). Digital technologies for mental health improvements in the COVID-19 pandemic: A scoping review. *BMC Public Health*, 23(1), 413. DOI: 10.1186/s12889-023-15302-w PMID: 36859184

Liu, H., Peng, H., Song, X., Xu, C., & Zhang, M. (2022). Using AI chatbots to provide self-help depression interventions for university students: A randomized trial of effectiveness. *Internet Interventions : the Application of Information Technology in Mental and Behavioural Health*, 27, 100495. DOI: 10.1016/j.invent.2022.100495 PMID: 35059305

Lopes, E., Jain, G., Carlbring, P., & Pareek, S. (2023). Talking Mental Health: A Battle of Wits Between Humans and AI. *Journal of Technology in Behavioral Science*, 9(4), 1–11. DOI: 10.1007/s41347-023-00359-6

Lueken, U., & Hahn, T. (2020). Personalized mental health: Artificial intelligence technologies for treatment response prediction in anxiety disorders. In *Personalized Psychiatry* (pp. 201–213). Academic Press. DOI: 10.1016/B978-0-12-813176-3.00017-1

Luxton, D. D. (2014). Artificial intelligence in psychological practice: Current and future applications and implications. *Professional Psychology, Research and Practice*, 45(5), 332–339. DOI: 10.1037/a0034559

Ly, K. H., Ly, A. M., & Andersson, G. (2017). A fully automated conversational agent for promoting mental well-being: A pilot RCT using mixed methods. *Internet Interventions : the Application of Information Technology in Mental and Behavioural Health*, 10, 39–46. DOI: 10.1016/j.invent.2017.10.002 PMID: 30135751

Mahato, S., Goyal, N., Ram, D., & Paul, S. (2020). Detection of depression and scaling of severity using six channel EEG data. *Journal of Medical Systems*, 44(7), 1–12. DOI: 10.1007/s10916-020-01573-y PMID: 32435986

Manríquez Roa, T., Biller-Andorno, N., & Trachsel, M. (2019). The ethics of artificial intelligence in psychotherapy.

Marks, I. M., Cavanagh, K., & Gega, L. (2007). Computer-aided psychotherapy: Revolution or bubble? *The British Journal of Psychiatry*, 191(6), 471–473. DOI: 10.1192/bjp.bp.107.041152 PMID: 18055948

McCarthy, J. (1989). *Artificial Intelligence*. Logic and Formalizing Common Sense.

McCorduck, P., & Cfe, C. (2004). *Machines who think: A personal inquiry into the history and prospects of artificial intelligence*. AK Peters/CRC Press. DOI: 10.1201/9780429258985

Meehan, A. J., Lewis, S. J., Fazel, S., Fusar-Poli, P., Steyerberg, E. W., Stahl, D., & Danese, A. (2022). Clinical prediction models in psychiatry: A systematic review of two decades of progress and challenges. *Molecular Psychiatry*, 27(6), 2700–2708. DOI: 10.1038/s41380-022-01528-4 PMID: 35365801

Miller, D. D., & Brown, E. W. (2018). Artificial intelligence in medical practice: The question to the answer? *The American Journal of Medicine*, 131(2), 129–133. DOI: 10.1016/j.amjmed.2017.10.035 PMID: 29126825

Miner, A. S., Milstein, A., Schueller, S., Hegde, R., Mangurian, C., & Linos, E. (2016). Smartphone-based conversational agents and responses to questions about mental health, interpersonal violence, and physical health. *JAMA Internal Medicine*, 176(5), 619–625. DOI: 10.1001/jamainternmed.2016.0400 PMID: 26974260

Moghadasi, M. N., Zhuang, Y., & Gellban, H. (2020, July). Robo: A counselor chatbot for opioid addicted patients. In *Proceedings of the 2020 2nd Symposium on Signal Processing Systems* (pp. 91-95). DOI: 10.1145/3421515.3421525

Mohr, D. C., Zhang, M., & Schueller, S. M. (2017). Personal sensing: Understanding mental health using ubiquitous sensors and machine learning. *Annual Review of Clinical Psychology*, 13(1), 23–47. DOI: 10.1146/annurev-clinpsy-032816-044949 PMID: 28375728

Mörch, C. M., Gupta, A., & Mishara, B. L. (2020). Canada protocol: An ethical checklist for the use of artificial Intelligence in suicide prevention and mental health. *Artificial Intelligence in Medicine*, 108, 101934. DOI: 10.1016/j.artmed.2020.101934 PMID: 32972663

National Research Council, Division on Earth, Life Studies, Board on Life Sciences, & Committee on A Framework for Developing a New Taxonomy of Disease. (2011). Toward precision medicine: building a knowledge network for biomedical research and a new taxonomy of disease.

Oliver, D., Spada, G., Colling, C., Broadbent, M., Baldwin, H., Patel, R., Stewart, R., Stahl, D., Dobson, R., McGuire, P., & Fusar-Poli, P. (2021). Real-world implementation of precision psychiatry: Transdiagnostic risk calculator for the automatic detection of individuals at-risk of psychosis. *Schizophrenia Research*, 227, 52–60. DOI: 10.1016/j.schres.2020.05.007 PMID: 32571619

Pandey, A., & Misra, M. (2023). Artificial Intelligence in Mental Health Care. In Yadav, D. K., & Gulati, A. (Eds.), *Artificial Intelligence and Machine Learning in Healthcare*. Springer. DOI: 10.1007/978-981-99-6472-7_8

Panesar, A., & Panesar, H. (2021). Artificial intelligence and machine learning in global healthcare. In *Handbook of Global Health* (pp. 1775–1813). Springer International Publishing. DOI: 10.1007/978-3-030-45009-0_75

Peng, D., Wang, Z., & Xu, Y. (2020). Challenges and opportunities in mental health services during the COVID-19 pandemic. *General Psychiatry*, 33(5), e100275. DOI: 10.1136/gpsych-2020-100275 PMID: 32914056

Perna, G., Grassi, M., Caldirola, D., & Nemeroff, C. B. (2018). The revolution of personalized psychiatry: Will technology make it happen sooner? *Psychological Medicine*, 48(5), 705–713. DOI: 10.1017/S0033291717002859 PMID: 28967349

Pham, K. T., Nabizadeh, A., & Selek, S. (2022). Artificial intelligence and chatbots in psychiatry. *The Psychiatric Quarterly*, 93(1), 249–253. DOI: 10.1007/s11126-022-09973-8 PMID: 35212940

Prabhakar, S. K., Rajaguru, H., & Sun-Hee, K. (2020). Schizophrenia EEG signal classification based on swarm intelligence computing. *Computational Intelligence and Neuroscience: CIN, 2020.*

Prescott, M. R., Sagui-Henson, S. J., Welcome Chamberlain, C. E., Castro Sweet, C., & Altman, M. (2022). Real world effectiveness of digital mental health services during the COVID-19 pandemic. *PLoS One*, 17(8), e0272162. DOI: 10.1371/journal.pone.0272162 PMID: 35980879

Prochaska, J. J., Vogel, E. A., Chieng, A., Baiocchi, M., Maglalang, D. D., Pajarito, S., Weingardt, K. R., Darcy, A., & Robinson, A. (2021). A randomized controlled trial of a therapeutic relational agent for reducing substance misuse during the COVID-19 pandemic. *Drug and Alcohol Dependence*, 227, 108986. DOI: 10.1016/j.drugalcdep.2021.108986 PMID: 34507061

Prochaska, J. J., Vogel, E. A., Chieng, A., Kendra, M., Baiocchi, M., Pajarito, S., & Robinson, A. (2021). A therapeutic relational agent for reducing problematic substance use (Woebot): Development and usability study. *Journal of Medical Internet Research*, 23(3), e24850. DOI: 10.2196/24850 PMID: 33755028

Rutledge, R. B., Chekroud, A. M., & Huys, Q. J. (2019). Machine learning and big data in psychiatry: Toward clinical applications. *Current Opinion in Neurobiology*, 55, 152–159. DOI: 10.1016/j.conb.2019.02.006 PMID: 30999271

Ryu, J., Heisig, S., & McLaughlin, C. (2022). A natural language processing approach reveals interpretable linguistic features of therapeutic alliance in psychotherapy. *iScience*, 24, 102751.

Sackett, D. L. (1997, February). Evidence-based medicine. *Seminars in Perinatology*, 21(1), 3–5. DOI: 10.1016/S0146-0005(97)80013-4 PMID: 9190027

SAMHSA. (2022). *Adaptations and Innovations for Delivering Mental Health and Substance Use Disorder Treatment Services During the COVID-19 Pandemic.* https://www.samhsa.gov/sites/default/files/dtac-adaptations-innovations-covid-19-pandemic.pdf

Sau, A., & Bhakta, I. (2017). Predicting anxiety and depression in elderly patients using machine learning technology. *Healthcare Technology Letters*, 4(6), 238–243. DOI: 10.1049/htl.2016.0096

Schmidhuber, J. (2015). Deep learning in neural networks: An overview. *Neural Networks*, 61, 85–117. DOI: 10.1016/j.neunet.2014.09.003 PMID: 25462637

Shatte, A. B., Hutchinson, D. M., & Teague, S. J. (2019). Machine learning in mental health: A scoping review of methods and applications. *Psychological Medicine*, 49(9), 1426–1448. DOI: 10.1017/S0033291719000151 PMID: 30744717

Singh, V., Sarkar, S., Gaur, V., Grover, S., & Singh, O. P. (2024). Clinical Practice Guidelines on using artificial intelligence and gadgets for mental health and well-being. *Indian Journal of Psychiatry*, 66(Suppl 2), S414–S419. DOI: 10.4103/indianjpsychiatry.indianjpsychiatry_926_23 PMID: 38445270

Skinner, A. L., Attwood, A., Baddeley, R., Evans-Reeves, K., Bauld, L., & Munafo, M. (2017). Digital phenotyping and the development and delivery of health guidelines and behaviour change interventions. *Addiction (Abingdon, England)*, 112(7), 1281–1285. DOI: 10.1111/add.13746 PMID: 28472848

Søvold, L. E., Naslund, J. A., Kousoulis, A. A., Saxena, S., Qoronfleh, M. W., Grobler, C., & Münter, L. (2021). Prioritizing the mental health and well-being of healthcare workers: An urgent global public health priority. *Frontiers in Public Health*, 9, 679397. DOI: 10.3389/fpubh.2021.679397 PMID: 34026720

Squires, M., Tao, X., Elangovan, S., Gururajan, R., Zhou, X., Acharya, U. R., & Li, Y. (2023). Deep learning and machine learning in psychiatry: A survey of current progress in depression detection, diagnosis and treatment. *Brain Informatics*, 10(1), 10. DOI: 10.1186/s40708-023-00188-6 PMID: 37093301

Tachmazidis, I., Chen, T., Adamou, M., & Antoniou, G. (2020). A hybrid AI approach for supporting clinical diagnosis of attention deficit hyperactivity disorder (ADHD) in adults. *Health Information Science and Systems*, 9(1), 1. DOI: 10.1007/s13755-020-00123-7 PMID: 33235709

Tajbakhsh, N., Shin, J. Y., Gurudu, S. R., Hurst, R. T., Kendall, C. B., Gotway, M. B., & Liang, J. (2016). Convolutional neural networks for medical image analysis: Full training or fine tuning? *IEEE Transactions on Medical Imaging*, 35(5), 1299–1312. DOI: 10.1109/TMI.2016.2535302 PMID: 26978662

Thieme, A., Belgrave, D., & Doherty, G. (2020). Machine learning in mental health: A systematic review of the HCI literature to support the development of effective and implementable ML systems. *ACM Transactions on Computer-Human Interaction*, 27(5), 1–53. DOI: 10.1145/3398069

Tikka, S. K., Singh, B. K., Nizamie, S. H., Garg, S., Mandal, S., Thakur, K., & Singh, L. K. (2020). Artificial intelligence-based classification of schizophrenia: A high density electroencephalographic and support vector machine study. *Indian Journal of Psychiatry*, 62(3), 273–282. DOI: 10.4103/psychiatry.IndianJPsychiatry_91_20 PMID: 32773870

Turing, A. M. (1950). Computing machinery and intelligence. *Mind*, 59(October), 433–460. DOI: 10.1093/mind/LIX.236.433

US Food and Drug Administration. (2020). *Qualification Process for Drug Development Tools Guidance for Industry and FDA Staff.* https://www.fda.gov/media/133511/download

Vaidyam, A. N., Wisniewski, H., Halamka, J. D., Kashavan, M. S., & Torous, J. B. (2019). Chatbots and conversational agents in mental health: A review of the psychiatric landscape. *Canadian Journal of Psychiatry*, 64(7), 456–464. DOI: 10.1177/0706743719828977 PMID: 30897957

Van Le, D., Montgomery, J., Kirkby, K. C., & Scanlan, J. (2018). Risk prediction using natural language processing of electronic mental health records in an inpatient forensic psychiatry setting. *Journal of Biomedical Informatics*, 86, 49–58. DOI: 10.1016/j.jbi.2018.08.007 PMID: 30118855

Walsh, D. (2023, June 21). *A Blueprint for Using AI in Psychotherapy*. Stanford HAI. https://hai.stanford.edu/news/blueprint-using-ai-psychotherapy

Waring, O. M., & Majumder, M. S. (2020). Introduction to digital phenotyping for global health. *Leveraging data science for global health*, 251-261.

Warrier, U., Warrier, A., & Khandelwal, K. (2023). Ethical considerations in the use of artificial intelligence in mental health. *The Egyptian Journal of Neurology, Psychiatry and Neurosurgery*, 59(1), 139. Advance online publication. DOI: 10.1186/s41983-023-00735-2

Wies, B., Landers, C., & Ienca, M. (2021). Digital mental health for young people: A scoping review of ethical promises and challenges. *Frontiers in Digital Health*, 3, 697072. DOI: 10.3389/fdgth.2021.697072 PMID: 34713173

World Health Organization. (2022). *Mental health and COVID-19: early evidence of the pandemic's impact: scientific brief, 2 March 2022* (No. WHO/2019 -nCoV/ Sci_Brief/Mental_health/2022.1). World Health Organization.

World Mental Health Report: transforming mental health for all. (2022). World Health Organization.

Zhou, S., Zhao, J., & Zhang, L. (2022). Application of artificial intelligence on psychological interventions and diagnosis: An overview. *Frontiers in Psychiatry*, 13, 811665. DOI: 10.3389/fpsyt.2022.811665 PMID: 35370846

Chapter 3
Chatbots as Tools for Psychoeducation and Self-Help in Mental Health

Archana Sowbarnika
https://orcid.org/0009-0006-8457-5312
Infiheal HeathTech Private Limited, India

Abhinanda Patra
https://orcid.org/0009-0003-3638-1482
Infiheal Healthtech Private Limited, India

Lavleen Kaur
https://orcid.org/0009-0006-0289-6412
Infiheal Healthtech Private Limited, India

Sruthi Suresh
https://orcid.org/0000-0002-2505-9872
Christ University, India

Srishti Srivastava
https://orcid.org/0009-0002-8773-2687
Infiheal Healthtech Private Limited, India

Drishti Chawla
https://orcid.org/0009-0008-3011-0514
Infiheal Healthtech Private Limited, India

ABSTRACT

The chapter highlights the role of mental health chatbots in solving problems in global mental health. It aims to explore how AI-powered conversational agents bridge the gap between growing demand and limited availability of mental health services. The authors explain advantages of chatbots, including accessibility, affordability, and user anonymity. They investigate the effectiveness of chatbots in improving treatment outcomes, meeting user needs, and improving operational efficiency. In addition, the chapter highlights the ability of chatbot as a knowledge sharer that seamlessly integrates information from various sources and keeps professionals up to date with

DOI: 10.4018/979-8-3693-3112-5.ch003

current events. It deals with psychoeducation in clinical and non-clinical populations, covering biological, cognitive, emotional, and behavioural aspects. The authors also discuss the potential of chatbots in screening and self-help. Finally, they emphasise the importance of collaboration between psychologists, physicians, and engineers to optimise the development of chatbots to respond dynamically to user needs.

BACKGROUND

Mental health comprises our emotional, psychological, and social well-being. It affects our thinking, feelings, perception of the world, and our actions. Hence, prioritising mental health is essential for overall well-being, influencing our quality of life, productivity, and resilience (Bezerra et al., 2018). Much like we care for our physical health through exercise and a balanced diet, attending to our mental health is crucial. It directly impacts cognitive functions, emotional connections, and the ability to navigate life's challenges. It also helps us determine how one handles stress, relationships with others, and possible healthy and unhealthy choices in life (Fusar-Poli et al., 2020). However, despite the importance of mental health, the numbers suggest an overall treatment gap for mental health disorders.

The overall treatment gap for mental disorders ranged from 70% to 92% across various disorders (Murthy, 2017). The National Mental Health Survey by the National Institute of Mental Health and Neurosciences reported an overall weighted prevalence for any mental health morbidity at 13.7% (Singh, 2019). According to Math et al. (2019), the number of mental health service providers is almost negligible compared to the demand, further highlighting the gravity of the situation. The ideal number of psychiatrists, psychologists, psychiatric social workers, and mental health nurses is 1/10,000 for developed countries. However, in India, the current numbers are: psychiatrists – 0.2/100,000, psychologists – 0.03/100,000, psychiatric social workers – 0.03/100,000, and mental health nurses – 0.05/100,000 population. Various innovative approaches are needed to bridge this huge gap.

Worldwide, mental health care faces a multitude of similar challenges, encompassing high costs, supply-side limitations, prolonged waiting times (often 2-8 weeks), frequent misdiagnosis of personality disorders as mood disorders, outdated treatment methods, low awareness, dissemination of incorrect information, absence of centralised records, lack of intermediary support between therapy sessions, lack of distress helplines, talk support and reminders. Additionally, social stigma, particularly prevalent among older generations, further complicates access to mental health services. The emergence of online solutions during the COVID-19 pandemic has mitigated stigma by offering services from the comfort of one's home, sometimes anonymously, resulting in increased demand. However, these solutions have yet to comprehensively address the broader spectrum of issues and supply-side constraints inherent in mental health care (Meghrajani et al., 2023; Moghimi et al., 2023; Wainberg et al., 2017).

In this scenario, digital interfaces are emerging as viable alternatives for reducing this gap and making mental health care and treatment accessible and affordable. Alongside smartphones, VR technology, and E-learning systems, artificial intelligence (AI) is an effective option. It can detect, predict, and assess mental health issues, thus working as a preventive measure for overall well-being (Ettman & Galea, 2023). A chatbot is a computer program that simulates human conversation using conversational artificial intelligence (CAI) techniques such as natural language processing (IBM, n.d.). Chatbots are typically freely available 24/7 for users to converse, obtain information, and access suitable recommendations. Currently, several mental health chatbots such as Anna, Woebot, Earkick, Virtua Health, Healo and Wysa exist. Many of these chatbots use generative AI and Natural language processing (NLP) to imitate human language and conversations.

Natural language processing (NLP) helps computers understand the meaning, intentions, and emotions in written text. It uses rules and algorithms inspired by how people use language to make sense of it all. With the help of NLP, generative AI models can understand and generate human-like text (Gupta, 2023). This enables chatbots to understand a user's query or statement, then formulate an appropriate response. Talviya (2023) highlights that it is also possible to employ machine learning algorithms to recognize user intents based on the input they receive. This involves categorising user queries into predefined categories or actions, allowing the chatbot to determine the user's purpose or goal. This aids in directing the conversation flow and providing relevant assistance to users. Because of this capacity to discern and recognize, chatbots can possibly differentiate between the degrees and severity of mental health issues of the user. High-risk cases can be connected to the nearest distress helpline, whereas moderate-risk cases can be matched to the right therapist based on their personality and preferences. Low-risk clients can be offered digital solutions - meditation audios, exercises, self-work-based pathways, mood trackers, reading lists, movie recommendations, relatable content (jokes, memes), as well as matching to support groups and peers.

Artificial intelligence also can take in information about various therapeutic modalities and modify responses accordingly. An example of this can be seen in the work of Andrade-Arenas et al. (2024), where they developed and evaluated a chatbot based on CBT principles. Eventually, both digital and talk support options in chatbots can incorporate the biopsychosocial perspective by connecting the latest research integrating fields like epigenetics and psychoneuroimmunology. Furthermore, a variety of therapeutic modalities, including Gestalt, acceptance and commitment therapy, solution-focused therapy, and trauma-informed approach, contribute to a holistic solution, drawing from Eastern mindfulness and Western psychology. In adopting a community-driven approach, chatbots can also foster an environment that encourages the exchange of best practices among therapists and mental health professionals. This collaboration can enhance therapy quality and record-keeping. The detailed history collected by a chatbot not only has the power to streamline record-keeping but can also reduce the time therapists spend, resulting in higher-quality care (Chen et al., 2023; Co et al., 2022). As a result of such features, chatbot services can aid in improving accessibility to mental health care by reducing the associated stigma and managing the shortage of mental health professionals. However, these services are not a replacement for therapy but aim to assist those with less severe issues or are to be used in addition to therapy (Perrone, 2024). Viduani et al. (2023) highlight that using chatbots in clinical settings is advantageous in increasing access to mental health care, facilitating data collection and management, and promoting patient disclosure. Nonetheless, it is also important to consider patient safety, privacy and confidentiality of data, and the management of emergencies in this context.

FEATURES OF A CHATBOT

The emergence of artificial intelligence (AI) chatbots has dramatically changed the way humans interact with computers in recent years. This technology has transformed industries such as customer service, healthcare, management, education, and almost all areas of our lives. Powered by state-of-the-art natural language processing (NLP) algorithms and machine learning, AI chatbots are not just a passing fad but they have established themselves as essential components of our online lives, which integrates in our daily routines and provides us with a wide range of tasks and questions (Kulkarni & Jaiswal, 2023). Chatbots have several different use cases, which can be classified under certain parameters – knowledge domain, service provided, goals, input processing and response generation method, human-aid, and build methods. Classification based on the input processing and response generation method takes into account the method of processing inputs and generating responses.

Three models are used to produce the appropriate responses – rule-based, retrieval-based, and generative (Bao et al., 2020). Rule-based chatbots can be commonly seen in online chat systems. They use preset rules to respond to user messages. It uses the system response based on a fixed predefined set of rules, based on recognizing lexical form of the input text without creating any new answers in the text. The knowledge used in these chatbots is hand-coded and organised and presented with conversational patterns. A more comprehensive rule database allows the chatbot to reply to more types of user input. However, this type of model is not robust to spelling and grammatical mistakes in the user input. In more human-like bots, multi-turn response selection takes into consideration previous parts of the conversation to select a response that is relevant to the whole conversation context. Some examples include chatbots that offer information about hours of business or assist with basic customer service inquiries (Oracle Cloud Infrastructure (OCI), n.d.).

Different from the rule-based model is the retrieval-based model which uses machine learning models, such as statistical NLP models and sometimes supervised neural networks, to interpret the user input and determine the most fitting response to retrieve. Like rule-based models, retrieval-based models rely on predefined responses, but they have the additional ability to self-learn and improve their selection of response over time (Codecademy, n.d.). The generative model generates answers in a better way than the other two models, based on current and previous user messages. These chatbots are more human-like that use machine learning algorithms and deep learning techniques (Bao et al., 2020).

Intersection of Chatbots and Mental Health

Conversational agents (CAs), or chatbots, have shown substantial promise in the realm of mental health care offering a wide range of functionalities to address various challenges faced by individuals. Powered by NLP, machine learning, and deep learning, these AI-based CAs possess expanding capabilities to process more complex information and thus allow for more personalised, adaptive, and sophisticated responses to mental health concerns. (Mesko, 2023). They assist with preliminary diagnosis, facilitate consultations, provide psychoeducation, and deliver treatment options while also simultaneously playing a role in offering social support and boosting mental resilience to the users (Li et al., 2023). These chatbots have the potential to address the needs of individuals with mental disorders, particularly those who may be hesitant to seek traditional therapy due to stigmatisation. They provide a safe and non-judgmental space for individuals to seek support and guidance, reducing stigma and improving mental hygiene.

There are already several chat-based AI platforms in the global market that identify mental health concerns, track moods, and deliver interventions like cognitive behavioural therapy. Some examples include Replika, a US-based virtual AI companion that facilitates emotional processing and connection in a safe environment. Xiaotian is from China and was built with professional deconstruction skills. Xiaotian listens, analyses, and guides conversations to clarify true feelings (XinhuaNet, 2021). Healo, a mental health chatbot by Infiheal, India, is focused on holistic mental healthcare. It employs an advanced personality assessment algorithm and risk profiling for triaging, and uses Generative AI for functionality like venting, advice, recommendations, and guided meditations. Various advantages of such chatbots include:

Accessibility, Affordability, Agency: A 2021 national survey by the American Psychiatric Association commissioned by Woebot Health, one of the leading therapeutic chatbot companies, in a study found that 22% of adults used a mental health chatbot, and 47% said they would be interested in using one if needed. Among the respondents who had tried a mental health chatbot, nearly 60% said they began to use during the COVID-19 pandemic, and 44% said they used chatbots exclusively and did not see a human therapist. "The most common reasons people cited as to why they used and/or might be interested in using a chatbot included that the tool was cheap, easy to use, and accessible anytime (24/7)." This does not imply that chatbots are surrogates for human-delivered psychotherapy, even in cases where they become more sophisticated. Darcy acknowledged "A tennis ball machine will never replace a human opponent, and a virtual therapist will not replace a human connection," she said. Instead, Chatbots support human clinicians by providing situational help to patients in between therapist appointments.

By using AI chatbots, individuals can access mental healthcare services from the convenience of their own homes through their mobile phones, without the need to schedule an appointment or travel to a clinic. This is particularly beneficial where mental health services are lacking, i.e. for individuals who live in remote areas, or for those who have difficulty accessing mental healthcare services due to financial or logistical reasons. Additionally, bots can provide support and guidance 24/7, allowing individuals to access help whenever and at the frequency they need it. Overall, the use of chatbots has the potential to greatly improve access to mental healthcare services, making them more widely available and easier to access for individuals around the globe (Yunus et al., 2020).

User-friendly Interface: Chatbots are the novel innovative and interactive way to communicate, especially with youngsters. For instance, Ash, an Australia, CBT-based App was designed to enhance teen mental health at schools. It was developed in response to the increasing number of youth struggling to cope with stress at school, feelings of depression and anxiety, and the lack of adequate help for their problems (Monash University, 2021). The ease of use and interface can help us open-up and connect more easily. Bots are human-like representations of information providers that are increasingly applied within popular private messenger services that most of us are already familiar with, such as Facebook Messenger, Kik, Telegram, Viber, and WhatsApp. Similarly, in mental health bots too, users type questions (i.e. queries) in natural language, and meaningful answers are returned. The chatbot parses the content of the user input (questions such as "Why do I have anxiety?") and intelligently responds by using advanced AI capabilities The chatbot conversations can be perceived as meaningful and trustworthy. Thus, chatbots provide a text-based conversational interface for information, which delivers immediate feedback in a human-like way. (Skjuve & Brandtzæg, 2017)

Free from Bias and Stigmas: One of the most profound impacts of AI in mental healthcare is its role in reducing stigma. For many, the mere act of seeking help can be daunting due to societal prejudices (for example, marginalised communities like people of colour and LGBTQ+ individuals,) and discrimination (based on categories like caste or socio-economic background). These are communities who become "othered" pushed away from the "margins" of mainstream society. They are excluded in various ways, such as, lowering participation in education, work and in healthcare access leading to lesser health and social outcomes (Robards et al., 2020; Shukla, 2022; Thapa et al., 2021). In this regard, chatbots offer more inclusive and acceptable space for stigmatised communities. AI driven platforms offer anonymity, allowing individuals to seek support without the fear of judgement. The Chatbot conversations can be perceived as meaningful and trustworthy. This is especially crucial for the youth and middle-aged population, who often grapple with societal pressures and are at ease with technology. Many people hesitate to seek traditional therapy because they feel uncomfortable discussing their issues with a stranger or fear the stigma associated with seeking mental health support. By providing a safe, non-judgmental space, AI tools are making mental health discussions mainstream (Intelliverse.ai, 2023).

Evidence-Based Therapy: Chatbots can be programmed to offer evidence-based therapeutic techniques such as cognitive-behavioural therapy (CBT). CBT is a common form of therapy used to treat mental health issues like anxiety and depression. By using chatbots, individuals can receive benefits of CBT in a convenient and accessible way. Some chatbots are fully automated and some use human interfaces. Woebot is a fully automated conversational agent developed by Woebot Labs in San Francisco. It treats depression and anxiety using a digital version of time-tested cognitive behaviour therapy Interpersonal psychotherapy (IPT), and dialectical behaviour therapy (DBT). In a feasibility study which compared 34 college students undergoing therapy with Woebot and 36 students who were a part of the information-only control group, it was found that after 2 weeks, participants in the Woebot group had shown a significant decrease in depression scores as measured by PHQ-9. Chatbots like Ellie almost serve as virtual therapists as they can detect subtleties in facial expressions, rates of speech, or length of pauses and respond accordingly. It also provides an option to meet an actual therapist (Singh, 2019).

Consistency and Reliability: Chatbots offer consistent and reliable support without the risk of human error. They track progress and provide reminders for self-care activities or appointments, ensuring that individuals stay on track with their mental health goals. Consistent support and reminders can help individuals stay motivated and engaged in their mental health journey. Wysa, a US based AI-guided CBT app, integrates meditation, yoga, and guided journaling activities. Healo by Infiheal, an India, also provides consistent support and reminders for self-care.

Increased Engagement and Empowerment: Chatbots can increase engagement and empowerment by encouraging individuals to take an active role in their mental health journey. Youper, a US based app utilises CBT, conducts daily check-ins, tracking users' moods, thoughts, and feelings. A study from Stanford University showed significant improvement in symptoms of depression and anxiety after just two weeks of using the Youper app (Youper, n.d.). Bots can provide rich psycho-education, educational resources, tools, and exercises that individuals can use to manage their symptoms and improve their mental wellness. Additionally, chatbots can provide encouragement and positive reinforcement to individuals, improving their motivation and overall treatment outcomes (Sachdeva, 2023).

Improved Crisis Management: How to prevent the next suicide is one of the most common and still highly complicated questions in the field of psychology and psychiatry. Indeed, it is a question of critical importance given that suicide poses a grave public health concern, with approximately 817,000 individuals dying by suicide annually. This staggering figure underscores the urgent necessity for a comprehensive investment in a broad array of suicide prevention strategies aimed at curtailing the global suicide prevalence. Chatbots can be used as a valuable tool for crisis management and suicide prevention as they can provide immediate support and resources to individuals in crisis, and can also alert emergency services or caregivers if necessary. Bots can help save lives by providing immediate support to those in distress (Sachdeva, 2023). An article published by research square suggests that GenAI has the potential to play a crucial role in promoting safe reporting practices, with implications for public health. The method involved two independent human reviewers and two AI systems, Claude.AI and ChatGPT-4, which assessed 40 suicide-related articles from online platforms based on the WHO's 15 criteria. The findings indicated strong agreement between ChatGPT-4 and the two human reviewers (0.81–0.87). Strong agreement was also found between Claude.AI and the two human reviewers (0.73–0.78) (Niederkrotenthaler et al., 2021).

From the above, it can be seen that various features of chatbots are of great help in supporting people with mental health issues. One can argue how it might be useful for psychoeducation, especially in clinical populations, and for self-help in general populations.

CHATBOTS AS A PSYCHOEDUCATIONAL TOOL FOR THE CLINICAL POPULATION

Psychoeducation is the process of providing information to the client and family to elicit their support in working together with the mental health professional. The main goals of psychoeducation include – (1) ensuring basic knowledge and competence of patients and their relatives about the illness, (2) providing insight into the illness, (3) promoting relapse prevention, and (4) engaging in crisis management and suicide prevention. By incorporating aspects of cognitive behaviour therapy, group therapy, and education, psychoeducation is considered to be an effective form of psychotherapy for both the clinical and non-clinical populations (Sarkhel et al., 2020). Anderson et al. (1980) highlighted that psychoeducation consisted of four essential elements – briefing the patients about their illness, problem-solving training, communication training, and self-assertiveness training. However, the timing and content of the psychoeducation sessions may vary based on the nature of the issue, the audience, and the focus of the session.

Role of Psychoeducation

The evidence-based practice of psychoeducation across mental health settings is effective due to its flexibility and range of elements included (Lukens & McFarlane, 2006). For clients experiencing schizophrenia, psychoeducation not only improves satisfaction with mental health services and treatment adherence but also helps reduce relapse and hospital readmission rates and enhance functioning and quality of life (Xia et al., 2011). It also helps reduce the recurrence of bipolar disorder and depression (Goodwin et al., 2016), increases positive attitude towards attention-deficit/hyperactivity disorder (Nussey et al., 2013) and has positive effects on stress and anxiety (Klainin-Yobas et al., 2016). Additionally, being a relatively low-risk psychosocial treatment, psychoeducation assists the clinical high-risk (CHR) population in preventative and early treatment interventions (McGorry et al., 2010) as well as reduces the stigma associated with psychiatric labels (Herrera et al., 2023). However, the accessibility of psychoeducation is limited due to factors such as perceptions about its significance, lack of knowledge and skills for its implementation, lack of training, and lack of adequate reimbursement for these services (Motlova et al., 2017).

Role of Chatbots in Psychoeducation

In recent years, there has been an increase in demand for mental health services. The simultaneous increase in the capabilities of artificial intelligence has led to the development of digital mental health intelligence (DMHI) to support diagnostics and screening, symptom management and behaviour change, and content delivery using chatbots (Boucher et al., 2021).

The use of chatbot-based psychoeducation is said to reduce the cost, time, and space constraints that prevent clients from receiving adequate treatment; however, the effectiveness of chatbot-supported psychoeducation needs to be considered simultaneously. A study by Selaskowski et al. (2023) examined the benefits of self-guided psychoeducation based on a chatbot for adults with attention-deficit hyperactivity disorder. The results of the randomised control trial indicated that both chatbot-based and conventional app self-guided psychoeducation were equally beneficial and safe for the participants. Another study by Jang et al. (2021) reported similar results for the chatbot application "Todaki". Participants in the study mentioned that they enjoyed the empathic and friendly character but perceived it to have an unnatural flow of conversation.

Several researchers have reviewed the effectiveness of chatbots in mental health. A systematic literature review by Vaidyam et al. (2019) examined ten studies that used chatbots offering primarily dynamic user input and output response for the clinical population. These studies were selected from six databases containing 1466 records based on the inclusion criteria. The results indicated that there was high satisfaction and potential for psychiatric use of chatbots across all studies. It was not only beneficial for psychoeducation and adherence but also increased accessibility to treatment by reducing stigma and cost. However, drawbacks were also reported, such as limited and time-inappropriate responses and blurring of therapeutic boundaries. There were mixed results regarding the lack of a human in such interactions, with some studies reporting higher disclosure of sensitive information in the absence of human involvement and others studies reporting the opposite. Overall, there was positive user satisfaction, indicating that clients found benefits and enjoyed using chatbot services.

A scoping review by Ahmed et al. (2023) examined the features of chatbots available for anxiety or depression. The review included forty-two studies by filtering six bibliographic databases, which returned 1302 citations. There were different methods of support offered by the chatbots, including traditional therapeutic counselling, unique features for depression and anxiety, empathetic phrasing, and care-receiving. The care-receiving chatbots, such as Vincent, Gloomy, and Perla, encourage users to practise self-reflection and self-compassion by facilitating a deeper level of understanding of their experiences. The findings indicated favourable patient outcomes and adoption of chatbots; however, limited quality research is available. Another review by Boucher et al. (2021) focused on AI-based chatbots and used a case study on Happify Health's AI chatbot, Anna. The authors highlighted that it is important to examine the perceptions and acceptance of professionals and clients regarding the use of the mental health services offered by chatbots. Further, the usage of these chatbots could also vary based on the user demographic profile. It is also imperative to understand user perceptions of the social attributes, empathy, and therapeutic interactions offered by the chatbot in comparison to those provided by human therapists. Finally, the safety and ethical implications of using chatbot-based mental health services need to be evaluated. Nonetheless, the authors mention that AI-based chatbots help reduce the workload and balance the shortage of mental health professionals. However, the widespread adoption of chatbot services and educating and working with mental health professionals will improve the quality and effectiveness of chatbot services.

Based on existing literature, the use of digital mental health interventions is increasing. Although there is limited evidence to support the effectiveness of all such DMHIs, the available research shows benefits in promoting understanding and treatment of issues faced by the clinical population. It also overcomes common obstacles to mental health services, such as the stigma surrounding labels, limited accessibility and availability of services, and the cost of availing services. However, ensuring standardised outcomes reporting is essential to provide a generalisable picture regarding the effectiveness of chatbot-based psychoeducation. Over the years, there could be an increase in the use of chatbots as essential tools to support mental health or as therapists themselves. Hence, promoting the use of chatbots and examining their benefits and challenges is the critical step to ensure their safe and effective usage.

Chatbots offering Psychoeducation

In the existing reign of digital mental health initiatives, several mental health chatbots are designed to support specific issues. Many of the chatbots, such as Woebot, Wysa, Youper, Healo, Todaki, and Ensemble, assist users in dealing with depression and anxiety-related problems. Some chatbots are also designed to provide mental health support and encourage users to practise self-care. The Vincent chatbot is a care receiver which aims to promote self-compassion among its users. Unlike other chatbots that provide helpful strategies, Vincent shares its challenges and asks for advice from the user. Lee et al. (2019) reported that participants in the care-receiving condition of the Vincent chatbot showed a significant increase in self-compassion in comparison to those in the care-giving condition of the chatbot. Earkick is another such chatbot specialising in providing personalised chats based on the users' unique needs and preferences, simultaneously ensuring privacy and confidentiality (Frey, 2024). Chatbots like Moodfit, Tess (Stephens et al., 2019), and Student Bodies (Dev et al., 1999) also offer psychoeducation to help users deal with body image issues, difficult emotions, procrastination, and rumination. Through the use of tracking and summary reports, users can have insights into their mental health and lifestyle and make required modifications (Valera, 2023).

CHATBOTS AS A SELF-HELP TOOL FOR THE GENERAL POPULATION

In contemporary parlance, self-help is a popular term often used to indicate a wide array of practices ranging from relaxing to invigorating and to bring about behavioural and attitudinal changes (for example, lifestyle changes, habit building, handling distress). This may involve self-help books, attending support and 12-step groups, and referring to popular internet forums or podcasts for advice, stress management techniques, and alternative medicine. In general, such methods can be applied to any facet of an individual's life- physical, psychological, financial, or professional. In the context of mental health, self-help can be seen as any preventive strategies and techniques a person might apply to manage their psychological well-being (Chang et al., 2021; Norcross, 2000).

Contrary to popular belief, the concept of self-help has been practised for a long time. Late 18th-century and early 19th-century history suggests that the self-help movement had a pluralistic approach. People joined each other in seeking support and bettering themselves in the face of a physical or mental illness, or even for cognitive betterment. It can be inferred that this aided in the birth of groups like Alcoholics Anonymous (AA) and Narcotics Anonymous (NA) (Flora et al., 2010).

In the age of digital intervention, self-help strategies can be applied seamlessly to both individual and group settings. They can be broadly divided into two categories: Guided (the individual has professional help while they still pursue the self-help material) and unguided (simple self-help strategies that can be used without professional help) (Jorm & Griffiths, 2006). Self-help has also been used interchangeably with self-care and self-management techniques, which will be discussed later. A significant overlap exists between what they entail, suggesting they can be grouped under one term (Town et al., 2023)

Need for Correct Self-help in the General Population

Despite the criticism from some professionals, self-help as an industry persists and is effective when compared to no-treatment control groups. (Mains & Scogin, 2003; Rosen, 1993). It can be argued that much of the burden of symptoms of anxiety, depression, or any other issue that is perceived as minor in general is attributable to subclinical symptoms. Using self-help strategies primarily in these scenarios can prevent further clinical development and can be encouraged (Jorm & Griffiths, 2006). Meta-analysis of Self-help in children and adolescents (Benett et al., 2019) echoes the same sentiment, claiming that it reduces the stigma around mental health issues. In a research paper (Biringer et al., 2016), a case is made for how learning about self-management techniques like positive activities, habits, and surrounding yourself with positive people can initiate recovery and promote self-efficacy before even stepping into mental health treatment sessions aided by professionals.

The need to disseminate proper and effective self-help techniques is evident from its popularity. It is often the "go-to" for individuals who are dealing with difficulties, especially the emotional kind, as there are barriers that prevent the general population from accessing basic mental health care. In India, Recent research by Bhargava and Mor (2024) shows that "about 200 million people are estimated to be living with poor mental health. Eight out of ten not receiving treatment further compounds the problem. Without interventions that together target mental health resilience, reduction, recognition, and recovery, we expect this burden of disease to increase by 35 percent..." (p.1). The percentage of mental health service workers is approximately 0.3 psychiatrists, 0.07 psychologists and 0.07 social workers per 100,000 people in India (The Economic Times, 2022). Similarly, there are financial, cultural, and social barriers like low affordability, lack of awareness, lack of accessibility and stigma (Andrade et al., 2013).

AI chatbots can bridge this gap between the general population and mental health professionals by providing evidence-based self-help and management techniques under many of its features, such as usability, personalisation capacity, acceptability, scalability, free-flowing conversations, and non-judgemental space (Aggarwal et al., 2023). As chatbots can be easily integrated into popular SNS platforms, They offer an immediate and less intimidating avenue for support. This is shown in the research of (Kamita et al., 2018), where they used LINE, a popular chat tool in Japan, to test their digital-SAT method through the chatbot.

Evidence of Effectiveness of Chatbots in the Context of Self-help

Multiple sources have found that digital predecessors to AI chatbots, such as computer-assisted therapy, smartphone apps, and wearable technologies, effectively aid mental health issues. The general mechanism of change these interventions follow is providing users with worksheets, self-reflective questions based on psychological theories, mood, habits and stress monitoring, and journaling. In a systematic meta-review (Hollis et al., 2017), multiple digital health interventions were looked at in children and adolescents. For depressive symptoms, some of these were positively associated with improvements in outcomes compared to waitlist and no intervention controls.

Project CATCH-IT incorporated behavioural activation, CBT, interpersonal psychotherapy, and a community resiliency concept model. 6 weeks post-intervention, the improvements were sustained and increased in both intervention groups at one-year follow-up for Project CATCH-IT.

PratenOnline delivered one-to-one chat room-based Solution-Focused Brief Therapy (SFBT). Over a quarter of young people receiving PratenOnline maintained clinically significant change at 4.5-month follow-up, compared to waitlist controls. Additionally, adolescents who used StressBusters (using cCBT theoretical base) reported improvements in depression and anxiety from post-intervention to 3-month follow-up. A multi-theoretical online intervention, Bounce Back Now for adolescents affected by natural disasters, resulted in improvements in PTSD and depressive symptoms at 12-month follow-up. Another systematic review and meta-analysis (Grist et al., 2018) found that technology-based interventions had a small positive impact compared to waitlist controls. Cognitive Behavioral Therapy (CBT) interventions showed a medium impact, while Attention Bias Modification (ABM) interventions had a negligible impact.

Regarding AI chatbots, these above-mentioned interventions can be incorporated easily because of AI's open and generative nature. Because of its relational and conversational capacity, more can be done when it comes to rapport building (Zhang et al., 2020), even across different cultures (Chin et al., 2023). Evidence of this has been shown across multiple fields that can arguably come under self-help: lifestyle changes, habit building, learning better, and managing addiction, depression and anxiety symptoms.

Management of Mental Health Issues. In a randomised controlled trial, the participants were randomly assigned to either a chatbot test group to receive a newly developed chatbot-delivered intervention or a bibliotherapy control group to receive a minimal level of bibliotherapy for symptoms of anxiety and depression. After the treatment, individuals belonging to the chatbot group showed a significant reduction in scores in questionnaires that measured general health and anxiety levels (PHQ-9 and GAD-7). Follow-up analysis suggested that the reduction of anxiety was significant only in the first four weeks (Liu et al., 2021). In their paper, which talked about the overview of freely available chatbots, Haque and Rubya (2023) mention how they have great potential to offer social and psychological support in situations where no support is available. This study involved apps like Woebot, Wysa, Youper, Stresscoach, and Serenity, which targeted Stress, anxiety, depression, self-care, relationship issues, and loneliness and provided access to self-care tools to users 24/7. Kamita et al. (2018) also suggest that Woebot, as part of an evaluation experiment, decreased depressive symptoms in students significantly. Text-based chatbots like ELIZA and MYLO led to emotional relief of anxiety, stress, and pain in general, Although MYLO focused more on problem-solving. In their subsequent studies, it was observed that in a two-week comparative study between the self-guided mental healthcare systems with and without a chatbot, the system with a chatbot showed higher stress reduction effects and continuity of use. The chatbot had the SAT counselling method integrated, created by Munakata (Kamita et al., 2020).

Lifestyle Changes. Multiple studies have found that AI chatbots were efficacious in promoting healthy lifestyles, including physical exercise and diet, smoking cessation, treatment or medication adherence, and reduction in substance misuse. In a study by Piao et al. (2020), the Healthy Lifestyle Coaching Chatbot program delivered through KakaoTalk (a popular messenger service in South Korea) resulted in effective habit formation for stair-climbing behaviour. Compared to the baseline, The participants's habit strength scores were positively impacted after four weeks of the intervention on the Self Rating Habit Index (SRHI).

A systematic review and meta-analysis by Singh et al. (2023) found that chatbots aided in significant lifestyle changes. Specifically, chatbots led to an extra 735 steps per day, one additional serving of fruit and vegetables, and an additional 45 minutes of sleep per night. They also found that text-based chatbots are more effective than speech or voice-based AI, which suggests that, at least for the time being, text-based communication is more conducive to achieving positive outcomes in health-related interventions. Further evidence of physical activity and diet programs can be seen in the study by Maher et al. (2020), where a virtual assistant-led lifestyle change program, driven by Chatbot Paola, was both doable and led to noticeable improvements in physical activity, diet, and body composition after 12 weeks. In the area of weight management, Tess, the behavioural coaching chatbot, has been successfully implemented to help support teens in a weight management program and can expand further (Stephens et al., 2019).

In the context of health intervention, CoachAI is a chatbot designed to help with creating and providing health programs for individuals or groups. It sends health activities regularly, like daily or weekly, or at times chosen by the coach. The one-month pilot study done by Fadhil et al. (2019) showed that users were satisfied with the bot, trusted it greatly, and were comfortable sharing personal details, like their stress levels. This suggests that using a conversational agent to support individuals who want to improve their lives is possible. However, the choice between using a virtual agent, a human agent, or a mix depends on the specific health context.

In the study by Prochaska et al. (2021) Woebot shows a promising impact when it comes to handling substance use. During an eight-week program, participants engaged with the app extensively, especially with modules on COVID-19, urge surfing, and substance use labels. Mood and craving ratings decreased significantly, while pain ratings remained stable. Among retained participants, confidence in resisting substance use increased significantly, and self-reported substance use decreased. Most participants would recommend the app, although less than half felt it met all their needs. Similarly, Participants in the study by Chun-Hung et al. (2023) had favourable acceptance and generally positive outcomes related to interventions for Methamphetamine usage. For smoking cessation, evidence of motivational interviewing (MI) working through chatbot has been found in the study by Brown et al. (2023). Using generative reflections of the MIbot boosts the conversation's impact on quitting smoking a week later, but asking questions alone can also have a significant effect. This suggests the need to improve the chatbot dialogue and provides a basis for comparing it with more advanced versions.

Overall, AI chatbots as tools to aid self-help efforts show great promise with its interventions for emotional problems being acceptable, engaging and with high usability (Balan et al., 2024). Although it is not without limitations, Users across studies have reported a lack of personal connection with chatbots, poor smartphone skills among the participants, impractical recommendations by the chatbot, and technical challenges such as those where the participants stopped receiving the chatbot messages. Users are greatly influenced by the quality of the relationship between humans and AI, how engaged they are with the content, and how effectively the content is communicated. This is still in the process of improvement when it comes to AI technology (Li et al., 2023). Meta-analyses have also found that guided or chatbots, which are already integrated or adjunct with a mental health professional, work better (Gellatly et al., 2007). Another major problem that remains is non-compliance or falling out of the program (Gould & Clum, 1993). Nevertheless, the majority of the research done in this area have a similar optimistic view- that it is indeed possible to use AI chatbots to aid self-help efforts for the general population and reach numbers that are not possible by the current physical resources.

CHATBOTS AS A TOOL FOR THERAPIST MATCHING

Why is it important to match with the right kind of therapist?

The client-counsellor relationship is perhaps the most important part of the healing process in therapy. The right fit can make the difference between therapy being positive, empowering, or frustratingly unproductive. When the user works with a therapist who is suitable for them and their needs, they create an alliance that can foster personal growth, improve their coping skills, and significantly improve the user's ability to deal with the challenges that brought them to therapy in the first place (France, 2016).

The question remains: how does the user know which therapist is right for them? Traditionally, this decision is made by asking for referrals from close ones, researching therapists nearby, contacting different therapists that we might be interested in and interviewing them, and looking for the therapist's professional orientationist and their education and licensure.

Even doing all these things does not lead to a therapist that matches with the personality. As personality is very subjective, there needs to be a fit and balance between one's personality and the potential therapist's personality for it to be an excellent therapeutic alliance. For instance, when an extremely introverted user meets an extroverted therapist, the therapist might not necessarily comprehend what it means to be in the shoes of an introverted individual. This does not negate their professional capabilities. However, if you, the user, are significantly different in their disposition and have a high someone who requires a sense of being heard, understood and nurtured, their clinical style might simply not align with your needs. Often, this intangible yet crucial factor can only be adequately assessed through an in-person interaction.

Moreover, this is where AI-driven therapist matching can be transformative. AI-driven therapist matching can simplify this process as the AI analyses your traits, preferences, and overall persona to highlight therapists who are predicted to be highly compatible fits. This personalised approach allows users to choose from a curated pool of professionals, ensuring compatibility and increasing the likelihood of a successful treatment relationship. A good client-clinician fit promises to lead to a better therapeutic alliance, better client functioning, reliable reductions in depressive symptoms, and positive change in many other client outcomes (Peacock et al., 2021).

In addition, this system not only saves users valuable time but also offers flexibility. If the user finds that the initial match is not quite right, they can explore other available therapists without starting the entire search process. This flexibility encourages users to try different matches until they find one that suits their needs.

In addition, users can provide feedback and additional information about their preferences and experiences, allowing the AI system to continuously refine its recommendations. This iterative process ensures that recommendations are adjusted over time, leading to more effective matches and, ultimately, better treatment outcomes.

How Chatbots can Match Client-Therapist using NLP and AI

Chatbots use natural language processing (NLP) and artificial intelligence (AI) to interact with users. The use of NLP techniques helps to analyse and understand the meaning of user inputs based on text. Research also shows that there is an upward trend in the detection of mental disorders using NLP (Zhang, 2022). By understanding the user's question or statement, the bot can formulate an appropriate response.

The chatbot recognises intention by applying NLU mechanisms to recognise user intents based on their input. This can involve categorising user queries into predefined categories or actions, analysing semantic patterns, extracting entities, and understanding context, allowing the chatbot to determine the user's purpose or goal. Intent recognition is essential for directing the conversation flow and providing relevant assistance to users.

Natural language processing can be used to develop conversational agents used for therapeutic intervention (D'Alfonso, 2020). They use contextual understanding techniques to remember previous interactions, user preferences, and relevant information exchanged during the conversation to ensure coherence and relevance in their responses. This allows chatbots to provide personalised and contextual responses, improving the user experience.

After understanding user intent and context, chatbots generate natural-sounding responses using natural language generation (NLG) techniques. NLG involves synthesising human-like language based on predefined patterns, rules or by using GenAI models. By generating consistent and contextual responses, chatbots can engage users in meaningful conversation and provide valuable help or information.

Functionality of Chatbots in Therapist Matching

Chatbots play a central role in the initial assessment of users' mental health needs, preferences and demographics by engaging in interactive conversations. This data collection process enables chatbots to personalise therapist recommendations effectively. Leveraging advanced algorithms, chatbots facilitate algorithmic matching between users and therapists, considering factors such as specialisation, location, availability, and treatment approach. This ensures precise and tailored matches, enhancing the overall user experience. Additionally, Chatbots are highly usable due to their simple interface and conversation-driven functionality (Holmes, 2019).

In addition, mental health chatbots are valuable resources that provide users with comprehensive information about therapists, including their credentials, specialities, availability, and session formats. This can help the user feel empowered to make informed decisions about their treatment options. Additionally, mental health chatbots can streamline the appointment process by seamlessly integrating with calendars and providing automatic booking tools. Users can easily view available appointments, select desired appointments and receive reminders, promoting greater engagement with therapy services.

In terms of efficiency, mental health chatbots excel at quickly assessing user needs and preferences, thus streamlining the therapist-matching process. This process saves considerable time compared to traditional methods, such as searching through directories or waiting for human assistance. Research has also shown that chatbots are an acceptable solution to offering mental health support (Koulouri, 2022).

Lastly, chatbots offer scalability benefits by efficiently handling many inquiries simultaneously. This scalability makes them well-suited for platforms serving diverse user bases, as they can adapt to growing demand without requiring additional resources. Overall, chatbots are a valuable asset in mental health services, offering efficiency, scalability, and personalised support.

Case Study, Therapist Matching: Healo, an Initiative by Infiheal

Infiheal's Healo Chatbot has attempted a novel approach to mental health support. Healo AI coach provides emotional guidance and provides psychoeducation to users. A significant point of difference is utilising conversational data for therapist-matching based on personality types. Healo uses advanced algorithms to create personalised connections between clients and therapists. Furthermore, it delves into the user's specific concerns, preferred communication style, desired therapeutic approach, and personality type to find the best fit.

On the therapist side, it considers things like therapeutic modalities, specialisations, and even the languages spoken. This AI algorithm-based matching aims to streamline the challenging process of finding the right therapist. By prioritising compatibility, Healo hopes to increase client satisfaction and, ultimately, improve overall therapeutic outcomes.

MENTAL HEALTH CHATBOTS: THE WAY FORWARD

Mental health chatbots are constantly evolving, and addressing their current limitations is a priority. One development problem is the capacity for crisis intervention. Future chatbots could be equipped with algorithms that detect signs of acute psychological distress or suicidal thoughts and respond with appropriate crisis advice or connect the user to emergency services.

The rapidly increasing research on chatbots in the field of clinical psychology and psychotherapy requires corrective measures. Issues like effectiveness, sustainability, and especially safety and subsequent tests of technology are elements that should be instituted as a corrective for future funding programs of chatbots in clinical psychology and psychotherapy (Bendig et al., 2019). Accessibility is another area that can be improved. Next-generation chatbots should provide disabled multimodal user interfaces such as voice control, screen readers or even haptic feedback for visually/hearing impaired users.

The inclusion of different regional languages can also make it easier. The linguistic capabilities of the chatbots have to be able to deal adequately with unexpected user input, provide high-quality responses, and show high variability in responses. To be useful for clinical practice, we have to find ways to harmonise chatbot content with individual treatment recommendations; that is, a personalisation of chatbot conversations is required (Abd-Alrazaq, 2021).

Chatbots can implement controls that limit over-use and instead encourage the augmentation of conversational AI with humans to address issues of over-reliance or technology dependency. Smart instructions can remind users that chat is not a substitute for professional mental health support. Ultimately, interdisciplinary, human-centred design that synthesises the perspectives of psychologists, clinicians, technologists, and end users is essential to unlocking the full transformative potential of mental health chatbots.

CONCLUSION

In conclusion, it is paramount that we remain steadfast in our goal of improving the quality of mental health care in the digital frontier. However, there are numerous advantages that come with mental health chatbots, as previously discussed in this chapter, like accessibility, affordability, and free from bias. However, if not trained properly, it can raise a variety of ethical concerns that might exacerbate or cause more harm to individuals experiencing mental health concerns. Hence, ethical considerations should be strictly addressed at every stage of developing and utilising this technology. Thus, by carefully understanding the nature and scope of AI around the

REFERENCES

Abd-Alrazaq, A. A., Alajlani, M., Ali, N., Denecke, K., Bewick, B. M., & Househ, M. (2021). Perceptions and opinions of patients about mental health chatbots: Scoping review. *Journal of Medical Internet Research. Journal of Medical Internet Research*, 23(1), e17828. DOI: 10.2196/17828 PMID: 33439133

Aggarwal, A., Tam, C. C., Wu, D., Li, X., & Qiao, S. (2023). Artificial intelligence–based chatbots for promoting health behavioral changes: Systematic review. *Journal of Medical Internet Research*, 25(1), e40789. DOI: 10.2196/40789 PMID: 36826990

Ahmed, A., Hassan, A., Aziz, S., Abd-Alrazaq, A. A., Ali, N., Alzubaidi, M., Al-Thani, D., Elhusein, B., Siddig, M. A., Ahmed, M., & Househ, M. (2023). Chatbot features for anxiety and depression: A scoping review. *Health Informatics Journal*, 29(1). Advance online publication. DOI: 10.1177/14604582221146719 PMID: 36693014

Anderson, C. M., Hogarty, G. E., & Reiss, D. J. (1980). Family treatment of adult schizophrenic patients: A psycho-educational approach. *Schizophrenia Bulletin*, 6(3), 490–505. DOI: 10.1093/schbul/6.3.490 PMID: 7403810

Andrade, L. H., Alonso, J., Mneimneh, Z., Wells, J. E., Al-Hamzawi, A., Borges, G., Bromet, E., Bruffaerts, R., de Girolamo, G., de Graaf, R., Florescu, S., Gureje, O., Hinkov, H. R., Hu, C., Huang, Y., Hwang, I., Jin, R., Karam, E. G., Kovess-Masfety, V., & Kessler, R. C. (2013). Barriers to mental health treatment: Results from the WHO World Mental Health (WMH) surveys. *Psychological Medicine*, 44(6), 1303–1317. DOI: 10.1017/S0033291713001943 PMID: 23931656

Andrade-Arenas, L., Yactayo-Arias, C., & Pucuhuayla-Revatta, F. (2024). therapy and emotional support through a chatbot. *International Journal of Online and Biomedical Engineering*, 20(2), 114–130. DOI: 10.3991/ijoe.v20i02.45377

Balan, R., Dobrean, A., & Poetar, C. R. (2024). Use of automated conversational agents in improving young population mental health: A scoping review. *NPJ Digital Medicine*, 7(1), 1–9. DOI: 10.1038/s41746-024-01072-1 PMID: 38503909

Bao, R., Zhang, A., & Li, S. (2020). COVID-19 pandemic and intrahepatic cholestasis of pregnancy: A case report. *BMC Pregnancy and Childbirth*, 20(1), 1–3. https://www.ncbi.nlm.nih.gov/pmc/articles/PMC7256567/

Bendig, E., Erb, B., Schulze-Thuesing, L., & Baumeister, H. (2022). The next generation: Chatbots in clinical psychology and psychotherapy to foster mental health – a scoping review. *Verhaltenstherapie*, 32(1, Suppl. 1), 64–76. DOI: 10.1159/000501812

Bennett, S., Cuijpers, P., Ebert, D., McKenzie, M., Coughtrey, A., Heyman, I., Manzotti, G., & Shafran, R. (2019). Practitioner review: Unguided and guided self-help interventions for common mental health disorders in children and adolescents: A systematic review and meta-analysis. *Journal of Child Psychology and Psychiatry, and Allied Disciplines*, 60(8), 828–847. DOI: 10.1111/jcpp.13010 PMID: 30775782

Bezerra, A. C. V., de Mendonça, R. D., Lamborda, T. C., & César, C. L. G. (2018). Trends in prevalence of overweight and obesity in adults in 26 Brazilian state capitals and the Federal District from 2006 to 2016. *BMC Public Health*, 18(1), 1–10. DOI: 10.1186/s12889-018-5235-x

Bhargava, I., & Mor, N. (2024, February 15). *The future of mental health: Emerging trends and innovations*. Economics Times. https://health.economictimes.indiatimes.com/news/industry/the-future-of-mental-health-emerging-trends-and-innovations/107673809

Biringer, E., Davidson, L., Sundfør, B., Lier, H. Ø., & Borg, M. (2016). Coping with mental health issues: Subjective experiences of self-help and helpful contextual factors at the start of mental health treatment. *Journal of Mental Health (Abingdon, England)*, 25(1), 23–27. DOI: 10.3109/09638237.2015.1078883 PMID: 26484831

Boucher, E. M., Harake, N. R., Ward, H. E., Stoeckl, S. E., Vargas, J., Minkel, J., Parks, A. C., & Zilca, R. (2021). Artificially intelligent chatbots in digital mental health interventions: a review. *Expert Review of Medical Devices, 18*(sup1), 37–49. DOI: 10.1080/17434440.2021.2013200

Brown, A., Kumar, A. T., Melamed, O., Ahmed, I., Wang, Y. H., Deza, A., Morcos, M., Zhu, L., Maslej, M., Minian, N., Sujaya, V., Wolff, J., Doggett, O., Iantorno, M., Ratto, M., Selby, P., & Rose, J. (2023). A motivational interviewing chatbot with generative reflections for increasing readiness to quit smoking: Iterative development study. *JMIR Mental Health*, 10(1), e49132. DOI: 10.2196/49132 PMID: 37847539

Chang, S., Sambasivam, R., Seow, E., Tan, G. C.-Y., Lu, S. H., Assudani, H., Chong, S. A., Subramaniam, M., & Vaingankar, J. A. (2021). "We are all trying to find a way to help ourselves": A look at self-help strategies among psychotherapy clients. *Frontiers in Psychology*, 12, 621085. Advance online publication. DOI: 10.3389/fpsyg.2021.621085 PMID: 34690850

Chen, Y., Lin, Q., Chen, X., Liu, T., Ke, Q., Yang, Q., Guan, B., & Ming, W. K. (2023). Need assessment for history-taking instruction program using chatbot for nursing students: A qualitative study using focus group interviews. *Digital Health*, 29(9), 20552076231185435. DOI: 10.1177/20552076231185435 PMID: 37426591

Chin, H., Song, H., Baek, G., Shin, M., Jung, C., Cha, M., Choi, J., & Cha, C. (2023). The potential of chatbots for emotional support and promoting mental well-being in different cultures: Mixed methods study. *Journal of Medical Internet Research*, 25, e51712. Advance online publication. DOI: 10.2196/51712 PMID: 37862063

Chun-Hung, L., Guan-Hsiung, L., Wu-Chuan, Y., & Yu-Hsin, L. (2023). Chatbot-assisted therapy for patients with methamphetamine use disorder: A preliminary randomized controlled trial. *Frontiers in Psychiatry*, 14, 1159399. Advance online publication. DOI: 10.3389/fpsyt.2023.1159399 PMID: 37484677

Co, M., Yuen, T. H. J., & Cheung, B. H. H. (2022). Using clinical history taking chatbot mobile app for clinical bedside teachings – A prospective case control study. *Heliyon*, 8(6), e09751. DOI: 10.1016/j.heliyon.2022.e09751 PMID: 35770149

Codecademy. (n.d.). *What are chatbots?*https://www.codecademy.com/article/what-are-chatbots

D'Alfonso, S. (2020). AI in mental health. *Current Opinion in Psychology*, 36, 112–117. DOI: 10.1016/j.copsyc.2020.04.005 PMID: 32604065

Dev, P., Winzelberg, A. J., Celio, A., & Taylor, C. B. (1999). Student bodies: Psycho-education communities on the web. *Proc AMIA Symp*, 510–514. PMID: 10566411

Ettman, C. K., & Galea, S. (2023). The potential influence of AI on population mental health. *JMIR Mental Health*, 10, e49936. DOI: 10.2196/49936 PMID: 37971803

Fadhil, A., Wang, Y., & Reiterer, H. (2019). Assistive conversational agent for health coaching: A validation study. *Methods of Information in Medicine, 58*(1), 9–23. DOI: 10.1055/s-0039-1688757

Flora, K., Raftopoulos, A., & Pontikes, T. (2010). A look at the evolution of the self-help movement. *Journal of Groups in Addiction & Recovery*, 5(3-4), 214–225. DOI: 10.1080/1556035X.2010.523349

France, B. (2016, November 23). *The importance of choosing the right therapist.* Medium. https://medium.com/@BenFrance/the-importance-of-choosing-the-right-therapist-5622d4f22a13

Frey, B. (2024, March 27). *Earkick: AI-powered mental health support.* Earkick. https://blog.earkick.com/earkick-ai-powered-mental-health-support/

Fusar-Poli, P., De Pablo, G. S., De Micheli, A., Nieman, D. H., Correll, C. U., Kessing, L. V., Pfennig, A., Bechdolf, A., Borgwardt, S., Arango, C., & van Amelsvoort, T. (2020). What is good mental health? A scoping review. *European Neuropsychopharmacology*, 31, 33–46. DOI: 10.1016/j.euroneuro.2019.12.105 PMID: 31901337

Gellatly, J., Bower, P., Hennessy, S., Richards, D., Gilbody, S., & Lovell, K. (2007). What makes self-help interventions effective in the management of depressive symptoms? Meta-analysis and meta-regression. *Psychological Medicine*, 37(9), 1217–1228. DOI: 10.1017/S0033291707000062 PMID: 17306044

Goodwin, G., Haddad, P., Ferrier, I., Aronson, J. K., Barnes, T. R. H., Cipriani, A., Coghill, D. R., Fazel, S., Geddes, J. R., Grunze, H., Holmes, E. A., Howes, O., Hudson, S., Hunt, N., Jones, I., Macmillan, I. C., McAllister-Williams, H., Miklowitz, D. R., Morriss, R., & Young, A. H. (2016). *Evidence-based guidelines for treating bipolar disorder*: Revised third edition recommendations from the British Association for Psychopharmacology. *Journal of Psychopharmacology, 30*(6), 495-553. DOI: 10.1177/0269881116636545

Gould, R., & Clum, G. (1993). A meta-analysis of self-help treatment approaches. *Clinical Psychology Review*, 13(2), 169–186. DOI: 10.1016/0272-7358(93)90039-O

Grist, R., Croker, A., Denne, M., & Stallard, P. (2018). Technology delivered interventions for depression and anxiety in children and adolescents: A systematic review and meta-analysis. *Clinical Child and Family Psychology Review*, 22(2), 147–171. DOI: 10.1007/s10567-018-0271-8 PMID: 30229343

Gupta, T. (2023, October 26). *The role of generative AI in natural language processing*. eLearning Industry. https://elearningindustry.com/role-of-generative-ai-in-natural-language-processing#:~:text=In%20the%20context%20of%20Natural,Pre%2Dtrained%20Transformer)%20series.

Haque, M. D. R., & Rubya, S. (2023). An overview of chatbot-based mobile mental health apps: Insights from app description and user reviews. *JMIR mHealth and uHealth*, 11, e44838. DOI: 10.2196/44838 PMID: 37213181

Herrera, S. N., Sarac, C., Phili, A., Gorman, J., Martin, L., Lyallpuri, R., Dobbs, M. F., DeLuca, J. S., Mueser, K. T., Wyka, K. E., Yang, L. H., Landa, Y., & Corcoran, C. M. (2023). Psychoeducation for individuals at clinical high risk for psychosis: A scoping review. *Schizophrenia Research*, 252, 148–158. DOI: 10.1016/j.schres.2023.01.008 PMID: 36652831

Hollis, C., Falconer, C. J., Martin, J., Whittington, C., Stockton, S., Glazebrook, C., & Davies, E. B. (2017). Annual research review: Digital health interventions for children and young people with mental health problems – a systematic and meta-review. *Journal of Child Psychology and Psychiatry, and Allied Disciplines*, 58(4), 474–503. DOI: 10.1111/jcpp.12663 PMID: 27943285

Holmes, S., Moorhead, A., Bond, R., Zheng, H., Coates, V., & Mctear, M. (2019). Usability testing of a healthcare chatbot: Can we use conventional methods to assess conversational user interfaces? *Proceedings of the 31st European Conference on Cognitive Ergonomics - ECCE 2019*. DOI: 10.1145/3335082.3335094

IBM. (n.d.). *What is a chatbot?*https://www.ibm.com/topics/chatbots

Intelliverse.ai. (2023, September 12). *How AI is making mental healthcare more accessible*. LinkedIn. https://www.linkedin.com/pulse/how-ai-making-mental-healthcare-more-accessible/

Jang, S., Kim, J.-J., Kim, S.-J., Hong, J., Kim, S., & Kim, E. (2021). Mobile app-based chatbot to deliver cognitive behavioral therapy and psychoeducation for adults with attention deficit: A development and feasibility/usability study. *International Journal of Medical Informatics*, 150, 104440. DOI: 10.1016/j.ijmedinf.2021.104440 PMID: 33799055

Jorm, A. F., & Griffiths, K. M. (2006). Population promotion of informal self-help strategies for early intervention against depression and anxiety. *Psychological Medicine*, 36(1), 3–6. DOI: 10.1017/S0033291705005659 PMID: 16356291

Kamita, T., Ito, T., Matsumoto, A., Munakata, T., & Inoue, T. (2018). A chatbot system for mental healthcare based on SAT counseling method. *Mobile Information Systems,* 9517321:1-9517321:11. DOI: 10.1155/2019/9517321

Kamita, T., Matsumoto, A., Sun, B., & Inoue, T. (2020). Promotion of continuous use of a self-guided mental healthcare system by a chatbot. *Companion Publication of the 2020 Conference on Computer Supported Cooperative Work and Social Computing,* 293–298. DOI: 10.1145/3406865.3418343

Klainin-Yobas, P., Ng, S. H., Stephen, P. D. M., & Lau, Y. (2016). Efficacy of psychosocial interventions on psychological outcomes among people with cardiovascular diseases: A systematic review and meta-analysis. *Patient Education and Counseling*, 99(4), 512–521. DOI: 10.1016/j.pec.2015.10.020 PMID: 27045976

Koulouri, T., Macredie, R. D., & Olakitan, D. (2022). Chatbots to support young adults' mental health: An exploratory study of acceptability. *ACM Transactions on Interactive Intelligent Systems*, 12(2), 1–39. DOI: 10.1145/3485874

Kulkarni, R., & Jaiswal, R. C. (2023). A survey on AI chatbots. *International Journal for Research in Applied Science and Engineering Technology*, 11(9), 1738–1744. DOI: 10.22214/ijraset.2023.55911

Li, H., Zhang, R., Lee, Y.-C., Kraut, R. E., & Mohr, D. C. (2023). Systematic review and meta-analysis of AI-based conversational agents for promoting mental health and well-being. *NPJ Digital Medicine*, 6(1), 1. Advance online publication. DOI: 10.1038/s41746-023-00979-5 PMID: 38114588

Liu, H., Peng, H., Song, X., Xu, C., & Zhang, M. (2021). Using AI chatbots to provide self-help depression interventions for university students: A randomized trial of effectiveness. *Internet Interventions : the Application of Information Technology in Mental and Behavioural Health*, 27, 100495. DOI: 10.1016/j.invent.2022.100495 PMID: 35059305

Lukens, E. P., & McFarlane, W. R. (2006). Psychoeducation as evidence-based practice: Considerations for practice, research, and policy. In Roberts, A. R., & Yeager, K. R. (Eds.), *Foundations of evidence-based social work practice* (pp. 291–313). Oxford University Press. DOI: 10.1093/oso/9780195305944.003.0022

Maher, C. A., Davis, C. R., Curtis, R. G., Short, C. E., & Murphy, K. J. (2020). A physical activity and diet program delivered by artificially intelligent virtual health coach: Proof-of-concept study. *JMIR mHealth and uHealth*, 8(7), e17558. DOI: 10.2196/17558 PMID: 32673246

Mains, J. A., & Scogin, F. R. (2003). The effectiveness of self-administered treatments: A practice-friendly review of the research. *Journal of Clinical Psychology*, 59(2), 237–246. DOI: 10.1002/jclp.10145 PMID: 12552632

Math, S. B., Gowda, G. S., Basavaraju, V., Manjunatha, N., Kumar, C. N., Enara, A., Gowda, M., & Thirthalli, J. (2019). Cost estimation for the implementation of the Mental Healthcare Act 2017. *Indian Journal of Psychiatry*, 61(10, Suppl 4), S650–S659. DOI: 10.4103/psychiatry.IndianJPsychiatry_188_19 PMID: 31040453

McGorry, P. D., Nelson, B., Goldstone, S., & Yung, A. R. (2010). Clinical staging: A heuristic and practical strategy for new research and better health and social outcomes for psychotic and related mood disorders. *Canadian Journal of Psychiatry*, 55(8), 486–497. DOI: 10.1177/070674371005500803 PMID: 20723276

Meghrajani, V. R., Marathe, M., Sharma, R., Potdukhe, A., Wanjari, M. B., & Taksande, A. B. (2023). A comprehensive analysis of mental health problems in India and the role of mental asylums. *Cureus*, 15(7), e42559. DOI: 10.7759/cureus.42559 PMID: 37637646

Meskó, B. (2023, August 10). *Top 10 health chatbots*. LinkedIn. https://www.linkedin.com/pulse/top-10-health-chatbots-bertalan-mesk%C3%B3-md-phd/

Moghimi, E., Stephenson, C., Gutierrez, G., Jagayat, J., Layzell, G., Patel, C., McCart, A., Gibney, C., Langstaff, C., Ayonrinde, O., Khalid-Khan, S., Milev, R., Snelgrove-Clarke, E., Soares, C., Omrani, M., & Alavi, N. (2023). Mental health challenges, treatment experiences, and care needs of post-secondary students: A cross-sectional mixed-methods study. *BMC Public Health*, 23(1), 655. DOI: 10.1186/s12889-023-15452-x PMID: 37020282

Monash University. (2021, March 19). *All you need is Ash: Chatbot designed to boost teen mental health at school.*https://www.monash.edu/news/articles/all-you-need-is-ash-chatbot-designed-to-boost-teen-mental-health-at-school

Motlova, L. B., Balon, R., Beresin, E. V., Brenner, A. M., Coverdale, J. H., Guerrero, A. P. S., Louie, A. K., & Roberts, L. W. (2017). Psychoeducation as an opportunity for patients, psychiatrists, and psychiatric educators: Why do we ignore it? *Academic Psychiatry*, 41(4), 447–451. DOI: 10.1007/s40596-017-0728-y PMID: 28536990

Murthy, R. S. (2017). National Mental Health Survey of India 2015-2016. *Indian Journal of Psychiatry*, 59(1), 21–26. DOI: 10.4103/psychiatry.IndianJPsychiatry_102_17 PMID: 28529357

Niederkrotenthaler, T., Eisenwort, B., Till, B., Sonneck, G., Tran, U. S., & Sonneck, G. (2021). Applying language models for suicide prevention: Evaluating news article adherence to WHO reporting guidelines. *Crisis*. Advance online publication. DOI: 10.1027/0227-5910/a000811

Norcross, J. C. (2000). Here comes the self-help revolution in mental heath. *Psychotherapy (Chicago, Ill.)*, 37(4), 370–377. DOI: 10.1037/0033-3204.37.4.370

Nussey, C., Pistrang, N., & Murphy, T. (2013). How does psychoeducation help? A review of the effects of providing information about Tourette syndrome and attention-deficit/hyperactivity disorder. *Child: Care, Health and Development*, 39(5), 617–627. DOI: 10.1111/cch.12039 PMID: 23461278

Oracle Cloud Infrastructure (OCI). (n.d.). *What is a chatbot?*https://www.oracle.com/in/chatbots/what-is-a-chatbot/

Peacock, S. M., Goodwin, I. H., Wood, R. K., McBride, C. J., Brock, A. C., Erekson, D. M., & Boyd, Z. M. (2021). *MATCH: Client-therapist matching with machine learning*. Brigham Young University.

Perrone, M. (2024, March 23). *Ready or not, AI chatbots are here to help with Gen Z's mental health struggles.* AP News. https://apnews.com/article/chatbots-mental-health-therapy-counseling-ai-73feb819ff52a51d53fee117c3207219

Piao, M., Ryu, H., Lee, H., & Kim, J. (2020). Use of the healthy lifestyle coaching chatbot app to promote stair-climbing habits among office workers: Exploratory randomized controlled trial. *JMIR mHealth and uHealth*, 8(5), e15085. DOI: 10.2196/15085 PMID: 32427114

Prochaska, J. J., Vogel, E. A., Chieng, A., Kendra, M., Baiocchi, M., Pajarito, S., & Robinson, A. (2021). A therapeutic relational agent for reducing problematic substance use (Woebot): Development and usability study. *Journal of Medical Internet Research*, 23(3), e24850. DOI: 10.2196/24850 PMID: 33755028

Robards, F., Kang, M., Luscombe, G., Hawke, C., Sanci, L., Steinbeck, K., Zwi, K., Towns, S., & Usherwood, T. (2020). Intersectionality: Social marginalisation and self-reported health status in young people. *International Journal of Environmental Research and Public Health*, 17(21), 8104. DOI: 10.3390/ijerph17218104 PMID: 33153094

Rosen, G. (1993). Self-help or hype? comments on psychology's failure to advance self-care. *Professional Psychology, Research and Practice*, 24(3), 340–345. DOI: 10.1037/0735-7028.24.3.340

Sachdeva, N. (2023, July 12). *Chatbots as virtual therapists: The future of mental health care*. Daffodil Software Engineering Insights. https://insights.daffodilsw.com/blog/chatbots-the-future-of-mental-health-care

Sarkhel, S., Singh, O. P., & Arora, M. (2020). Clinical practice guidelines for psychoeducation in psychiatric disorders general principles of psychoeducation. *Indian Journal of Psychiatry*, 62(8, Suppl 2), S319–S323. DOI: 10.4103/psychiatry.IndianJPsychiatry_780_19 PMID: 32055073

Selaskowski, B., Reiland, M., Schulze, M., Aslan, B., Kannen, K., Wiebe, A., Wallbaum, T., Boll, S., Lux, S., Philipsen, A., & Braun, N. (2023). Chatbot-supported psychoeducation in adult attention-deficit hyperactivity disorder: Randomised controlled trial. *BJPsych Open*, 9(6), e192. DOI: 10.1192/bjo.2023.573 PMID: 37827996

Shukla, D. (2022, April 20). *Why mental healthcare is less accessible to marginalized communities*. MedicalNewsToday. https://www.medicalnewstoday.com/articles/why-mental-healthcare-is-less-accessible-to-marginalized-communities

Singh, B., Olds, T., Brinsley, J., Dumuid, D., Virgara, R., Matricciani, L., Watson, A., Szeto, K., Eglitis, E., Miatke, A., Simpson, C. E. M., Vandelanotte, C., & Maher, C. (2023). Systematic review and meta-analysis of the effectiveness of chatbots on lifestyle behaviours. *NPJ Digital Medicine*, 6(1), 1–10. DOI: 10.1038/s41746-023-00856-1 PMID: 37353578

Singh, O. P. (2019). Chatbots in psychiatry: Can treatment gap be lessened for psychiatric disorders in India. *Indian Journal of Psychiatry*, 61(3), 225. DOI: 10.4103/0019-5545.258323 PMID: 31142896

Skjuve, M. B., & Brandtzæg, P. B. (2017). Chatbots as a new user interface for providing health information to young people. In Andersson, Y., Dahlquist, U., & Ohlsson, J. (Eds.), *Youth and news in a digital media environment – Nordic-Baltic perspectives*. Nordicom.

Stephens, T. N., Joerin, A., Rauws, M., & Werk, L. N. (2019). Feasibility of pediatric obesity and prediabetes treatment support through Tess, the AI behavioral coaching chatbot. *Translational Behavioral Medicine*, 9(3), 440–447. DOI: 10.1093/tbm/ibz043 PMID: 31094445

Talaviya, A. (2023, November 6). *Machine learning algorithms used in creating AI chatbots*. Medium. https://medium.com/@avikumart_/machine-learning-algorithms-used-in-creating-ai-chatbots-3bac9fe27cb9

Thapa, R., van Teijlingen, E., Regmi, P. R., & Heaslip, V. (2021). Caste exclusion and health discrimination in South Asia: A systematic review. *Asia-Pacific Journal of Public Health*, 33(8), 828–838. DOI: 10.1177/10105395211014648 PMID: 34024157

The Economic Times. (2022, October 10). *World Mental Health Day: 60-70 mn people in India suffer from common mental disorders; stigmatisation, financial barriers prevent timely treatment.* https://economictimes.indiatimes.com/magazines/panache/world-mental-health-day-60-70-mn-people-in-india-suffer-from-common-mental-disorders-stigmatisation-financial-barriers-prevent-timely-treatment/articleshow/104289268.cms?from=mdr

Town, R., Hayes, D., March, A., Fonagy, P., & Stapley, E. (2023). Self-management, self-care, and self-help in adolescents with emotional problems: A scoping review. *European Child & Adolescent Psychiatry*, •••, 1–28. DOI: 10.1007/s00787-022-02134-z PMID: 36641785

Vaidyam, A. N., Wisniewski, H., Halamka, J. D., Kashavan, M. S., & Torous, J. B. (2019). Chatbots and conversational agents in mental health: A review of the psychiatric landscape. *Canadian Journal of Psychiatry*, 64(7), 456–464. DOI: 10.1177/0706743719828977 PMID: 30897957

Valera, S. (2023, March 8). *Best mood tracker apps.* Verwell Mind. https://www.verywellmind.com/best-mood-tracker-apps-5212922

Viduani, A., Cosenza, V., Araújo, R. M., & Kieling, C. (2023). Chatbots in the field of mental health: Challenges and opportunities. In Passos, I. C., Rabelo-da-Ponte, F. D., & Kapczinski, F. (Eds.), *Digital mental health*. Springer. DOI: 10.1007/978-3-031-10698-9_8

Wainberg, M. L., Scorza, P., Shultz, J. M., Helpman, L., Mootz, J. J., Johnson, K. A., Neria, Y., Bradford, J. E., Oquendo, M. A., & Arbuckle, M. R. (2017). Challenges and opportunities in global mental health: A research-to-practice perspective. *Current Psychiatry Reports*, 19(5), 28. DOI: 10.1007/s11920-017-0780-z PMID: 28425023

Xia, J., Merinder, L. B., & Belgamwar, M. R. (2011). Psychoeducation for schizophrenia. *Cochrane Database of Systematic Reviews*, 15(6), CD002831. Advance online publication. DOI: 10.1002/14651858.CD002831.pub2 PMID: 21678337

XinhuaNet. (2021, July 16). *China launches new space station core module.*http://www.xinhuanet.com/english/2021-07/16/c_1310064630.htm

Youper. (n.d.). *Effectiveness.* Youper. https://www.youper.ai/effectiveness

Yunus, A. P., Masago, Y., Hijioka, Y., & Saito, Y. (2020). Evaluation of PM2.5 exposure and its impact on premature mortality in South and Southeast Asia. *Environmental Research Letters*, 15(7), 074025. Advance online publication. DOI: 10.1088/1748-9326/ab9375

Zhang, J., Oh, Y. J., Lange, P., Yu, Z., & Fukuoka, Y. (2020). Artificial intelligence chatbot behavior change model for designing artificial intelligence chatbots to promote physical activity and a healthy diet: Viewpoint. *Journal of Medical Internet Research*, 22(9), e22845. DOI: 10.2196/22845 PMID: 32996892

Zhang, T., Schoene, A. M., Ji, S., & Ananiadou, S. (2022). Natural language processing applied to mental illness detection: A narrative review. *NPJ Digital Medicine*, 5(1), 46. DOI: 10.1038/s41746-022-00589-7 PMID: 35396451

KEY TERMS AND DEFINITIONS

Care-Receiving Chatbots: Unlike other chatbots that provide helpful strategies, care-receiving chatbots like Vincent share their challenges and ask for advice from the user.

Cognitive-Behaviour Therapy: A type of therapy modality that targets negative schemas and brings about positive changes in the thoughts, feelings, and behaviours of individuals.

Conversational Agents: A conversational agent is any dialogue system that conducts natural language processing (NLP) and responds automatically using human language.

Generative Artificial Intelligence: Generative artificial intelligence (AI) models are AI platforms that generate a variety of outputs based on massive training datasets, neural networks, deep learning architecture, and prompts from users.

Habit Building: A process through which a sequence of behaviours becomes routine.

Psychoeducation: The process of providing information to the client and family to elicit their support in working with the mental health professional.

Self-Help: Any strategy or technique that an individual applies to deal with emotional or physical distress.

Self-Management: The process through which one manages and regulates their emotions and thought patterns.

Stress Reduction: The process or a set of techniques which reduces the everyday stress an individual might feel.

Chapter 4
AI in Mental Healthcare: Exploring Technology Acceptance, Emotional and Cognitive Innovation, and Cultural Influences

Vishnu Achutha Menon
https://orcid.org/0000-0003-4028-3685
Institute for Educational and Developmental Studies, India

ABSTRACT

This study conducted a comprehensive investigation across Karnataka involving 575 college students to explore their perceptions and acceptance of artificial intelligence (AI) in mental healthcare. The research utilized a mixed-methods approach, incorporating the Technology Acceptance Model (TAM 2) to assess technology acceptance levels, the Cognitive and Sensory Innovativeness scale to measure innovative approaches in adopting AI technologies, an affective scale to evaluate emotional responses, and specific inquiries into participants' perceptions of AI. Stratified random sampling ensured representation across various colleges and demographics within Karnataka. Data analysis employed correlation and regression analyses in SPSS to examine relationships between variables, including technology acceptance, cognitive and sensory innovativeness, affective responses, and perceptions of AI's cultural impact in mental healthcare.

DOI: 10.4018/979-8-3693-3112-5.ch004

INTRODUCTION

Artificial Intelligence (AI) has increasingly found applications in revolutionizing mental healthcare globally, with India emerging as a significant adopter of AI-driven solutions. Specifically, chatbots have garnered attention for their potential to enhance accessibility, affordability, and effectiveness in addressing mental health challenges. In India, where mental health resources are often scarce relative to the population size, chatbots represent a promising technological intervention. These AI-powered systems simulate human-like conversation through text or voice interfaces, providing users with immediate, round-the-clock support for various mental health concerns. The general scenario in India reflects a growing acceptance and utilization of chatbots in mental healthcare. Organizations, both public and private, are leveraging chatbot technology to extend mental health services beyond traditional clinical settings. This approach not only addresses the stigma associated with seeking psychological help but also caters to the diverse linguistic and cultural needs across the country.

The integration of chatbots into mental healthcare aligns with India's digital health initiatives, aiming to make healthcare more inclusive and accessible nationwide. With advancements in natural language processing (NLP) and machine learning, these chatbots can offer personalized interventions, ranging from mood tracking and self-help techniques to crisis intervention and therapy referrals. However, challenges such as data privacy concerns, the need for regulatory frameworks, and ensuring the efficacy of AI-driven interventions remain critical considerations. As research continues to validate the effectiveness of chatbots in diverse cultural contexts and clinical settings, their role in augmenting mental healthcare delivery in India is poised to expand significantly.

AI-driven chatbots operate at the intersection of Natural Language Processing (NLP) and Machine Learning (ML), leveraging sophisticated algorithms to facilitate human-like interactions. When a user engages with a chatbot, the NLP component, known as Natural Language Understanding (NLU), plays a pivotal role. It meticulously parses the user's input—be it text or voice—to discern the underlying intent and extract pertinent information using advanced techniques like tokenization, part-of-speech tagging, and named entity recognition. This initial step forms the foundation for the chatbot's response strategy. Following NLU, the chatbot's dialog management system takes charge. This system is responsible for comprehending the context of the conversation, maintaining continuity across exchanges, and navigating through multiple user intents seamlessly. It dynamically decides how best to respond based on a combination of predefined rules, learned patterns from previous interactions, and real-time user input. This phase is crucial for ensuring that the chatbot's responses are not only accurate but also contextually relevant and aligned with the user's needs. Once the dialog strategy is determined, the chatbot employs

Natural Language Generation (NLG) to craft its replies in a manner that mirrors natural human communication. NLG transforms structured data or pre-defined templates into coherent sentences that convey information clearly and effectively to the user. This process is augmented by the chatbot's ability to learn and adapt over time, thanks to its integration with Machine Learning models. Through exposure to extensive datasets and continuous training, chatbots refine their understanding of language nuances, improve response accuracy, and expand their capacity to handle a wide range of user queries and scenarios.

AI-driven chatbots are not standalone entities but are intricately linked with backend systems and databases. This integration allows them to fetch real-time information, execute tasks such as booking appointments or retrieving personalized recommendations, and provide up-to-date responses based on the latest data available. The seamless integration with backend systems enhances the chatbot's utility and ensures that it remains a valuable tool for users seeking efficient, round-the-clock assistance. As these chatbots are deployed across various platforms—ranging from websites and mobile applications to messaging services—they undergo continual monitoring and optimization. User interactions are monitored to analyze patterns, identify areas for improvement, and gather feedback that informs further enhancements. This iterative process ensures that AI-driven chatbots evolve iteratively, becoming increasingly adept at understanding user needs, fostering engagement, and delivering tangible value in diverse contexts of use. The general objective of this study is to investigate the influence of technology acceptance on various dimensions of innovativeness and cultural perceptions related to AI in mental healthcare contexts.

REVIEW OF LITERATURE

The study investigates mental healthcare professionals' perceptions and acceptance of AI technology in psychotherapeutic practices (Alimour et al., 2024). Therapists' willingness to integrate AI-based tools like virtual counselors or AI-driven diagnostic systems into their practice is influenced by their familiarity with technology, perceived efficacy of AI interventions, and the extent to which they believe these tools can enhance patient outcomes. A mental health professional who regularly uses AI tools to monitor patient progress might perceive these technologies as beneficial and reliable, whereas a professional with limited exposure to AI might exhibit skepticism. The study explores people's perceptions of openness, concerns, and benefits regarding AI-driven healthcare technologies, finding trust in healthcare and technology are key correlates (Antes et al., 2021). Patients who trust their healthcare providers and the technology used are more likely to engage with AI-based health interventions. This trust can be influenced by factors such as the transparency of AI algorithms, the perceived accuracy of AI diagnostics, and the endorsement of these technologies by respected healthcare professionals. A patient who is aware of the rigorous testing and validation of an AI mental health app may feel more confident in using it compared to one who doubts the app's credibility.

The study examines factors predicting acceptance of mental health apps, including technological and sociocultural factors like stigma and prior experience (Kim et al., 2022). Individuals with prior positive experiences using digital health tools are more likely to adopt mental health apps. Conversely, those who perceive a high level of stigma around mental health issues may be hesitant to use such apps, fearing judgment or misunderstanding from their peers. A young adult who has successfully used fitness apps might be more open to trying a mental health app, whereas another individual who feels mental health should be addressed privately might avoid these digital solutions. This paper examines the role of cultural dimensions in technology acceptance models, but does not specifically address AI in mental healthcare (Jan et al., 2024). Cultural factors such as collectivism versus individualism can influence how technology is perceived and adopted. In collectivist cultures, where community and social harmony are emphasized, there might be a greater reliance on human interactions and traditional methods of therapy. Individualistic cultures might be more open to the autonomy and privacy provided by AI mental health tools. An American college student may readily embrace a self-help AI app, while a student from a more collectivist society might prefer group therapy sessions facilitated by human therapists. Immersive virtual environment experience of ChatGPT on student engagement in online scriptwriting among media students shows that the AI has more impact on students (Kunnumpurath, Menon, et al., 2024). Students who engage with ChatGPT in a virtual classroom setting for scriptwriting tasks report higher levels of engagement and creativity. The interactive nature of the AI, combined with its ability to provide instant feedback and suggestions, helps students refine their scripts more efficiently and fosters a collaborative learning environment. A media student might find ChatGPT's instant feedback invaluable for iterating on script ideas quickly, leading to more polished final projects.

Rapid adoption can be attributed to several factors, such as its intuitive interface, robust technological infrastructure, and adaptability across various educational contexts. Against the backdrop of the global pandemic, which has mandated a widespread transition to remote learning, Zoom has emerged as a pivotal tool for educators endeavoring to transcend geographical constraints and engage with students in virtual classrooms (Thomas et al., 2024). Zoom's user-friendly interface, combined with features like breakout rooms and screen sharing, has made it easier for educators to conduct interactive and collaborative sessions. During the pandemic, a university professor might use Zoom to host live lectures, facilitate group discussions, and provide real-time feedback, thereby maintaining a high level of student engagement despite the physical separation.

The paper examines how cultural factors influence mental health help-seeking behaviors, highlighting the need for culturally sensitive approaches in mental health technology design (Ahmed et al., 2024). In cultures where mental health issues are stigmatized, individuals may be less likely to seek help from AI-driven mental health tools unless these tools are designed to ensure privacy and confidentiality. A culturally sensitive AI mental health app might include features that respect cultural norms and provide support in a manner that aligns with users' values and beliefs, such as incorporating traditional healing practices or providing content in multiple languages. The study examines predictors of psychology students' and early practitioners' intention to use two specific AI-enabled mental health tools (Kleine et al., 2023). Factors such as perceived ease of use, perceived usefulness, and personal innovativeness in information technology (PIIT) were found to significantly influence the intention to use these tools. A psychology student who finds an AI-enabled mental health tool user-friendly and believes it will enhance their clinical skills is more likely to integrate it into their practice.

Self-esteem and workplace communication were statistically significant, affirming the reliability of these associations. Linear regression analyses further elucidated the relationships between self-esteem and specific workplace behaviors for new digital environments in Karnataka among female media professionals (Kunnumpurath, Prasad, et al., 2024). Higher self-esteem was associated with better communication skills in digital environments, suggesting that female media professionals who feel confident in their abilities are more effective in virtual teamwork and collaboration. A female media professional with high self-esteem might be more proactive in participating in virtual meetings and sharing ideas, thereby contributing more effectively to team projects. The paper examines the social implications of AI chatbots in mental healthcare mobile apps, noting their potential benefits and limitations (Gamble, 2020). AI chatbots can provide immediate support and guidance to users, making mental health resources more accessible. However, they may also lack the empathy and nuanced understanding that human therapists provide, potentially limiting their effectiveness in addressing complex emotional issues. A user might appreciate the convenience and availability of an AI chatbot for managing anxiety but might find it insufficient for dealing with deep-seated trauma. This paper examines user perceptions of intelligent conversational agents in mental healthcare, identifying factors influencing their adoption and use (Prakash, 2020). For instance, users' trust in the technology, the perceived reliability of the AI's responses, and the overall user experience play crucial roles in adoption. A user who trusts the AI to provide accurate and helpful advice is more likely to use it regularly, whereas a user who experiences inconsistent or unhelpful responses may abandon the tool. This paper identifies perceptions and needs regarding AI adoption in healthcare but does not directly address the influence of technology acceptance on innovativeness and cultural perceptions related to AI in mental healthcare (Chew & Achananuparp, 2022). While the paper highlights the general willingness to adopt AI in healthcare settings, it does not delve into how cultural attitudes towards innovation and technology might shape the acceptance and use of AI in mental health contexts. A healthcare professional in a tech-forward culture might eagerly adopt AI tools, while one in a culture with a cautious approach to new technologies might be more skeptical.

Graham et al. (2019) provide an overview of the potential and limitations of using AI in mental healthcare but do not directly address the influence of technology acceptance on innovativeness and cultural perceptions related to AI in mental healthcare. While they highlight the advancements AI can bring to diagnosis and treatment, they lack an analysis of how cultural attitudes towards technology might affect its adoption in different communities. Lee et al. (2021) discuss the potential of AI to improve mental healthcare, including clinical applications, challenges, and the need for "artificial wisdom" to enable more compassionate and ethical care. AI can assist in the early diagnosis of mental health conditions through predictive analytics, but the challenge remains in ensuring these tools are used ethically and compassionately, balancing technological efficiency with human empathy. Kelly et al. (2023) review factors that contribute to the acceptance of artificial intelligence, including perceived usefulness, performance expectancy, attitudes, trust, and effort expectancy. Healthcare providers are more likely to use AI tools if they find them useful, trust their accuracy, and believe they can improve patient outcomes without requiring excessive effort to learn and use. AlQudah et al. (2021) provide a systematic review of factors affecting technology acceptance in healthcare but do not specifically address the influence of technology acceptance on innovativeness and cultural perceptions related to AI in mental healthcare. While they cover general acceptance factors like ease of use and perceived benefits, they do not explore how these factors might vary across different cultural contexts or how they might influence the adoption of innovative AI solutions in mental health.

Ho et al. (2023) propose an analytical framework to study the acceptance of emotional AI based on the Technology Acceptance Model and Moral Foundation Theory. For instance, their framework could be used to analyze how users perceive the benefits and ethical implications of emotional AI, such as AI-driven mental health apps that recognize and respond to users' emotional states. The framework might evaluate how factors like perceived usefulness, ease of use, and ethical concerns influence the acceptance of such technologies. An AI app that effectively identifies signs of depression in a user's speech and offers timely support might be well-received if users believe it is both beneficial and ethically designed to protect their privacy. Olawade et al. (2024) review the current trends and future prospects of integrating

AI into mental healthcare, including ethical considerations. They discuss how AI can enhance mental health diagnostics and treatment plans but also emphasize the need for ethical guidelines to ensure patient privacy and data security. They might examine the potential for AI to provide personalized mental health care through continuous monitoring and data analysis, offering examples such as AI systems that adjust treatment recommendations based on real-time patient data. However, they also caution against potential ethical pitfalls, such as biases in AI algorithms and the importance of maintaining human oversight in AI-assisted care.

Srite and Karahanna (2006) found that espoused national cultural values moderate the relationships between technology acceptance beliefs and behavioral intention. For instance, in cultures that value individualism, people might be more inclined to adopt AI technologies that offer personalized mental health solutions. In such contexts, AI tools providing tailored interventions based on individual data might be highly attractive. Conversely, in collectivist cultures, there might be a preference for AI tools that facilitate community support and shared decision-making. An AI platform that enables group therapy sessions or community support networks might see higher acceptance in these settings. Ojha (2023) examines how technological innovations can improve the accessibility and affordability of mental healthcare but does not directly address the influence of technology acceptance on innovativeness and cultural perceptions related to AI in mental healthcare. While Ojha highlights how AI can make mental health services more accessible to underserved populations through mobile apps and teletherapy, there is no exploration of how cultural factors might affect the acceptance and use of these technologies. An example could be an AI-driven mental health service providing affordable therapy sessions via smartphone apps to remote areas. However, the study does not delve into whether cultural attitudes towards technology or mental health stigma in these regions impact the adoption of such innovations.

Tam et al. (2021) examine perceptions of using an AI-supported mental health app within the Canadian military community but do not address the hypotheses about technology acceptance and innovativeness. While they might explore how military personnel view the utility and reliability of the app, they do not delve into how these perceptions influence broader acceptance or innovative use of AI in mental healthcare. Hirunyawipada and Paswan (2006) examine how consumer innovativeness and perceived risk impact the adoption of new high-tech products but do not address AI in mental healthcare. Their study might show that consumers who are more innovative and willing to take risks are quicker to adopt new technologies, yet it does not specifically apply these findings to AI-driven mental health solutions. Wei et al. (2024) examine factors that influence consumer adoption of healthcare technologies but do not specifically address AI in mental healthcare. Their research might identify general barriers and facilitators to adopting healthcare tech, such as cost, ease of use, and perceived benefits, without focusing on AI's unique aspects in mental health contexts. While they might find that users prefer technologies that are easy to integrate into their daily routines, this insight is not applied to AI mental health tools. Torous et al. (2021) provide a comprehensive overview of the growing field of digital psychiatry, including the relevance of recent technological advances and the current evidence for their use in mental health contexts. They might discuss the benefits of digital tools like mobile health apps and telepsychiatry platforms in improving access to mental health care, offering evidence of their effectiveness in various clinical settings. However, they do not specifically focus on how acceptance of these technologies is influenced by cultural or innovative factors related to AI. Anton and Jones (2017) propose a framework to address organizational readiness and clinician acceptance of technology-enhanced mental health treatments but do not directly investigate the influence of technology acceptance on innovativeness and cultural perceptions related to AI in mental healthcare. Their framework might include strategies for preparing mental health organizations to implement new technologies and for training clinicians to use these tools effectively. However, it does not explore how cultural attitudes towards innovation or specific beliefs about AI impact the adoption and use of these technologies in mental health settings.

Rogan et al. (2024) review mental health professionals' views on the use of passive sensing and AI in mental healthcare, identifying barriers, facilitators, and consequences. They may highlight concerns about data privacy and the accuracy of AI assessments as barriers, while recognizing the potential for AI to enhance patient monitoring and early intervention as facilitators. The consequences might include improved patient outcomes but also ethical considerations around patient consent and autonomy. Thordardottir et al. (2019) review facilitators and barriers to acceptance and use of innovative assistive technologies among people with cognitive impairments and their caregivers. They might find that ease of use, perceived usefulness, and the level of caregiver support are key facilitators, while high costs, lack of training, and concerns about reliability are significant barriers. This can be applied to mental healthcare by considering how these factors similarly affect the adoption of AI-driven mental health tools for individuals with cognitive impairments. Chan and Honey (2022) explore consumer perceptions of mobile mental health apps but do not address the influence of technology acceptance on innovativeness and cultural perceptions related to AI in mental healthcare. Their study might show that users appreciate the convenience and accessibility of mobile mental health apps, yet it does not examine how cultural attitudes or openness to new technologies influence these perceptions. Tao et al. (2020) synthesize existing studies on user acceptance of consumer-oriented health information technologies using the Technology Acceptance Model but do not address AI in mental healthcare. They might conclude that perceived ease of use and perceived usefulness are critical for user acceptance of health information technologies. However, their review does not specifically focus on how these factors apply to AI-based mental health tools, nor does it consider the impact of cultural perceptions on the acceptance and use of such technologies.

Papadopoulos and Kouloglioti (2018) review the influence of culture on attitudes towards humanoid and animal-like robots but do not address specific hypotheses about technology acceptance and AI in mental healthcare. Their study might reveal that certain cultures prefer animal-like robots due to their perceived friendliness and less threatening appearance, while others may favor humanoid robots for their familiarity and advanced capabilities. However, this research does not extend to how these cultural preferences impact the acceptance of AI in mental health applications. Menon et al. (2023) report that digital knowledge, social media dependency, and Facebook intensity are high in urban localities, with South Kerala showing significantly higher rates of social media dependency compared to North and Central regions of Kerala. This study could imply that regions with higher social media usage might be more open to digital mental health interventions, although it does not specifically investigate the acceptance of AI technologies in mental healthcare. Boonstra et al. (2018) examine challenges in using mobile phone sensor technology for mental health research, including battery life, trust, and privacy concerns. They might find that participants are hesitant to use mobile health apps due to fears about data privacy and the potential for constant monitoring to drain their phone batteries. These findings highlight significant barriers to the adoption of AI-driven mental health tools but do not address the broader context of technology acceptance and cultural perceptions. Yadav and Hasija (2022) discuss how AI techniques can be leveraged to improve mental healthcare, including risk modeling, screening tools, and virtual therapists. They may illustrate how AI can predict mental health crises by analyzing patient data or provide continuous support through virtual therapists. However, their paper does not directly address the hypotheses about how technology acceptance influences innovativeness and cultural perceptions related to AI in mental healthcare.

Mittal et al. (2023) provide a comprehensive review of the use of AI in mental healthcare, highlighting its potential for analysis, diagnosis, treatment, and monitoring. They may discuss how AI algorithms can analyze large datasets to identify patterns in mental health conditions, offer personalized treatment recommendations, and monitor patient progress over time. However, their review does not directly address the influence of technology acceptance on innovativeness and cultural perceptions related to AI in mental healthcare. Alanzi et al. (2023) study generational differences in the acceptance of AI-powered mental health virtual assistants. They might explore how different age groups perceive and interact with virtual assistants designed to provide mental health support. Their findings could reveal that younger generations, more accustomed to digital technologies, are more accepting of AI-driven mental health tools compared to older generations who may have reservations about relying on technology for healthcare. This study contributes to understanding how generational attitudes influence the adoption of innovative AI solutions in mental health contexts.

Hypotheses

1. Higher levels of technology acceptance will be positively associated with more positive affective responses towards AI-driven innovations in mental healthcare.
2. Higher levels of technology acceptance will predict greater cognitive innovativeness in adopting and utilizing AI technologies for mental health support.
3. Individuals with higher technology acceptance scores will demonstrate increased sensory innovativeness in their utilization of AI applications in mental healthcare.
4. Increased technology acceptance will be positively correlated with stronger perceptions of cultural influence from AI in mental healthcare settings.

METHODOLOGY

In a comprehensive study conducted across Karnataka, 575 college students were surveyed to investigate their perceptions and acceptance of artificial intelligence (AI) in mental healthcare. The data collection instruments included demographic information, the Technology Acceptance Model (TAM 2) to gauge technology acceptance levels, the Cognitive and Sensory Innovativeness scale to measure innovative approaches in adopting AI technologies, an Affective scale to assess emotional responses, and specific inquiries into their perceptions of AI. The study employed a stratified random sampling technique to ensure representation across different colleges and demographics within Karnataka. Data analysis was conducted using statistical methods in SPSS. Initially, correlation analyses were performed to examine the relationships between variables such as technology acceptance, cognitive and sensory innovativeness, affective responses towards AI, and perceptions of AI in mental healthcare. Subsequently, regression analyses were employed to identify predictive relationships, exploring how technology acceptance influences cognitive and sensory innovativeness, affective responses, and overall perceptions of AI.

Variables taken for the study and definitions

1. Usage of AI (Technology Adoption): Refers to the extent to which individuals or groups integrate and utilize artificial intelligence (AI) technologies in various domains, such as mental health. It encompasses the adoption rates, patterns of use, and acceptance levels of AI applications within specific contexts (Davis, 1989).

2. Affective: In the context of AI and mental health, affective refers to emotional responses and experiences triggered by interactions with AI systems. It focuses on how AI technologies influence users' emotional states, mood regulation, and overall emotional well-being (Pham & Avnet, 2004).
3. Cognitive Innovativeness: Denotes the capacity and inclination of individuals to adopt innovative cognitive strategies and approaches facilitated by AI technologies. It involves the exploration and application of novel thinking patterns, problem-solving techniques, and cognitive enhancements arising from interactions with AI systems (Venkatraman & Price, 1990).
4. Sensory Innovativeness: Describes the exploration and utilization of sensory-based interventions and experiences enabled by AI technologies. It includes the use of sensory stimuli (e.g., visual, auditory, tactile) to enhance mental health support and therapeutic outcomes, promoting sensory exploration and engagement (Venkatraman & Price, 1990).
5. Cultural Influence of AI: Examines how the integration and adoption of AI technologies in mental healthcare shape cultural norms, values, and practices within specific social contexts. It explores perceptions of AI's cultural impact, including changes in attitudes, behaviors, and societal responses influenced by technological advancements in AI (Gerlich, 2023).

RESULTS

The correlation analysis reveals significant relationships among technology acceptance, affective response, cognitive innovativeness, sensory innovativeness, and cultural influence of AI. Technology acceptance shows a strong positive correlation with cognitive innovativeness ($r = .950$), sensory innovativeness ($r = .865$), and cultural influence of AI ($r = .868$), indicating that individuals who are more cognitively and sensory innovative and who perceive a strong cultural influence of AI are highly likely to accept technology. Affective responses to technology also show a moderate to strong positive correlation with cognitive innovativeness ($r = .606$), sensory innovativeness ($r = .862$), and cultural influence of AI ($r = .631$), suggesting that emotional responses are linked to both cognitive and sensory innovation as well as cultural perceptions of AI. Furthermore, cognitive innovativeness is strongly correlated with sensory innovativeness ($r = .742$) and cultural influence of AI ($r = .912$), highlighting a close relationship between these factors. Sensory innovativeness and cultural influence of AI are also strongly correlated ($r = .731$), indicating that sensory innovators are likely to perceive a significant cultural impact of AI. The descriptive statistics provide insights into the distribution of scores among the 575 participants. Technology acceptance scores range from 36 to 60, with an average score of 47.27 and a standard deviation of 4.69. Affective scores range from 9 to 15, with an average of 12.23 and a standard deviation of 1.38. Cognitive innovativeness scores range from 24 to 40, with a mean of 31.44 and a standard deviation of 3.21. Sensory innovativeness scores also range from 24 to 40, with an average of 32.18 and a standard deviation of 3.22. Cultural influence of AI scores range from 15 to 25, with a mean of 19.80 and a standard deviation of 2.06. These statistics suggest a moderate level of variability in responses, with the mean scores indicating general tendencies in the sample.

The regression analyses reveal compelling relationships between technology acceptance and several key variables: affective responses, cognitive innovativeness, sensory innovativeness, and cultural influence of AI. For affective responses, the regression model demonstrates that technology acceptance explains a substantial 39.7% of the variance, with a significant positive effect (Beta = 0.630, $p < .001$). This indicates that higher levels of technology acceptance correspond to more positive affective responses towards AI-driven innovations in mental healthcare. The model's fit is robust, as indicated by the high Adjusted R Square of 39.6% and a low standard error of the estimate (1.06873), suggesting that the observed data points closely align with the predicted values. Moving to cognitive innovativeness, the regression analysis shows an impressive 90.3% of the variance explained by technology acceptance, with a highly significant positive effect (Beta = 0.950, $p < .001$). This finding underscores that individuals with higher technology acceptance scores tend to exhibit greater cognitive innovativeness in embracing and utilizing AI technologies for mental health support. The model's fit is excellent, supported by an Adjusted R Square of 90.3% and a small standard error of the estimate (1.00176), indicating precise predictions within the dataset.

Similarly, for sensory innovativeness, the regression model explains 74.8% of the variance, with technology acceptance showing a significant positive effect (Beta = 0.865, $p < .001$). This suggests that individuals who are more accepting of technology also tend to be more innovative in sensory aspects related to AI applications in mental healthcare. The model's high Adjusted R Square of 74.8% and a standard error of the estimate (1.61802) illustrate a strong fit, indicating the model's reliability in predicting sensory innovativeness scores based on technology acceptance levels. Concerning the cultural influence of AI, the regression analysis reveals that technology acceptance explains 75.3% of the variance, with a significant positive effect (Beta = 0.868, $p < .001$). This indicates that higher technology acceptance is associated with a stronger perception of AI's cultural influence in mental healthcare contexts. The model's fit is robust, with an Adjusted R Square of 75.3% and a low standard error of the estimate (1.02439), affirming the accuracy of predictions regarding cultural perceptions influenced by technology acceptance.

DISCUSSION

Chatbots for mental health have seen significant growth in India due to advancements in artificial intelligence and increasing demand for accessible mental health support. These chatbots serve various purposes, offering timely interventions, emotional support, and therapeutic techniques through virtual conversations. They engage users in dialogue, providing coping strategies for anxiety, stress relief, mindfulness exercises, and psychoeducation about mental health conditions. They also monitor users' moods and behaviors over time, offering feedback and insights into patterns affecting mental health. Some examples used in India include Wysa, InnerHour, ePsyClinic, YourDost, and Woebot, which provide interactive, CBT-based approaches to improving emotional well-being through chat interactions. These chatbots reflect a growing trend in leveraging technology to make mental health support accessible and effective across India, catering to diverse emotional and psychological needs.

Chatbots for mental health care offer a convenient and accessible platform, available for free download, making them widely accessible to users seeking support. They deliver information efficiently in short, focused sessions, catering to individuals looking for quick insights and guidance without the formality of traditional therapy sessions. Many users appreciate that interacting with chatbots doesn't feel like undergoing therapy; instead, it feels like a supportive conversation, suitable for a diverse range of age groups. The ability to check in for timely support and engage with educational modules enhances their utility, providing users with structured learning and interactive feedback. However, chatbots for mental health care have their limitations. They cannot replace professional therapy or provide long-term treatment, which may leave some users seeking more intensive support. Some users find it challenging to consider using chatbots during periods of heightened stress or anxiety, feeling that their structured responses don't always align with their immediate emotional needs. The requirement to fit responses into pre-scripted categories can feel limiting, leading to frustration when chatbots struggle to understand nuanced situations or provide tailored advice. While convenient, interacting with chatbots lacks the empathetic engagement of speaking to a real person, which some users find essential for deeper emotional support. Additionally, the beginner-level information provided can be repetitive and uninspiring, detracting from their overall effectiveness for sustained engagement and learning.

This study reveals several key findings regarding the relationship between technology acceptance and AI applications in mental healthcare. Firstly, it shows that higher levels of technology acceptance are associated with more positive affective responses towards AI, indicating that individuals who embrace technology tend to perceive AI interventions as emotionally supportive within the mental health context. Secondly, increased technology acceptance scores are linked to greater cognitive innovativeness, illustrating how accepting individuals are more inclined to adopt and creatively utilize AI technologies for mental health support, fostering innovative cognitive approaches. Thirdly, individuals with higher technology acceptance scores exhibit enhanced sensory innovativeness in their use of AI applications, underscoring technology acceptance's role in encouraging exploration and utilization of sensory-focused AI tools in mental healthcare settings. Lastly, higher technology acceptance correlates positively with stronger perceptions of cultural influence from AI in mental healthcare, suggesting that technology-accepting individuals perceive a more pronounced cultural impact of AI interventions in reshaping mental health practices and perceptions. These findings collectively highlight the significant role of technology acceptance in shaping emotional, cognitive, sensory, and cultural aspects of AI integration within mental healthcare contexts.

CONCLUSION

The study reveals significant relationships between technology acceptance and key aspects of AI innovation in mental healthcare. Higher technology acceptance correlates strongly with positive affective responses, enhanced cognitive and sensory innovativeness, and a heightened perception of AI's cultural influence. These findings underscore the critical role of technology acceptance in shaping advancements in mental healthcare, emphasizing its influence on emotional engagement, innovative adoption of AI technologies, and cultural perceptions within this evolving field.

REFERENCES

Ahmed, N., Liu, X., Al-Hazwani, I., & Huang, E. M. (2024). Cultural dimensions and mental health technology: A systematic review of hofstede's dimensions in shaping mental health experiences. *Extended Abstracts of the CHI Conference on Human Factors in Computing Systems.*

Alanzi, T., Alsalem, A. A., Alzahrani, H., Almudaymigh, N., Alessa, A., Mulla, R., AlQahtani, L., Bajonaid, R., Alharthi, A., Alnahdi, O., & Alanzi, N. (2023). AI-powered mental health virtual assistants acceptance: An empirical study on influencing factors among generations X, Y, and Z. *Cureus*. Advance online publication. DOI: 10.7759/cureus.49486 PMID: 38156169

Alimour, S. A., Alnono, E., Aljasmi, S., Farran, H. E., Alqawasmi, A. A., Alrabeei, M. M., Shwedeh, F., & Aburayya, A. (2024). The quality traits of artificial intelligence operations in predicting mental healthcare professionals' perceptions: A case study in the psychotherapy division. *Journal of Autonomous Intelligence*, 7(4). Advance online publication. DOI: 10.32629/jai.v7i4.1438

AlQudah, A. A., Al-Emran, M., & Shaalan, K. (2021). Technology acceptance in healthcare: A systematic review. *Applied Sciences (Basel, Switzerland)*, 11(22), 10537. DOI: 10.3390/app112210537

Antes, A. L., Burrous, S., Sisk, B. A., Schuelke, M. J., Keune, J. D., & DuBois, J. M. (2021). Exploring perceptions of healthcare technologies enabled by artificial intelligence: An online, scenario-based survey. *BMC Medical Informatics and Decision Making*, 21(1), 221. Advance online publication. DOI: 10.1186/s12911-021-01586-8 PMID: 34284756

Anton, M. T., & Jones, D. J. (2017). Adoption of technology-enhanced treatments: Conceptual and practical considerations. *Clinical Psychology : a Publication of the Division of Clinical Psychology of the American Psychological Association*, 24(3), 223–240. DOI: 10.1111/cpsp.12197 PMID: 28966479

Boonstra, T. W., Nicholas, J., Wong, Q. J. J., Shaw, F., Townsend, S., & Christensen, H. (2018). Using mobile phone sensor technology for mental health research: Integrated analysis to identify hidden challenges and potential solutions. *Journal of Medical Internet Research*, 20(7), e10131. DOI: 10.2196/10131 PMID: 30061092

Chan, A. H. Y., & Honey, M. L. L. (2022). User perceptions of mobile digital apps for mental health: Acceptability and usability - An integrative review. *Journal of Psychiatric and Mental Health Nursing*, 29(1), 147–168. DOI: 10.1111/jpm.12744 PMID: 33604946

Chew, H. S. J., & Achananuparp, P. (2022). Perceptions and needs of Artificial intelligence in health care to increase adoption: Scoping review. *Journal of Medical Internet Research*, 24(1), e32939. DOI: 10.2196/32939 PMID: 35029538

Davis, F. D. (1989). Perceived usefulness, perceived ease of use, and user acceptance of information technology. *Management Information Systems Quarterly*, 13(3), 319. DOI: 10.2307/249008

Gamble, A. (2020). Artificial intelligence and mobile apps for mental healthcare: A social informatics perspective. *Proceedings of the International Conferences on Internet Technologies & Society (ITS 2020) and Sustainability, Technology and Education (STE 2020).*

Gerlich, M. (2023). Perceptions and acceptance of artificial intelligence: A multi-dimensional study. *Social Sciences (Basel, Switzerland)*, 12(9), 502. DOI: 10.3390/socsci12090502

Graham, S., Depp, C., Lee, E. E., Nebeker, C., Tu, X., Kim, H.-C., & Jeste, D. V. (2019). Artificial intelligence for mental health and mental illnesses: An overview. *Current Psychiatry Reports*, 21(11), 116. Advance online publication. DOI: 10.1007/s11920-019-1094-0 PMID: 31701320

Hirunyawipada, T., & Paswan, A. K. (2006). Consumer innovativeness and perceived risk: Implications for high technology product adoption. *Journal of Consumer Marketing*, 23(4), 182–198. DOI: 10.1108/07363760610674310

Ho, M.-T., Mantello, P., & Ho, M.-T. (2023). An analytical framework for studying attitude towards emotional AI: The three-pronged approach. *MethodsX*, 10(102149), 102149. DOI: 10.1016/j.mex.2023.102149 PMID: 37091958

Jan, J., Alshare, K. A., & Lane, P. L. (2024). Hofstede's cultural dimensions in technology acceptance models: A meta-analysis. *Universal Access in the Information Society*, 23(2), 717–741. DOI: 10.1007/s10209-022-00930-7

Kelly, S., Kaye, S.-A., & Oviedo-Trespalacios, O. (2023). What factors contribute to the acceptance of artificial intelligence? A systematic review. *Telematics and Informatics*, 77(101925), 101925. DOI: 10.1016/j.tele.2022.101925

Kim, H. M., Xu, Y., & Wang, Y. (2022). Overcoming the mental health stigma through m-health apps: Results from the healthy minds study. *Telemedicine Journal and e-Health*, 28(10), 1534–1540. DOI: 10.1089/tmj.2021.0418 PMID: 35254886

Kleine, A.-K., Kokje, E., Lermer, E., & Gaube, S. (2023). Attitudes toward the adoption of 2 artificial intelligence–enabled mental health tools among prospective psychotherapists: Cross-sectional study. *JMIR Human Factors*, 10, e46859. DOI: 10.2196/46859 PMID: 37436801

Kunnumpurath, B., Menon, V. A., & Paul, A. (2024). ChatGPT and virtual experience: Student engagement in online script writing - an experimental investigation among media students. In *Advances in Computational Intelligence and Robotics* (pp. 32–50). IGI Global.

Kunnumpurath, B., Prasad, A., Menon, V. A., & Thomas, J. (2024). Cultivating self-esteem: Exploring the intersection of culture, neurocognition, and behavior among female media professionals. In *Cognitive Behavioral Neuroscience in Organizational Settings* (pp. 65–82). IGI Global. DOI: 10.4018/979-8-3693-1858-4.ch004

Lee, E. E., Torous, J., De Choudhury, M., Depp, C. A., Graham, S. A., Kim, H.-C., Paulus, M. P., Krystal, J. H., & Jeste, D. V. (2021). Artificial intelligence for mental health care: Clinical applications, barriers, facilitators, and artificial wisdom. *Biological Psychiatry: Cognitive Neuroscience and Neuroimaging*, 6(9), 856–864. DOI: 10.1016/j.bpsc.2021.02.001 PMID: 33571718

Menon, V. A., Prasad, A., Puthur, L. A., K K, S., & Joseph, L. (2023). Social media dependency and Facebook usage among the older adults of Kerala. *Studies in Media and Communication*, 11(4), 202. DOI: 10.11114/smc.v11i4.6060

Mittal, A., Dumka, L., & Mohan, L. (2023). A comprehensive review on the use of artificial intelligence in mental health care. *2023 14th International Conference on Computing Communication and Networking Technologies (ICCCNT).*

Ojha, A. K. (2023). Technological innovations in mental health: Enhancing access and affordability for improved well-being. *Journal of Mental Health Issues and Behavior*, 33(33), 5–11. DOI: 10.55529/jmhib.33.5.11

Olawade, D. B., Wada, O. Z., Odetayo, A., David-Olawade, A. C., Asaolu, F., & Eberhardt, J. (2024). Enhancing mental health with Artificial Intelligence: Current trends and future prospects. *Journal of Medicine, Surgery, and Public Health*, 3(100099), 100099. DOI: 10.1016/j.glmedi.2024.100099

Papadopoulos, I., & Koulouglioti, C. (2018). The influence of culture on attitudes towards humanoid and animal-like robots: An integrative review. *Journal of Nursing Scholarship*, 50(6), 653–665. DOI: 10.1111/jnu.12422 PMID: 30242796

Pham, M. T., & Avnet, T. (2004). Ideals and oughts and the reliance on affect versus substance in persuasion. *The Journal of Consumer Research*, 30(4), 503–518. DOI: 10.1086/380285

Prakash, A. V. (2020). Intelligent Conversational Agents in Mental Healthcare Services: A Thematic Analysis of User Perceptions Authors. *Pacific Asia Journal of the Association for Information Systems, 12.*

Rogan, J., Bucci, S., & Firth, J. (2024). Health care professionals' views on the use of passive sensing, AI, and machine learning in mental health care: Systematic review with meta-synthesis. *JMIR Mental Health*, 11, e49577. DOI: 10.2196/49577 PMID: 38261403

Srite & Karahanna. (2006). The role of espoused national cultural values in technology acceptance. *MIS Quarterly: Management Information Systems, 30*(3), 679. DOI: 10.2307/25148745

Tam-Seto, L., Wood, V. M., Linden, B., & Stuart, H. (2021). Perceptions of an AI-supported mobile app for military health in the Canadian armed forces. *Military Behavioral Health*, 9(3), 247–254. DOI: 10.1080/21635781.2020.1838364

Tao, D., Wang, T., Wang, T., Zhang, T., Zhang, X., & Qu, X. (2020). A systematic review and meta-analysis of user acceptance of consumer-oriented health information technologies. *Computers in Human Behavior*, 104(106147), 106147. DOI: 10.1016/j.chb.2019.09.023

Thomas, L. P., Menon, V. A., Thomas, J., Ali, K. A. A., Soman, K. K., & Kumar, T. K. S. (2024). Towards a model: Exploring fatigue factors in ZOOM online classes. *2024 International Conference on Current Trends in Advanced Computing (ICCTAC).* DOI: 10.1109/ICCTAC61556.2024.10581300

Thordardottir, B., Malmgren Fänge, A., Lethin, C., Rodriguez Gatta, D., & Chiatti, C. (2019). Acceptance and use of innovative Assistive Technologies among people with cognitive impairment and their caregivers: A systematic review. *BioMed Research International*, 2019, 1–18. DOI: 10.1155/2019/9196729 PMID: 30956989

Torous, J., Bucci, S., Bell, I. H., Kessing, L. V., Faurholt-Jepsen, M., Whelan, P., Carvalho, A. F., Keshavan, M., Linardon, J., & Firth, J. (2021). The growing field of digital psychiatry: Current evidence and the future of apps, social media, chatbots, and virtual reality. *World Psychiatry; Official Journal of the World Psychiatric Association (WPA)*, 20(3), 318–335. DOI: 10.1002/wps.20883 PMID: 34505369

Venkatraman, M. P., & Price, L. L. (1990). Differentiating between cognitive and sensory innovativeness. *Journal of Business Research*, 20(4), 293–315. DOI: 10.1016/0148-2963(90)90008-2

Wei, X., Cao, Y., Peng, X., & Prybutok, V. (2024). A meta-analysis of technology acceptance in healthcare from the consumer's perspective. *Health Marketing Quarterly*, 41(2), 1–22. DOI: 10.1080/07359683.2024.2316425 PMID: 38421028

Yadav, K., & Hasija, Y. (2022). Artificial intelligence and technological development in behavioral and mental healthcare. *2022 International Conference for Advancement in Technology (ICONAT)*. DOI: 10.1109/ICONAT53423.2022.9726100

Chapter 5
Tracing the Development and Influence of Chatbots in Contemporary Healthcare Systems

Aashiq Khan
https://orcid.org/0000-0003-4532-8774
School of Educational Science, Anhui Normal University, Wuhu, China

Irum Zeb
School of Education, Huazhong University of Science and Technology, China

Shuanghu Fang
School of Educational Science, Anhui Normal University, Wuhu, China

ABSTRACT

This chapter explores the transformative impact of chatbot technology in healthcare. It details the evolution from simple scripts to advanced AI systems that improve patient-provider interactions. Chatbots enhance healthcare accessibility, efficiency, and quality by providing services like appointment scheduling, real-time consultations, and patient data management. The text highlights their crucial role during the COVID-19 pandemic in information dissemination and remote patient management. However, challenges such as privacy, security, and ethical concerns are also discussed, with insights on mitigating these risks to ensure ethical technology use. This overview aims are to inform healthcare professionals, technologists, and policymakers about safely integrating AI in healthcare.

DOI: 10.4018/979-8-3693-3112-5.ch005

INTRODUCTION

In recent times, there has been a notable surge in the adoption of e-healthcare services, primarily attributed to their user-friendliness and the superior quality of patient care they facilitate (Mbunge et al., 2022; Sharma & Kumar, 2022). These services represent a significant shift in the healthcare sector towards a digitalized framework, utilizing cutting-edge technology and information systems to streamline the interaction and procedural dynamics between patients and medical personnel. E-health, at its core, is an innovative electronic system profoundly reliant on the continual advancements in technological and artificial intelligence domains (Al-Mistarehi et al., 2023; Alshammari et al., 2022). This system encompasses a wide array of tools, including secure storage and management of patient and medication data. It integrates electronic health records (EHRs), telemedicine platforms, mobile health applications, and numerous other digital solutions, all aimed at enhancing patient care and providing tailored services (Shafi et al., 2023).

The evolution of hospital and clinical systems has facilitated more precise diagnoses and the provision of timely medical treatments. The healthcare industry's trajectory is increasingly intertwined with developments in technology and artificial intelligence methodologies (Alabdulatif et al., 2023; Mijwil & Shukur, 2022). This integration has significantly refined the healthcare environment, extending the spectrum of digital services accessible to patients. In the realm of computer science, artificial intelligence has emerged as a particularly prominent field, drawing considerable attention in recent times, especially with the introduction of human-mind-simulating applications such as ChatGPT (Deiana et al., 2023; Wang et al., 2023). It involves complex concepts associated with logic, and learning, and comprises algorithms that undergo training on extensive datasets, which might include an array of images or diverse signal types. This scientific discipline is characterized by its focus on intelligent computational behavior, manifesting in the design of computerized tools that replicate human cognitive functions, encompassing learning, reasoning, and self-correction (Mijwil et al., 2023). Consequently, this enables computers to generate specific decisions based on overarching rules that are shaped by their training in a given environmental context.

The paramount advantage of e-healthcare lies in its exceptional capability to establish a centralized and secure repository containing comprehensive patient data, readily accessible to healthcare professionals and physicians (Tanwar et al., 2020). Electronic health records (EHRs) empower medical staff with real-time access to patient information, enabling them to review patients' medical histories, diagnoses, medications, and treatment plans with utmost accuracy and convenience (Chen et al., 2014). Telemedicine emerges as one of the key offerings of e-healthcare, facilitating remote consultations and monitoring. This transcends geographical limitations, augments communication with patients, and significantly improves their health outcomes (Garattini et al., 2021). These advancements are largely attributable to artificial intelligence techniques that have been instrumental in creating a virtual environment conducive to efficiently executing a myriad of tasks (Alowais et al., 2023).

The integration of artificial intelligence in the medical field is rapidly gaining momentum. There has been a marked increase in scientific research focused on incorporating AI technologies into healthcare, underscoring both the significance and rapid evolution of this area. It is anticipated that AI practices will soon become commonplace in various health sector settings, including hospitals, laboratories, and clinics (Sukums et al., 2023). A notable focus of AI in healthcare is medical imaging, which involves the processing and interpretation of images for diagnostic purposes. AI techniques enhance the precision and quality of diagnoses. They excel in automatically identifying complex patterns within images, filtering out noise, and facilitating the creation of 3D models from specific tissue images. As technological advancements continue, the ongoing integration of electronic healthcare solutions promises to further refine healthcare workflows, improve patient outcomes, and contribute substantially to the efficiency and effectiveness of contemporary healthcare systems.

CHATBOT TECHNOLOGY

Chatbot technology has emerged as a pivotal instrument in the advancement of the healthcare sector (Javaid et al., 2023). These digital tools are integral in shaping electronic medical services and augmenting the efficiency of healthcare professionals. Chatbots facilitate real-time interactions between patients and physicians with notable accuracy, creating a secure environment within hospital and clinic systems (Suppadungsuk et al., 2023). They provide essential information regarding symptoms, medications, and medical appointments, and play a significant role in educating patients and training healthcare staff in patient interaction strategies. Chatbots, a type of artificial intelligence (AI), have become increasingly essential in various sectors, including healthcare. The importance of chatbots in healthcare became more evident during the COVID-19 pandemic. As noted by (Torous et al., 2021), the pandemic hastened the adoption of telehealth and mobile mental health technologies, such as chatbots. These tools provide accessible and scalable solutions that enhance traditional healthcare methods, marking a significant shift towards digital psychiatry and the integration of chatbots in mental health services. The pandemic also highlighted the critical role of telemedicine, as demonstrated in a study by Reitzle et al. (2021) which examined the perceived accessibility of healthcare services during the pandemic in Germany and the impact of telemedicine. In this environment, chatbots were pivotal, offering remote healthcare access and facilitating the dissemination of information. Chatbots have also been applied in specific medical domains. For instance, a study by Li et al. (2024) explored the use of ChatGPT-4 for answering frequent questions about abdominoplasty, showcasing chatbots' potential in plastic surgery consultations.

Chatbots are revolutionizing the healthcare industry by improving decision-making and assisting with medical diagnostics. These artificial intelligence (AI) powered applications facilitate communication between patients and healthcare practitioners, prioritize cases based on severity, and do virtual illness categorization. Chatbots simplify difficult medical training and operational activities like patient tracking and appointment booking by reducing the stress on healthcare professionals and improving resource efficiency in hospitals and clinics. Their round-the-clock accessibility enhances patients' access to information, lowering worry about medical problems and encouraging preventative care. By automating processes like scheduling appointments and managing medical records, chatbots also improve administrative efficiency and free up medical professionals to focus on providing direct patient care. The extensive use of chatbots, however, brings up privacy and ethical issues, such as data openness and equal access to technology. To fully utilize chatbots' potential to transform healthcare delivery, enhance service quality, and guarantee patient-centered care, these problems must be resolved.

PURPOSE OF THE CHAPTER

This chapter aims to outline the history and significant impact of chatbots in healthcare. It highlights the evolution from simple rule-based systems to sophisticated AI-driven technologies and their integration into healthcare practices. The analysis covers how chatbots have transformed patient interaction, enhanced administrative efficiency, and provided clinical support. Additionally, the chapter discusses the benefits, such as increased accessibility and cost-effectiveness, alongside challenges like ethical concerns and privacy issues. It also considers chatbots' potential to reshape patient care and public health initiatives. Overall, the chapter provides a thorough understanding of chatbots' role in healthcare, targeting health professionals, technologists, and policymakers.

EARLY DEVELOPMENT OF CHATBOTS: FROM ELIZA TO MORE ADVANCED SYSTEMS

The development of chatbots began in the middle of the 20th century, which was a turning point in computer science and artificial intelligence. ELIZA, developed in the 1960s by Weizenbaum (1966) at the MIT Artificial Intelligence Laboratory, was one of the first innovations. ELIZA was a game-changer because it mimicked dialogue using a "pattern matching" and replacement method that created the appearance of comprehension without requiring context awareness (Costa, 2018). The development of ELIZA encouraged more research into interactions between humans and computers. It was a pivotal early experiment that showed how robots might mimic human speech by reacting to textual inputs in ways that appeared human (da Fona Costa & Cesar Jr, 2018). After ELIZA, chatbot technology advanced dramatically due to developments in machine learning and natural language processing (NLP). As a result, increasingly complex chatbots that can learn from conversations and provide more nuanced, context-aware replies have been created.

Zhongxuan He's work, "From ELIZA to ChatGPT. The Evolution of Chatbots in Public Health," shows the development from basic models to sophisticated AI-driven systems such as ChatGPT. It highlights recent developments. These days, these sophisticated chatbots are essential in many domains, including public health (He, 2023).The development of AI and chatbot technologies from ELIZA to the sophisticated chatbots of today highlights a noteworthy progression in these fields, augmenting their capabilities and expanding their use in several sectors, especially healthcare.

MILESTONES IN CHATBOT TECHNOLOGY RELEVANT TO HEALTH CARE

Many noteworthy turning points have occurred in the development of chatbot technology in the healthcare industry, indicating the increasing sophistication and use of these instruments in the medical domain. The creation of chatbots for mental health needs particularly amid the COVID-19 pandemic was one of the major turning points. Research by Jackson-Triche et al. (2023) details the planning and execution of a chatbot program intended to help staff members of a sizable academic medical institution obtain mental health evaluation and treatment by triaging them. This breakthrough demonstrated chatbots' ability to deliver prompt and effective mental health support a crucial requirement during the pandemic. The use of chatbot technology in cancer is a noteworthy development in healthcare technology. A comprehensive evaluation on chatbots for cancer and health care applications utilizing AI and machine learning was carried out by Xu et al. (2021). The research emphasized the use of chatbots to cancer therapy in a number of areas, such as patient support, monitoring, diagnosis, treatment, and workflow efficiency. This accomplishment shows how adaptable chatbots are in managing delicate and intricate medical fields like cancer.

Another significant development is the fusion of AI-powered chatbots with conventional medical procedures. Singh et al. (2023) talked about the creation of Healing Hands, an AI-powered chatbot made to offer individualized medical advice and research-backed suggestions for at-home treatments for a variety of medical issues. This development demonstrates how chatbots can provide individualized health advice and revitalize established medical procedures (Singh et al., 2023). In addition, a significant advancement in the dissemination of post-COVID-19 information is the development of chatbot technology. The development of the RAFAEL platform and chatbot, which was intended to handle the information and management needs linked to post-COVID-19 in children and adults, was detailed by Nehme et al. (2023). This advancement emphasizes how chatbots can be used to handle sudden health emergencies. Together, these achievements show how chatbot technology has advanced significantly in the healthcare industry, from simple informative tools to complex systems that can handle complicated medical data and offer individualized treatment.

THE TRANSITION FROM SIMPLE SCRIPTED BOTS TO AI-DRIVEN, NTERACTIVE SYSTEMS

The development of chatbot technology from straightforward programmed bots to complex interactive systems powered by artificial intelligence represents a major turning point in the area of AI and its applications in many industries, including healthcare.

At first, chatbots were mostly written programs that followed a predetermined set of guidelines and replies. The early bots' capacity to interpret user queries and provide dynamic responses was constrained. However, chatbot technology has undergone a paradigm leap with the introduction of AI and deep learning. Laymouna et al. (2024) offer a thorough examination of chatbots powered by AI and deep learning, showcasing its uses in a range of industries, including healthcare. Compared to their scripted predecessors, these sophisticated chatbots effectively engage users by using natural language comprehension. The interaction capabilities of chatbot systems were further improved by the incorporation of explainable AI (XAI). The Case-based Reasoning (CBR) paradigm is utilized by Wijekoon et al. to create iSee, an interactive platform that makes it easier to reuse explanation tactics in XAI. This advancement in chatbot technology has increased customer happiness and trust while also enabling chatbots to more successfully support AI-assisted decision-making processes (Wijekoon et al., 2024). The use of AI-powered chatbots in classrooms has completely changed how students engage with the content. The Curriculum-Driven EduBot, introduced by Li et al. (2023), is a methodology for creating a chatbot that helps students improve their conversational skills by combining methodical material with interactive features. According to Li et al. (2023), this example shows how chatbots may offer personalized and dynamic interactions. Moreover, the advancement of chatbots has been marked by their growing capacity to communicate with people more efficiently and naturally. In their discussion of the need for chatbots in the modern, fast-paced world, Rane (2023) emphasized the crucial role artificial intelligence (AI), and more specifically Natural Language Processing (NLP), has played in this development. The emergence of multiple chatbot kinds, such as text-to-text, text-to-speech, and speech-to-speech, showcases the extensive range of uses and proficiencies of these artificial intelligence-powered platforms (Rane et al., 2022).A major technical achievement, the shift from basic programmed bots to AI-driven interactive systems allows for more intelligent, efficient, and tailored interactions across a range of industries, including healthcare.

KEY TECHNOLOGIES BEHIND CHATBOTS

The development and operation of chatbots, particularly in healthcare environments, depend heavily on three key technologies that form their technological foundations: artificial intelligence (AI), machine learning (ML), and natural language processing (NLP). Modern chatbots rely on artificial intelligence (AI) to mimic human-like interactions. AI plays a crucial part in chatbot functioning as it enables chatbots to effectively extract and understand information in response to user questions, as demonstrated by a study on open domain question answering systems (Chowdhary & Chowdhary, 2020). A branch of AI called machine learning gives chatbots the ability to learn from data and get better over time. Chatbots can adjust to new information and improve their replies based on prior exchanges with the aid of machine learning techniques.

For instance, machine learning has been applied in the banking industry to create chatbots that efficiently comprehend and respond to customer demands (Bhise et al., 2022). By bridging the gap between human speech and machine comprehension, natural language processing (NLP) enables chatbots to comprehend and process human language. This includes linguistic translation and speech recognition. According to a survey on NLP, chatbots need to be able to analyze natural language data quickly, which is essential for a variety of applications, including healthcare

(George et al., 2021). Additionally, a research on the use of natural language processing (NLP) in emergency medicine chatbots shows how these technologies may be effectively applied to anticipate triage outcomes, highlighting their usefulness in crucial healthcare circumstances (Barak-Corren et al., 2024). Together, AI, ML, and NLP not only make chatbots function fundamentally better but also propel continuous development and adaptation, increasing their efficacy in a variety of industries, most notably healthcare.

CHATBOTS IN HEALTH CARE: A CHRONOLOGICAL OVERVIEW OF INITIAL APPLICATIONS

The initial applications of chatbots in healthcare marked a significant shift in the delivery and management of services, laying the groundwork for the sophisticated AI-driven chatbots now prevalent in the sector. Initially, these chatbots focused primarily on basic patient interactions and disseminating information. A systematic review by Xu et al. (2021), examined chatbot technology in various medical fields, including oncology, providing a historical overview of their development and roles in diagnosis, treatment, monitoring, patient support, and workflow efficiency. Although not directly related to chatbots, the evolution of healthcare financing and management techniques provides context for understanding the environment in which healthcare chatbots emerged. Gray (1984) detailed capital financing techniques for healthcare facilities, offering insights into the features, applications, and costs associated with these methods, helping to frame the technological advancements in healthcare, including chatbots. Additionally, the historical overview of volunteer practices in healthcare, discussed by Leshkevich and Motozhanets (2022), while not directly linked to chatbots, provides insights into the evolution of healthcare systems and the increasing need for technological solutions to enhance healthcare delivery and volunteer management. Together, these early applications and developments set the stage for integrating chatbots into more complex healthcare processes, leading to the current state where chatbots play a crucial role in patient care, administrative tasks, and healthcare management.

GROWTH AND EXPANSION OF CHATBOTS IN DIFFERENT HEALTH CARE DOMAINS

The growth and expansion of chatbots across various healthcare domains have been noteworthy, with applications extending from primary care to specialized medical fields. In school-based healthcare, chatbots have gained traction, assisting in the delivery of primary and mental health care among other services in schools, especially in underserved communities. Skjuve et al. (2021), highlighted this expansion over the past two decades, suggesting the need for innovative technologies like chatbots to support these services. During the COVID-19 pandemic, the significance of chatbots became more pronounced. Karmakar (2024), assessed the user experience and satisfaction with healthcare chatbots in China during the Omicron wave, noting an increased dependency on chatbots for health information and self-diagnosis, particularly among the youth during this health crisis. In the specialized field of critical care nephrology, chatbots have been explored for their potential to enhance patient care. Suppadungsuk et al. (2024) investigated their use in managing acute kidney injury and in systems like alert mechanisms and continuous renal replacement therapy, indicating a move toward integrating chatbots in more specialized and critical healthcare settings. Another growing area for chatbot applications is digital mental health. Bhatnagr et al. (2024), reviewed the potential of AI-driven chatbots to transform this sector, emphasizing the importance of ethical and trustworthy AI algorithms in mental health care, which underscores the expanding role of chatbots in this field. These examples showcase the diverse and evolving roles of chatbots in healthcare, from general information sharing and pandemic response to specialized applications in critical care and mental health. Their continued development highlights their potential to improve healthcare delivery and patient outcomes.

TIMELINE OF SIGNIFICANT CHATBOT DEPLOYMENTS AND THEIR IMPACTS IN HEALTH CARE

The deployment of chatbots in healthcare has marked significant advancements and impacts across various domains. Initially significant in telehealth and remote healthcare services, chatbots have been studied for their complexity and user interaction. Biro et al. (2023) investigated how a healthcare chatbot's design affects user trust and perceived effectiveness, highlighting the critical early integration of these tools. Furthering their utility in patient healthcare, chatbots have become pivotal in regions with dense populations and limited medical resources. Abisha et al. (2024) described an AI-based medical chatbot in India that was developed to provide immediate medical information, help locate specialists, and facilitate appointment scheduling, showcasing their role in improving access to healthcare services. During the COVID-19 pandemic, chatbots were extensively used for screening and monitoring, as noted by Chagas et al. (2023), who evaluated a COVID-19 chatbot in Brazil that helped in assessing symptom severity and providing reliable health information, underscoring their value in managing public health crises. Additionally, the role of chatbots in mobile health clinics, though indirectly, is supported by a study from Series et al. (2023), which provides a business framework for deploying mobile health services, aiding in the strategic use of chatbots in such settings. These deployments illustrate how chatbots have evolved from basic tools to complex systems that effectively manage medical information, enhance patient interaction, and address public health emergencies.

INFLUENCE OF CHATBOTS ON IMPROVING PATIENT ENGAGEMENT AND COMMUNICATION IN HEALTH CARE DELIVERY

The integration of chatbots in healthcare has significantly influenced patient engagement and communication, enhancing the overall delivery of healthcare services. Sands and Wald (2014), emphasized the transformation of healthcare delivery through increased consumer engagement and health data transparency. They advocated for new data streams to improve self-management and shared decision-making, where chatbots play a pivotal role by providing accessible, personalized health information to enhance patient-centered care. Tai-Seale et al. (2019) discussed how technology-enabled consumer engagement could improve the patient journey across the care continuum. In this integration, chatbots serve as crucial tools for engaging patients more effectively, supporting their healthcare journey by facilitating better interaction with care processes. In the realm of palliative care, Consolo et al. (2024), explored healthcare professionals' perspectives on the use of digital technologies, including chatbots, in routine palliative care delivery. The study noted that digital technologies are increasingly accepted and utilized for coordinating work processes, enhancing patient-centered care, and improving communication, particularly in overcoming spatial and temporal challenges in outpatient care, thereby contributing to more responsive palliative care. Additionally, Sieck et al. (2022), investigated the role of healthcare organizations in fostering patient engagement. The study highlighted the importance of tools that facilitate communication between patients and clinicians, where chatbots can significantly enhance interactions by providing a user-friendly and interactive platform. Collectively, these studies demonstrate the beneficial impact of chatbots on patient engagement and communication within healthcare. By providing an efficient means to access information and facilitating active participation in their own healthcare journey, chatbots empower patients and streamline the delivery of healthcare services.

Figure 1. The role of health care organizations

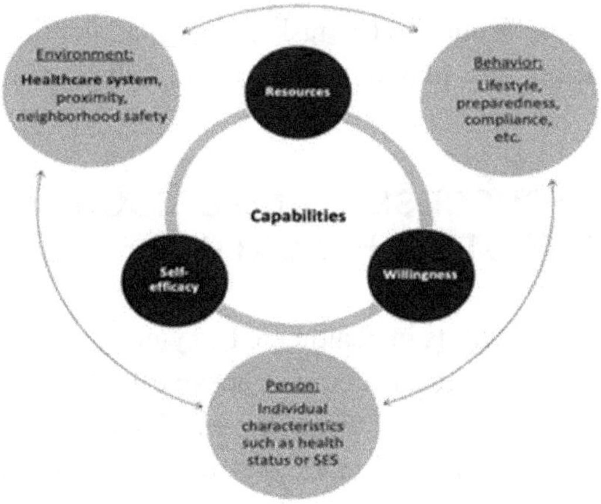

INFLUENCE OF CHATBOTS ON ENHANCING HEALTH CARE ACCESSIBILITY AND REDUCING DISPARITIES

Chatbots have significantly enhanced healthcare accessibility and mitigated disparities, especially in regions where traditional healthcare systems struggle with the crucial role of empathy, compassion, and healthcare trust values that are sometimes overshadowed by the push for efficiency. The integration of artificial intelligence, including chatbots, promises a balance between these values and operational efficiency. Chatbots help streamline workflows and enhance the accuracy of diagnoses and treatments, potentially allowing healthcare professionals to devote more time to the human aspects of care (Kerasidou, 2020). the transformative impact of advances in artificial intelligence (AI) and machine learning (ML) on the healthcare industry. These technologies, including chatbots, are revolutionizing care delivery, improving patient outcomes, and optimizing healthcare systems. By automating administrative tasks, enhancing decision-making, and improving patient engagement, AI and ML help reduce disparities in healthcare access (Naveed et al., 2024). While (Newell & Jordan, 2015) primarily focused on patient-centered communication with nurses in hospitals, their findings highlight the importance of effective communication in healthcare a domain where chatbots can make a significant contribution. Chatbots provide consistent, accessible, and personalized communication, improving the overall patient experience. Chatbots, as an AI application, address many contemporary healthcare challenges by providing easily accessible information, aiding clinical decision-making, and reducing healthcare access disparities (Morley et al., 2020). Collectively, these insights underscore chatbots' potential to enhance healthcare accessibility, streamline administrative tasks, support clinical decisions, and improve patient communication, thus playing a vital role in reducing healthcare disparities.

CASE STUDIES: SUCCESSES AND LESSONS LEARNED FROM KEY CHATBOTS IN HEALTH CARE

The deployment of chatbots in healthcare has yielded valuable insights through various case studies, which offer a comprehensive look at the development, implementation, and impact of these technologies. These studies reveal the lessons learned and best practices that have emerged from the deployment of key chatbots. In the realm of integrated care and technology implementation, a case study on the Health TAPESTRY program, focusing on the health of older adults supported by the Health TAPESTRY application (TAP-App). This study provides an in-depth look at the development and implementation phases of the TAP-App, highlighting the critical importance of adapting technology to support functional integration in healthcare settings (Di Pelino et al., 2022). the implementation of integrated health systems interventions, such as the Facility-Based Integrated Management of Childhood Illness and Insecticide Treated Nets in Bangladesh. The findings underscored the role of community engagement, effective data use, and the benefits of small-scale testing in ensuring successful implementation and extensive coverage of these health interventions (Huda et al., 2024). In another study, (Bamgboje-Ayodele et al., 2022) detailed the adaptation and implementation of an integrated care pathway for electronic patient-reported outcomes (ePROs) in routine oncology care. This case study emphasized the importance of engaging stakeholders and highlighted the decision-making processes necessary for the optimal implementation of ePROs, stressing the need for continuous dialogue and systematic problem resolution.

Lastly, the use of implementation frameworks to integrate the web-based application Care Heroes into clinical practice at two memory clinics. This study aimed to enhance caregiver-physician communication in dementia care and provided insights into the challenges and effective strategies for integrating new health information technology to support communication in this critical care area (Brown et al., 2023).

Together, these case studies demonstrate the varied applications of chatbots and related technologies in healthcare. They highlight the necessity of stakeholder engagement, the adaptability of technology to meet healthcare needs, and systematic planning in the successful implementation of these technologies. The lessons learned from these studies offer valuable guidance for future deployments of chatbots and similar technologies in healthcare environments.

CHALLENGES AND ETHICAL CONSIDERATIONS IN CHATBOTS: ADDRESSING ACCURACY, PRIVACY, SECURITY, AND ETHICAL IMPLICATIONS IN PATIENT CARE

The integration of chatbots in healthcare introduces several challenges and ethical considerations, especially concerning accuracy, privacy, security, and the broader ethical implications of AI in patient care. In the field of urology, the potential of AI-driven chatbots, discussing both the benefits and limitations. The study underscores concern regarding the accuracy of chatbot diagnoses and recommendations, privacy and security issues surrounding patient data, and the necessity for these systems to comply with legal standards. The research also pointed out resistance from both patients and healthcare professionals towards adopting new technologies (Talyshinskii et al., 2024).

Addressing AI more broadly in medicine (Mehta et al., 2023) analyzed its significant impact, including the challenges and ethical considerations it brings. The study emphasized ethical issues related to privacy, security, and the risk of increasing healthcare inequities. Furthermore, it highlighted the widespread mistrust in AI-enabled healthcare among the public and medical professionals, stressing the importance of transparency and ethical practices, particularly in cardiovascular care. In the specialized area of critical care nephrology, it was investigated the use of chatbots, reveals concerns related to their accuracy, reliability, data protection, transparency, potential for algorithmic biases, and ethical issues. The study stresses the critical need for human judgment and intervention in complex medical scenarios, acknowledging the limitations of AI in such contexts (Suppadungsuk et al., 2023). From an ethical standpoint in AI-enabled medical care, a literature review identifies key ethical barriers and facilitators from the perspectives of patients and healthcare providers in cardiovascular care. The review found major trust barriers, including concerns over data privacy, security, potential patient harm, and fears of AI supplanting the human aspects of care. It also highlighted the need for strict data privacy measures and thorough validation processes to foster ethical and trustworthy AI-enabled medical care (Mooghali et al., 2023). Collectively, these studies illustrate the complex challenges and ethical considerations associated with deploying chatbots and AI in healthcare. Addressing these issues is crucial for the successful and ethical integration of these technologies in patient care.

CONCLUSION

In sum, the evolution and integration of chatbot technology in healthcare have marked a significant transformation in patient care and administrative efficiency. Chatbots, leveraging advancements in artificial intelligence, have not only improved the immediacy and accuracy of patient-provider communications but also broadened access to medical information and services, especially in underserved or remote areas. Their role during the COVID-19 pandemic as essential tools in telemedicine and patient engagement has underscored their potential in managing health crises. However, the widespread adoption of this technology raises crucial concerns about privacy, data security, and the ethical use of AI in healthcare. These challenges necessitate rigorous standards and continuous scrutiny to ensure that the deployment of chatbots aligns with the overarching goals of ethical medical practice and equitable patient care. Addressing these concerns is vital as we continue to advance towards a more digitalized and AI-integrated healthcare environment, promising to reshape healthcare delivery for enhanced patient outcomes and operational efficiency.

ACKNOWLEDGMENT

We would like to express our sincere gratitude to Professor Shuanghu Fang from the School of Educational Science, Anhui Normal University, Wuhu, China, for his invaluable guidance and support in the development of this book chapter. His expertise and insights have greatly enriched our work.

REFERENCES

Abisha, D., Mahalakshmi, M., Pritiga, T., & Thanusiya, M. (2024). Revolutionizing Rural Healthcare in India: AI-Powered Chatbots for Affordable Symptom Analysis and Medical Guidance. 2024 International Conference on Inventive Computation Technologies (ICICT).

Alabdulatif, A., Al Asqah, M., Moulahi, T., & Zidi, S. (2023). Leveraging artificial intelligence in blockchain-based E-health for safer decision making framework. *Applied Sciences (Basel, Switzerland)*, *13*(2), 1035. DOI: 10.3390/app13021035

Alowais, S. A., Alghamdi, S. S., Alsuhebany, N., Alqahtani, T., Alshaya, A. I., Almohareb, S. N., Aldairem, A., Alrashed, M., Bin Saleh, K., Badreldin, H. A., Al Yami, M. S., Al Harbi, S., & Albekairy, A. M. (2023). Revolutionizing healthcare: The role of artificial intelligence in clinical practice. *BMC Medical Education*, *23*(1), 689. DOI: 10.1186/s12909-023-04698-z PMID: 37740191

Alshammari, N., Sarker, M. N. I., Kamruzzaman, M., Alruwaili, M., Alanazi, S. A., Raihan, M. L., & AlQahtani, S. A. (2022). Technology-driven 5G enabled e-healthcare system during COVID-19 pandemic. *IET Communications*, *16*(5), 449–463. DOI: 10.1049/cmu2.12240

Bamgboje-Ayodele, A., Avery, S., Pearson, J., Mak, M., Smith, K., Rincones, O., Vinod, S., Bray, V., Ducinoska, I., McCarthy, K., Williamson, K., Delaney, G. P., & Girgis, A. (2022). Adapting an integrated care pathway for implementing electronic patient reported outcomes assessment in routine oncology care: Lessons learned from a case study. *Journal of Evaluation in Clinical Practice*, *28*(6), 1072–1083. DOI: 10.1111/jep.13688 PMID: 35470525

Barak-Corren, Y., Wolf, R., Rozenblum, R., Creedon, J. K., Lipsett, S. C., Lyons, T. W., Michelson, K. A., Miller, K. A., Shapiro, D. J., Reis, B. Y., & Fine, A. M. (2024). Harnessing the Power of Generative AI for Clinical Summaries: Perspectives From Emergency Physicians. *Annals of Emergency Medicine*, *84*(2), 128–138. DOI: 10.1016/j.annemergmed.2024.01.039 PMID: 38483426

Bhatnagr, P., Rajesh, A., & Misra, R. (2024). Continuous intention usage of artificial intelligence enabled digital banks: A review of expectation confirmation model. *Journal of Enterprise Information Management, 37*(6), 1763–1787. DOI: 10.1108/JEIM-11-2023-0617

Bhise, A., Munshi, A., Rodrigues, A., & Sawant, V. (2022). Overview of AI in education. In *Artificial Intelligence in Higher Education* (pp. 31–62). CRC Press. DOI: 10.1201/9781003184157-2

Biro, J., Linder, C., & Neyens, D. (2023). The effects of a health care chatbot's complexity and persona on user trust, perceived usability, and effectiveness: Mixed methods study. *JMIR Human Factors, 10*(1), e41017. DOI: 10.2196/41017 PMID: 36724004

Brown, E. L., Ruggiano, N., Allala, S. C., Clarke, P. J., Davis, D., Roberts, L., Framil, C. V., Muñoz, M. T. H., Hough, M. S., & Bourgeois, M. S. (2023). Developing a Memory and Communication App for Persons Living With Dementia: An 8-Step Process. *JMIR Aging, 6*, e44007. DOI: 10.2196/44007 PMID: 36920462

Chagas, B. A., Pagano, A. S., Prates, R. O., Praes, E. C., Ferreguetti, K., Vaz, H., Reis, Z. S. N., Ribeiro, L. B., Ribeiro, A. L. P., Pedroso, T. M., Beleigoli, A., Oliveira, C. R. A., & Marcolino, M. S. (2023). Evaluating user experience with a Chatbot designed as a public health response to the COVID-19 pandemic in Brazil: Mixed methods study. *JMIR Human Factors, 10*(1), e43135. DOI: 10.2196/43135 PMID: 36634267

Chen, Y., Lorenzi, N., Nyemba, S., Schildcrout, J. S., & Malin, B. (2014). We work with them? Healthcare workers interpretation of organizational relations mined from electronic health records. *International Journal of Medical Informatics, 83*(7), 495–506. DOI: 10.1016/j.ijmedinf.2014.04.006 PMID: 24845147

Chowdhary, K., & Chowdhary, K. (2020). Natural language processing. *Fundamentals of artificial intelligence*, 603-649.

Consolo, L., Basile, I., Colombo, S., Rusconi, D., Pasquot, L., Campa, T., Caraceni, A., & Lusignani, M. (2024). Exploring patient perspectives on electronic patient-reported outcome measures in home-based cancer palliative care: A qualitative study. *Digital Health, 10*. DOI: 10.1177/20552076241249962 PMID: 38665884

da Fona Costa, L., & Cesar Jr, R. M. (2018). *Shape classification and analysis: theory and practice*. Crc Press. DOI: 10.1201/9781315222325

Deiana, G., Dettori, M., Arghittu, A., Azara, A., Gabutti, G., & Castiglia, P. (2023). Artificial intelligence and public health: Evaluating ChatGPT responses to vaccination myths and misconceptions. *Vaccines*, *11*(7), 1217. DOI: 10.3390/vaccines11071217 PMID: 37515033

Di Pelino, S., Lamarche, L., Carr, T., Datta, J., Gaber, J., Oliver, D., Gallagher, J., Dragos, S., Price, D., & Mangin, D. (2022). Lessons learned through two phases of developing and implementing a technology supporting integrated care: Case study. *JMIR Formative Research*, *6*(4), e34899. DOI: 10.2196/34899 PMID: 35404253

Garattini, L., Badinella Martini, M., & Zanetti, M. (2021). More room for telemedicine after COVID-19: Lessons for primary care? *The European Journal of Health Economics*, *22*(2), 183–186. DOI: 10.1007/s10198-020-01248-y PMID: 33231825

George, A. S., Muralikrishnan, G., Ninan, L. R., Varrier, P. S., & Dhanya, L. (2021). Survey on the design and development of Indian language chatbots. 2021 International Conference on Communication, Control and Information Sciences (ICCISc).

He, Z. (2023). From ELIZA to ChatGPT: The Evolution of Chatbots in Public Health. *XRDS: Crossroads. The ACM Magazine for Students*, *29*(3), 59–59.

Huda, F. A., Mathewos, K., Mahmood, H. R., Faruk, O., Hirschhorn, L. R., & Binagwaho, A. (2024). Examining the implementation of facility-based integrated management of childhood illness and insecticide treated nets in Bangladesh: Lessons learned through implementation research. *BMC Pediatrics*, *23*(S1, Suppl 1), 653. DOI: 10.1186/s12887-023-04389-0 PMID: 38413880

Jackson-Triche, M., Vetal, D., Turner, E.-M., Dahiya, P., & Mangurian, C. (2023). Meeting the behavioral health needs of health care workers during COVID-19 by leveraging chatbot technology: Development and usability study. *Journal of Medical Internet Research*, *25*, e40635. DOI: 10.2196/40635 PMID: 37146178

Javaid, M., Haleem, A., & Singh, R. P. (2023). ChatGPT for healthcare services: An emerging stage for an innovative perspective. *BenchCouncil Transactions on Benchmarks. Standards and Evaluations*, *3*(1), 100105.

Kerasidou, A. (2020). Artificial intelligence and the ongoing need for empathy, compassion and trust in healthcare. *Bulletin of the World Health Organization*, *98*(4), 245–250. DOI: 10.2471/BLT.19.237198 PMID: 32284647

Laymouna, M., Ma, Y., Lessard, D., Schuster, T., Engler, K., & Lebouché, B. (2024). Roles, Users, Benefits, and Limitations of Chatbots in Health Care: Rapid Review. *Journal of Medical Internet Research*, *26*, e56930. DOI: 10.2196/56930 PMID: 39042446

Leshkevich, T., & Motozhanets, A. (2022). Social perception of artificial intelligence and digitization of cultural heritage: Russian context. *Applied Sciences (Basel, Switzerland)*, *12*(5), 2712. DOI: 10.3390/app12052712

Li, W., Chen, J., Chen, F., Liang, J., & Yu, H. (2024). Exploring the potential of ChatGPT-4 in responding to common questions about abdominoplasty: An AI-based case study of a plastic surgery consultation. *Aesthetic Plastic Surgery*, *48*(8), 1571–1583. DOI: 10.1007/s00266-023-03660-0 PMID: 37770637

Li, Y., Qu, S., Shen, J., Min, S., & Yu, Z. (2023). Curriculum-Driven Edubot: A Framework for Developing Language Learning Chatbots Through Synthesizing Conversational Data. *arXiv preprint arXiv:2309.16804*.

Mbunge, E., Batani, J., Gaobotse, G., & Muchemwa, B. (2022). Virtual healthcare services and digital health technologies deployed during coronavirus disease 2019 (COVID-19) pandemic in South Africa: A systematic review. *Global Health Journal (Amsterdam, Netherlands)*, *6*(2), 102–113. DOI: 10.1016/j.glohj.2022.03.001 PMID: 35282399

Mehta, A., Kumar, H., Yazji, K., Wireko, A. A., Nagarajan, J. S., Ghosh, B., Nahas, A., Ojeda, L. M., Anand, A., & Sharath, M. (2023). Effectiveness of artificial intelligence-assisted colonoscopy in early diagnosis of colorectal cancer: A systematic review. *International Journal of Surgery*, *109*(4), 946–952. DOI: 10.1097/JS9.0000000000000285 PMID: 36917126

Mijwil, M. M., Hiran, K. K., Doshi, R., Dadhich, M., Al-Mistarehi, A.-H., & Bala, I. (2023). ChatGPT and the future of academic integrity in the artificial intelligence era: A new frontier. *Al-Salam Journal for Engineering and Technology*, *2*(2), 116–127. DOI: 10.55145/ajest.2023.02.02.015

Mijwil, M. M., & Shukur, B. S. (2022). A scoping review of machine learning techniques and their utilisation in predicting heart diseases. *Ibn AL-Haitham Journal For Pure and Applied Sciences*, *35*(3), 175–189. DOI: 10.30526/35.3.2813

Mooghali, M., Stroud, A. M., Yoo, D. W., Barry, B. A., Grimshaw, A. A., Ross, J. S., Zhu, X., & Miller, J. E. (2023). Barriers and Facilitators to Trustworthy and Ethical AI-enabled Medical Care From Patient and Healthcare Provider Perspectives: A Literature Review. medRxiv, 2023.2010. 2002.23296447.

Morley, J., Machado, C. C., Burr, C., Cowls, J., Joshi, I., Taddeo, M., & Floridi, L. (2020). The ethics of AI in health care: A mapping review. *Social Science & Medicine*, *260*, 113172. DOI: 10.1016/j.socscimed.2020.113172 PMID: 32702587

Naveed, M., Majeed, M., Jabeen, K., Hanif, N., Naveed, R., Saleem, S., & Khan, N. (2024). Plant Disease Diagnosis with Artificial Intelligence (AI). In *Microbial Data Intelligence and Computational Techniques for Sustainable Computing* (pp. 217-234). Springer.

Nehme, M., Schneider, F., Perrin, A., Sum Yu, W., Schmitt, S., Violot, G., Ducrot, A., Tissandier, F., Posfay-Barbe, K., & Guessous, I. (2023). The Development of a Chatbot Technology to Disseminate Post–COVID-19 Information: Descriptive Implementation Study. *Journal of Medical Internet Research, 25*, e43113. DOI: 10.2196/43113 PMID: 37195688

Newell, S., & Jordan, Z. (2015). The patient experience of patient-centered communication with nurses in the hospital setting: A qualitative systematic review protocol. *JBI Evidence Synthesis, 13*(1), 76–87. PMID: 26447009

Rane, M. S., Robertson, M. M., Westmoreland, D. A., Teasdale, C. A., Grov, C., & Nash, D. (2022). Intention to vaccinate children against COVID-19 among vaccinated and unvaccinated US parents. *JAMA Pediatrics, 176*(2), 201–203. DOI: 10.1001/jamapediatrics.2021.5153 PMID: 34870702

Rane, N. (2023). ChatGPT and similar Generative Artificial Intelligence (AI) for building and construction industry: Contribution, Opportunities and Challenges of large language Models for Industry 4.0, Industry 5.0, and Society 5.0. *Opportunities and Challenges of Large Language Models for Industry, 4*.

Reitzle, L., Schmidt, C., Färber, F., Huebl, L., Wieler, L. H., Ziese, T., & Heidemann, C. (2021). Perceived access to health care services and relevance of telemedicine during the COVID-19 pandemic in Germany. *International Journal of Environmental Research and Public Health, 18*(14), 7661. DOI: 10.3390/ijerph18147661 PMID: 34300110

Sands, D., & Wald, J. (2014). Transforming health care delivery through consumer engagement, health data transparency, and patient-generated health information. *Yearbook of Medical Informatics, 23*(01), 170–176. DOI: 10.15265/IY-2014-0017 PMID: 25123739

Series, T. L. H. S., Williams, A., Lee, J., Kadakia, K., Cupito, A., Cocchiola, M., Chukwurah, C. S., Chua, P. S., Bailey, A., & Ahmed, M. (2023). Digital health COVID-19 impact assessment: Lessons learned and compelling needs. In *Emerging Stronger from COVID-19: Priorities for Health System Transformation*. National Academies Press.

Shafi, I., Fatima, A., Afzal, H., Díez, I. T., Lipari, V., Breñosa, J., & Ashraf, I. (2023). A Comprehensive Review of Recent Advances in Artificial Intelligence for Dentistry E-Health. *Diagnostics (Basel), 13*(13), 2196. DOI: 10.3390/diagnostics13132196 PMID: 37443594

Sharma, A., & Kumar, R. (2022). A constrained framework for context-aware remote E-healthcare (CARE) services. *Transactions on Emerging Telecommunications Technologies, 33*(8), e3649. DOI: 10.1002/ett.3649

Sieck, C. J., Nicks, S. E., Salem, J., DeVos, T., Thatcher, E., & Hefner, J. L. (2022). Addressing Equity and Social Needs: The New Frontier of Patient Engagement Research. In *Responding to the Grand Challenges in Health Care via Organizational Innovation* (Vol. 21, pp. 151-165). Emerald Publishing Limited.

Singh, J., Bansal, A., Mittal, S., & Kumari, A. C. (2023). Revitalizing Traditional Health Practices with HealingHands: An AI powered Chatbot. 2023 International Conference on Computational Intelligence and Sustainable Engineering Solutions (CISES).

Sukums, F., Mzurikwao, D., Sabas, D., Chaula, R., Mbuke, J., Kabika, T., Kaswija, J., Ngowi, B., Noll, J., Winkler, A. S., & Andersson, S. W. (2023). The use of artificial intelligence-based innovations in the health sector in Tanzania: A scoping review. *Health Policy and Technology, 12*(1), 100728. DOI: 10.1016/j.hlpt.2023.100728

Suppadungsuk, S., Thongprayoon, C., Miao, J., Krisanapan, P., Qureshi, F., Kashani, K., & Cheungpasitporn, W. (2023). Exploring the Potential of Chatbots in Critical Care Nephrology. *Medicines (Basel, Switzerland), 10*(10), 58. DOI: 10.3390/medicines10100058 PMID: 37887265

Suppadungsuk, S., Thongprayoon, C., Nikravangolsefid, N., Singh, W., Cheungpasitporn, W., Dong, Y., & Kashani, K. B. (2024). Magnesium Derangement among Critically Ill Patients with Acute Kidney Injury: An Association with Acute Kidney Disease. *Nephron, 148*(8), 553–562. DOI: 10.1159/000539674 PMID: 38861941

Tai-Seale, M., Downing, N. L., Jones, V. G., Milani, R. V., Zhao, B., Clay, B., Sharp, C. D., Chan, A. S., & Longhurst, C. A. (2019). Technology-enabled consumer engagement: Promising practices at four health care delivery organizations. *Health Affairs, 38*(3), 383–390. DOI: 10.1377/hlthaff.2018.05027 PMID: 30830826

Talyshinskii, A., Naik, N., Hameed, B. Z., Juliebø-Jones, P., & Somani, B. K. (2024). Potential of AI-driven chatbots in urology: Revolutionizing patient care through artificial intelligence. *Current Urology Reports, 25*(1), 9–18. DOI: 10.1007/s11934-023-01184-3 PMID: 37723300

Tanwar, S., Parekh, K., & Evans, R. (2020). Blockchain-based electronic healthcare record system for healthcare 4.0 applications. *Journal of Information Security and Applications, 50*, 102407. DOI: 10.1016/j.jisa.2019.102407

Torous, J., Bucci, S., Bell, I. H., Kessing, L. V., Faurholt-Jepsen, M., Whelan, P., Carvalho, A. F., Keshavan, M., Linardon, J., & Firth, J. (2021). The growing field of digital psychiatry: Current evidence and the future of apps, social media, chatbots, and virtual reality. *World Psychiatry; Official Journal of the World Psychiatric Association (WPA), 20*(3), 318–335. DOI: 10.1002/wps.20883 PMID: 34505369

Wang, C., Liu, S., Yang, H., Guo, J., Wu, Y., & Liu, J. (2023). Ethical considerations of using ChatGPT in health care. *Journal of Medical Internet Research, 25*, e48009. DOI: 10.2196/48009 PMID: 37566454

Weizenbaum, J. (1966). ELIZA—A computer program for the study of natural language communication between man and machine. *Communications of the ACM, 9*(1), 36–45. DOI: 10.1145/365153.365168

Wijekoon, A., Wiratunga, N., Corsar, D., Martin, K., Nkisi-Orji, I., Palihawadana, C., Caro-Martínez, M., Díaz-Agudo, B., Bridge, D., & Liret, A. (2024). iSee: Advancing Multi-Shot Explainable AI Using Case-based Recommendations. *arXiv preprint arXiv:2408.12941*. DOI: 10.3233/FAIA241057

Xu, L., Sanders, L., Li, K., & Chow, J. C. (2021). Chatbot for health care and oncology applications using artificial intelligence and machine learning: Systematic review. *JMIR Cancer, 7*(4), e27850. DOI: 10.2196/27850 PMID: 34847056

Chapter 6
A Conversation With ChatGPT on Its Role in Teaching and Learning Real-World Problem Solving in School Mathematics: A Personal Experience

Murad E. Jurdak
American University of Beirut, Lebanon

ABSTRACT

The purpose of this chapter is to describe and analyze the author's conversation with ChatGPT's on teaching and learning real-world problem solving in school mathematics. The chapter is motivated by three considerations. First, extend existing research on ChatGPT by exploring its capability to generate and solve mathematical problems that contextualize the user's specified clues. These capabilities include problem-solving, real-world contextualization, and advanced language understanding. Second, extend the research on ChatGPT to include its role in teaching and learning real-world problem solving in school mathematics. Third, vet ChatGPT's proclaimed problem-solving capabilities against the author's experience in researching, publishing, teaching, and learning mathematical problem solving.

DOI: 10.4018/979-8-3693-3112-5.ch006

INTRODUCTION

The conversation with ChatGPT started with a question about its identity. Below is its response:

Question 1. Who are you? Briefly introduce Chat GPT to those who do not know you.

ChatGPT:

I am ChatGPT, a sophisticated artificial intelligence language model developed by OpenAI. My primary function is to understand and generate human-like text based on the prompts and questions I receive. I've been trained on a vast amount of text from the internet, which allows me to provide information, answer questions, generate text in various styles, and assist with a wide range of tasks. My capabilities span from explaining complex concepts to providing creative writing and assisting with problem-solving. I'm designed to be a versatile and helpful AI companion for a variety of tasks and inquiries, which makes it a unique and valuable tool for a wide variety of applications.

The purpose of this article is to describe and analyze the author's conversation with ChatGPT's on teaching and learning real-world problem solving in school mathematics. The article is motivated by three considerations. First, extend existing research on ChatGPT by exploring its capability to generate and solve mathematical problems that contextualize the user's specified clues. These capabilities include problem-solving, real-world contextualization, and advanced language understanding. Second, extend the research on ChatGPT to include its role in teaching and learning real-world problem solving in school mathematics. Third, vet ChatGPT's proclaimed problem-solving capabilities against the author's experience in researching, publishing, teaching, and learning mathematical problem solving.

ChatGPT's Capabilities in Real-world Problem Solving

In its response to the question on how it differs from other existing artificial generative intelligence tools (see question 2), ChatGPT explains that its problem-solving capabilities are designed to assist with problem-solving tasks across various domains. It can provide step-by-step guidance, explanations, and strategies to help users solve complex real-world problems. Furthermore, ChatGPT explains that its capability of real-world contextualization provides responses that are framed within real-world scenarios. It can provide examples and explanations about users' specific situations and needs. Finally, ChatGPT's advanced language understanding is based on its utilization of state-of-the-art natural language processing techniques, which enable it to better understand and generate human-like text. It can handle a wide range of topics and provide coherent, contextually relevant responses.

Question 2: How does ChatGPT differ from other existing generative intelligence tools?

ChatGPT

ChatGPT differs from other existing generative intelligence tools in several key ways:

1. *Advanced Language Understanding*: ChatGPT utilizes state-of-the-art natural language processing techniques, which enable it to better understand and generate human-like text. It can handle a wide range of topics and provide coherent, contextually relevant responses.
2. *Vast Training Data*: ChatGPT has been trained on a vast and diverse dataset sourced from the internet. This extensive training data allows it to have a broader knowledge base, covering a wide array of domains and topics.
3. *Problem-Solving Capabilities*: ChatGPT is designed to assist with problem-solving tasks across various domains. It can provide step-by-step guidance, explanations, and strategies to help users solve complex real-world problems.
4. *Interdisciplinary Insights*: ChatGPT can draw connections between different fields of knowledge, promoting interdisciplinary thinking and demonstrating how knowledge from various domains can be applied in practical scenarios.
5. *Real-World Contextualization*: ChatGPT excels at contextualizing responses within real-world scenarios. It can provide examples and explanations in a way that relates to users' specific situations and needs.
6. *Personalization*: ChatGPT can adapt its responses to individual user needs and levels of expertise. It can provide tailored explanations and information based on user input.
7. *Continuous Learning and Updates*: ChatGPT can be regularly updated with new information and knowledge, ensuring that it stays current and relevant for users' needs.
8. *Ethical Considerations*: OpenAI, the organization behind ChatGPT, has implemented ethical guidelines and safety measures to minimize the generation of harmful or biased content, making it a more responsible AI tool.
9. *Versatility*: ChatGPT is versatile and can be applied to a wide range of tasks, from answering questions and explaining concepts to generating creative content and assisting with problem solving.

While other generative intelligence tools may possess some of these characteristics, ChatGPT's combination of advanced language understanding, problem-solving capabilities, extensive training data, and a focus on safety and ethical considerations makes it a unique and valuable tool for a wide variety of applications.

The Author's Background in Real-world Problem-solving

In this article, the author plays the role of narrator as well as participant on whose experience, ChatGPT's role in problem solving is vetted. To better understand the conversation with ChatGPT, the author provides a brief background of his professional experience in real-world problem solving in school mathematics. I have just retired from my tenured professor position after 50 years of uninterrupted service in the education department of the American University of Beirut. I participated and contributed, in different capacities, to all ICME's conferences between 1980 and 2021. I have done significant scholarly work in real-world problem solving in school mathematics, including a published book, entitled *Learning and Teaching Real-world Problem Solving in School Mathematics* (Jurdak, 2016) and three journal articles in this area (Jurdak, 1999, 2001, and 2006). This article focuses on the encounter between the most recent and most sophisticated generative artificial intelligence tool and an 'old' hand in learning and teaching real-world problem solving in school mathematics.

Research on ChatGPT's Role in problem solving in School Mathematics

A search using the keywords (ChatGPT, problem solving, mathematics) yielded a few journal articles all published in 2023. Dao & Le (2023) analyzed ChatGPT's mathematics abilities in responding to multiple-choice questions for the Vietnamese National High School Graduation certificate. They concluded that ChatGPT had difficulty correctly answering questions on topics including derivatives and applications, spatial geometry, and spatial calculus. Frieder et al (2023) investigated whether ChatGPT could be a helpful assistant to professional mathematicians by emulating cases that arise in mathematicians' daily professional activities. They reported that ChatGPT can be used most successfully as a mathematical assistant for querying facts, acting as a mathematical search engine and knowledge base interface. It can additionally be used for undergraduate-level mathematics but fails on graduate-level difficulty. Shakarian et al (2023) studied ChatGPT's performance on math word problems and reported that performance can vary greatly depending on specific problem requirements. Rodrigues Vasconcelos & dos Santos (2023) investigated the potential of ChatGPT and Bing Chat as 'objects-to-think' resources that foster reflective and critical thinking, and concept comprehension in enhancing STEM education. The study concludes that ChatGPT and Bing Chat as 'objects-to-think-with' offer promising avenues to revolutionize STEM education through a constructionist lens, fostering engagement in inclusive and accessible learning environments. Wardat et al (2023) examined the perspectives of various educational stakeholders on the use of artificial intelligence in teaching mathematics. They reported that ChatGPT lacks a deep understanding of geometry and cannot effectively correct misconceptions and the accuracy and effectiveness of ChatGPT solutions may depend on the complexity of the equation, input data, and the instructions given to ChatGPT.

All the above-cited articles have addressed the performance of ChatGPT in solving mathematical problems, which is only one of its proclaimed problem-solving capabilities. This article extends existing research on ChatGPT by exploring its capability to generate and solve mathematical problems that contextualize the user's specified clues. In addition, this article extends existing knowledge on the pedagogy of mathematics by exploring ChatGPT's capability of generating simulated lessons to teach the problems it generates.

METHODOLOGY

This research follows a qualitative single-subject (the author's) case study design. It interrogates ChatGPT about selected issues pertaining to its role in learning and teaching real-world problem solving in school mathematics. The author interrogates ChatGPT on the following issues pertaining to its role in learning and teaching real-world problem solving in school mathematics:

1. Generation of a real-world problem involving uncertainty and a possible scenario for teaching it to grade 12 students.
2. Generation of a real-world problem in the context of the workplace and a possible scenario for teaching it to grade 12 students.
3. Generation of a real-world STEM-related problem in the context of the workplace and a possible scenario for teaching it to grade 12 students.
4. Planning and solving a real-world mathematically related policy implementation problem.
5. ChatGPT's capacity to reflect on its solution to a real-world problem.

DATA AND ANALYSIS

The data of this study are the logs of the author's interactions with ChatGPT. ChatGPT's responses in the section titled "Conversation with ChatGPT" are reported without editing. However, sometimes I asked follow-up clarifications.

A qualitative analysis was undertaken to identify the features of ChatGPT's capabilities in real-world problem solving. ChatGPT's features in questions 3 to 7 were categorized into four pre-determined categories: Features of ChatGPT's generated problem, features of ChatGPT's problem's context, ChatGPT's framing of the problem's solution, and ChatGPT's teaching of the problem. The features within each category were compared across five problems. The emerging pattern provided the basis for formulating the theme that characterizes the features of that category.

Conversation with ChatGPT

Question 3: This problem (given as a response to this same question without specifying the student grade level) *is very open and complex and the guidance you gave is too general and complex and may lead to frustration and hence aborting the problem-solving process. Could you give a simpler problem that require mathematics and has much less uncertainty and more likely to be solvable by grade 12?*

ChatGPT

Certainly! Let's consider a problem that involves mathematical decision-making and uncertainty:

Problem: You are a high school student planning to buy a ticket for a school event that includes a raffle. The raffle offers a chance to win a gift card, but you're not sure if it's worth the cost of the ticket. The ticket costs $5, and the gift card is worth $50. However, the probability of winning the gift card is not provided. How can you determine if buying a ticket is a good decision from a mathematical perspective?

ChatGPT's Assistance:

Student: "I'm trying to decide if I should buy a ticket for the school event raffle. The ticket costs $5, and the prize is a $50 gift card. But I don't know the chance of winning. What should I do?"

ChatGPT: "This is a situation where you can use expected value to make a decision. The expected value is the average amount you can expect to win per ticket, considering all possible outcomes. To calculate it, multiply the value of the prize by the probability of winning it and subtract the cost of the ticket."

Student: "Got it! But how can I calculate the expected value without knowing the probability of winning?"

ChatGPT: "Since the probability of winning isn't provided, you can estimate a reasonable range of probabilities based on your judgment. For instance, you might assume a low, medium, and high estimate, like 5%, 10%, and 20%. Calculate the expected value for each estimate and see how they compare to the ticket cost."

Student: "Okay, I'll give that a try. What do I do next?"

ChatGPT: "Calculate the expected value for each estimate of probability. For instance, if you assume a 10% chance of winning, the expected value would be (0.10 * $50) - $5 = $0. Subtracting the ticket cost ensures you're accounting for your investment. Compare the expected values to the ticket cost: if the expected value is greater than $5, it might be a good decision; if it's less, you might consider not buying the ticket."

Student: "This is helpful! I'll estimate probabilities and calculate the expected values to see if buying a ticket is worthwhile."

ChatGPT: "Exactly! Remember, this approach helps you make a decision based on the available information. Keep in mind that real-world decisions involve uncertainties, so it's important to consider both the mathematical aspect and your personal preferences."

In this example, ChatGPT guides the student through using the concept of expected value to make a decision involving uncertainty. The student estimates a range of probabilities and calculates the expected values to determine whether buying a ticket is a mathematically sound choice. This problem introduces mathematical decision-making and helps the student apply probabilistic thinking to a real-world scenario.

Question 4: Could you give me a problem in workplace context that requires math for its solution and is appropriate for grade 12?

ChatGPT

Certainly! Here's a workplace-related problem that requires mathematical skills and is suitable for a grade 12 level:

Problem: You work in a manufacturing company that produces electronic components. The production process involves testing each component for quality assurance. You've been tasked with optimizing the testing process to reduce both testing time and costs. Currently, each component is individually tested, and the testing process takes 10 minutes per component. The testing equipment costs $30 per hour to operate. The company produces 500 components per day. Management wants to maintain a 99% confidence level for the quality assurance. How can you use statistical concepts to determine the minimum number of components to test daily while meeting the confidence level requirement?

ChatGPT's Assistance:

Student: "I'm working on a problem in my workplace where I need to optimize testing processes. Can you help?"

ChatGPT: "Of course! This involves statistical sampling. To determine the minimum number of components to test daily, you'll need to calculate the sample size required for a given confidence level. Have you heard of confidence intervals and sample size calculations?"

Student: "Yes, we covered those in class. But how do I apply them here?"

ChatGPT: "Great! You'll want to calculate the sample size required for a 99% confidence level. To do this, you need to know the population size (number of components produced daily) and the margin of error (tolerance for confidence interval). Do you have those values?"

Student: "Yes, the company produces 500 components per day, and we want a margin of error of $\pm 1\%$."

ChatGPT: "Perfect. You'll use the formula for sample size calculation: $n = Z^2 \cdot p \cdot (1-p)/E^2$ where n is the sample size, Z is the Z-score for the desired confidence level (2.576 for 99% confidence), p is the estimated proportion of components that might fail (use 0.5 for maximum uncertainty), and E is the margin of error as a proportion."

Student: "Got it. I can plug in the values and calculate the sample size. Once I have that, how does it help optimize the testing process?"

ChatGPT: "The calculated sample size represents the number of components you need to test daily to maintain the desired confidence level. Since testing each component takes 10 minutes, you can calculate the total testing time for the sample size. This will help you compare the current testing time to the optimized time, considering both confidence requirements and cost."

Student: "So, by calculating the sample size and total testing time, I can propose a more efficient testing process that meets quality assurance standards?"

ChatGPT: "Exactly! By using statistical concepts and mathematical calculations, you can provide a data-driven solution that balances confidence level, testing time, and cost. This demonstrates the practical application of mathematics in workplace optimization."

In this example, ChatGPT guides the grade 12 student through a workplace-related problem that involves statistical sampling and sample size calculation. The student learns how to apply mathematical concepts to optimize a real-world testing process while meeting quality assurance requirements.

Question 5: Could you give me a STEM-related problem situation in workplace context that requires math for its solution and is appropriate for grade 12?

ChatGPT

Certainly! Here's a STEM-related workplace problem that involves mathematical skills and is suitable for a grade 12 level:

Problem: You are an engineer working for a renewable energy company that specializes in solar panel installations. Your team is designing a solar power system for a client's residential rooftop. The goal is to maximize energy output while considering the available rooftop area, panel efficiency, and local sunlight conditions. The client's rooftop has dimensions of 8 meters by 10 meters. Each solar panel you plan to use is 1.5 meters by 1 meter and has an efficiency of 18%. How can you calculate the maximum number of panels that can be installed on the rooftop and estimate the potential energy output of the system using mathematical concepts?

ChatGPT's Assistance:

Student: "I'm working on an engineering project involving solar panel installations. Can you help me with the calculations?"

ChatGPT: "Absolutely! To determine the maximum number of panels that can be installed, you'll need to calculate the total area of the rooftop and the area occupied by each panel. Have you covered area calculations before?"

Student: "Yes, we have. The rooftop is 8 meters by 10 meters, and each panel is 1.5 meters by 1 meter."

ChatGPT: "Great! Calculate the total area of the rooftop and the area of a single solar panel. Then, divide the total rooftop area by the panel area to find the maximum number of panels that can be installed."

Student: "I can do that. Once I know the number of panels, how can I estimate the energy output?"

ChatGPT: "The energy output of a solar panel system is usually measured in kilowatt-hours (kWh). You'll need to consider the panel's efficiency, the sunlight conditions, and the peak solar radiation for your location. Have you learned about calculating energy output from solar panels?"

Student: "Yes, we have. The panels are 18% efficient. Can you guide me on the calculations?"

ChatGPT: "Certainly. The energy output (in kWh) is given by the formula: $E=A \cdot P \cdot H \cdot PR$, where E is the energy output, A is the total area of panels (number of panels times panel area), P is the panel efficiency as a decimal (18% as 0.18), H is the peak solar radiation for your location, and PR is the performance ratio (usually around 0.75 for residential systems)."

Student: "I understand the formula. How do I find the peak solar radiation and the performance ratio?"

ChatGPT: "You can obtain the peak solar radiation data for your location from weather databases or solar radiation maps. The performance ratio considers factors like shading, temperature, and wiring losses. A value of 0.75 is a common estimate for residential systems."

Student: "Got it. So, by plugging in the values and calculating, I can estimate the potential energy output of the solar system."

ChatGPT: "Exactly! This calculation will help you determine the energy generation capacity of the proposed solar panel system, considering the available rooftop space and panel efficiency. It's a great way to apply mathematical concepts in real-world engineering projects."

In this example, ChatGPT assists the grade 12 student in solving a STEM-related workplace problem involving solar panel installations. The student uses mathematical concepts to calculate the maximum number of panels that can be installed and estimate the potential energy output of the system.

Question 6: A country decided to use a mathematical principle to draw the boundaries of the electoral zones for the sake of fairness. The principle is: Using the five regional capitals (A, B, C, D, E) as designated centers of the zones, any distinct population community (village, town, city...) belongs to a zone if it is closer to that zone center than any other centers. Develop a plan for drawing the boundaries of the five zones.

ChatGPT:

Designing electoral zones based on the principle of using regional capitals as centers requires a systematic approach to ensure fairness and accurate representation. Here's a plan for drawing the boundaries of the five zones using this principle:

1. Data Collection and Preliminary Analysis:
    - Gather geographical data that includes the locations of the five regional capitals (A, B, C, D, E) and the population communities in the country.
    - Calculate the distances between each population community and the five regional capitals
2. Center Assignment:
    - For each population community, identify the closest regional capital center based on distance.
    - Assign each population community to the zone corresponding to the closest regional capital.
3. Zone Boundary Formation:
    - Starting from each regional capital, create a boundary by including all population communities that are closer to that capital than to any other capital.
    - Repeat this process for all five regional capitals, ensuring that no community is assigned to multiple zones.
4. Check for Equitability:
    - Analyze the population distribution across the zones. Ensure that the zones have a balanced population to maintain fairness in representation.
    - Adjust zone boundaries if necessary to achieve more equitable population distribution
5. Consultation and Review:
    - Engage with relevant stakeholders, such as local governments, communities, and experts, to gather feedback on the proposed zone boundaries.

- Review the boundaries to identify any potential issues related to geography, transportation, or community cohesion.

6. Public Input and Transparency:
   - Conduct public consultations and gather input from citizens to ensure transparency and inclusivity in the boundary-drawing process.
   - Communicate the rationale behind the boundaries and the principle used to draw them.
7. Finalization and Implementation:
   - Incorporate feedback from stakeholders and the public to make final adjustments to the zone boundaries, if needed.
   - Prepare an official document outlining the boundaries, including maps and detailed descriptions.
   - Implement the finalized boundaries for the electoral zones.
8. Regular Review and Adjustment:
   - Establish a system for regular review and adjustment of the electoral zone boundaries as population distribution changes over time.
   - Use updated population data to ensure continued fairness and representation.
9. Legal and Ethical Considerations:
   - Ensure that the boundary-drawing process adheres to legal and ethical standards, including principles of non-discrimination and equal representation.
   - Address any potential concerns related to gerrymandering or manipulation of boundaries for political advantage.
10. Education and Outreach:
    - Educate citizens, communities, and officials about the new electoral zones and the principles used in their creation.
    - Provide resources and information to help voters understand which zone they belong to and the significance of the new boundaries.

By following this plan, the country can create electoral zones that are based on the principle of fairness and accurate representation, promoting equitable distribution of political power while minimizing bias and manipulation.

Question 7: Is there a practical way of calculating the distances?

ChatGPT

To identify the boundaries of each of the five zones based on the given rule, where towns or cities belong to a zone if they are closer to the capital of that zone than the capitals of the remaining zones, you can use a method that involves creating Voronoi polygons or Thiessen polygons. Voronoi polygons divide a space into regions based on proximity to a set of points. In your case, the capitals A, B, C, D, and E will be the points around which the Voronoi polygons are constructed. Here's a step-by-step approach to identifying the boundaries of each zone:

1. **Mark the Capital Locations:** Plot the locations of capitals A, B, C, D, and E on a map.
2. **Create Voronoi Diagram:** Use the capital locations as seed points to create Voronoi polygons. Each point on the map will belong to the zone associated with the nearest capital. This will create the initial division of the country into zones based on proximity to the capitals.
3. **Refine the Boundaries:** The initial Voronoi polygons might not accurately reflect geographic features or distances. You can refine the boundaries to make them more intuitive and aligned with geographical and transportation considerations. This step might involve adjusting the boundaries manually while ensuring that each town or city is closer to the capital of its designated zone than to the capitals of the other zones.
4. **Verify and Adjust:** Once you have refined the boundaries, it's important to verify the results. Check if each town or city is indeed closer to the capital of its designated zone. If needed, make further adjustments to ensure that the rule is consistently applied.

If you have access to GIS (Geographic Information Systems) software, it can be a valuable tool for creating and visualizing the Voronoi polygons and refining the boundaries based on geographic data and accurate distance measurements.

DISCUSSION

The findings of the qualitative analysis are reported under the headings of four predetermined categories used in the qualitative analysis:

1. Features of ChatGPT's generated problem
2. Features of ChatGPT's generated problem's context
3. ChatGPT's framing of the problem's solution
4. ChatGPT's simulated teaching of the problem

Features of ChatGPT's Generated Problem

The emerging theme from the qualitative analysis suggests that ChatGPT's generated real-world problem is a mathematized model of a real situation but does not involve the process through which the real-world situation is transformed into a mathematical model. Niss et al. (2007) define mathematization as a process that involves four components: Identification of a real-world situation that raises a question (issue), transforming the situation into the mathematical domain, solving the problem in the mathematical domain, and translating the solution to the real-world. In other words, ChatGPT's formulation of the problems is a direct description of the mathematical problem of the real-world situation. ChatGPT's generated problems are different from the 'messy' problems that human agents face in the real world. ChatGPT's real-world problems are what Jurdak (2006) calls situated problems i.e., problems that are situated in the real-world context but formulated to suit the school context. Jurdak (2006) differentiates between situated problem solving and decision-making in real life:

The situated problem solving in the school context is an activity within the school community, which results in a written solution using mostly mathematical tools and constrained by school rules, norms, and expectations; whereas decision-making in real life is a complex activity that occurs within the larger social context, and which results in a decision constrained by the acceptable social and personal rules and using all available mathematical and non-mathematical tools (p. 297).

ChatGPT's is capable to generate a problem in natural language but is not capable to process graphic or spatial data. This is a limitation in mathematics which often uses graphic and spatial media in representing problems and their solutions. ChatGPT's limitation in geometry was noted by Dao & Le (2023) and Wardat et al (2023).

Features of ChatGPT's Generated Problem's Context

ChatGPT generates a context for the real-world problem commensurate with the nature and number of contextual clues the user provides. If the specification of the requested real-world problem is not specific in terms of contextual clues, ChatGPT generates a problem with a non-specific context. For example, in question 3, I started by asking ChatGPT for a real-world problem that involves handling uncertainty without specifying any context. It generated a very open and complex problem with general guidance for solving. However, when I requested a real-world problem appropriate for grade 12 students, it generated a problem with a very appropriate context (buying a ticket for a school event, question 3). Another remarkable feature of ChatGPT is its capability to infer context from textual clues *implied* in the question provided by the user. This is demonstrated in question 6 in which I asked for developing a plan for determining electoral zones, but not for the solution of the problem (see question 7). In its generated plan (question 6), ChatGPT was able to infer some sociopolitical aspects not explicitly stated in the user-posed question such as:

- Incorporate feedback from stakeholders and the public to make final adjustments to the zone boundaries, if needed.
- Ensure that the zones have a balanced population to maintain fairness in representation.
- Engage with relevant stakeholders, such as local governments, communities, and experts, to gather feedback on the proposed zone boundaries.

ChatGPT's Framing of the Problem's Solution

ChatGPT's framing of the solution follows a certain pattern. The solution to a real-world problem starts with a paragraph that outlines the general strategy for solving the problem, without providing any justification for strategy choice. This is followed by a systematic presentation of the steps of the solution in a precise and concise mathematical discourse, interjected with natural language when needed. No justifications are given for the steps. ChatGPT ends the solution by stating the learning outcomes of solving the problem. ChatGPT solves the real-world problem mathematically but does not indicate how the solution would be implemented in a real-world situation.

An exception to this pattern is the solution given in question 7 (determining electoral zones). ChatGPT generated a solution that computes distances between population centers (Voronoi polygons) to determine the closest center for each population community. I have often used this problem in my methodology course to demonstrate how a seemingly complex problem may be solved by using simple geometric concepts. The geometrical solution for this problem involves constructing (on a map of the country) the perpendicular bisector of each segment that joins each pair of centers and determining visually the electoral zone for each center, using the property that a perpendicular bisector of a segment divides the plane into two regions that are closer to either one of the extremities of the segment. Why did ChatGPT fail to generate the geometrical solution? The answer is that ChatGPT can only process computational tools in natural language. This is another example of the limitations of ChatGPT's ability to process spatial or visual data.

ChatGPT's Simulated Teaching of the Generated Problem

In the simulated lessons in questions 2 to 7, ChatGPT projects itself as a teacher-centered educator whose mission is to transfer knowledge on problem solving in a systematic way governed mainly by a purely mathematical perspective. The content and sequence of instruction follow mathematical rather than pedagogical considerations. The interaction between ChatGPT and students is limited to questions by the teacher about students' background knowledge, and by students about clarification of concepts and procedures introduced by the teacher. Students are more likely to be receivers than partners in knowledge acquisition. Teachers may learn from such an approach the mathematical considerations of sequencing a lesson on problem solving.

CONCLUDING REMARKS

ChatGPT's capabilities of problem solving, and contextualization provide unique and highly impactful opportunities for learning and teaching real-world problem solving. ChatGPT's capacity to enable users to generate problems with such a wide range of real-world contexts at such a high speed exceeds the capability of any individual human agent. Mathematics educators, teacher educators, and curriculum developers are likely to utilize ChatGPT as tool to upscale the learning and teaching of real-world problem-solving in school mathematics- a sub-domain of mathematics education that has been, for a long time, a highly desired goal but a difficult one to achieve. ChatGPT's ability to generate unlimited number of problems and their solutions in response to a user's question expressed in language open many opportunities to cross the cultural boundary that exists between the real world and school systems (Jurdak 2016). ChatGPT's makes the crossing of the boundary between the two cultural worlds through generating problems that are situated in the real world but are amenable to the constraints of the school system. One remarkable potential of ChatGPT is its ability to predict sociocultural and sociopolitical contextual clues that are not explicitly stated by the user.

ChatGPT's problem solving, and contextualization capabilities exhibit a few limitations and drawbacks when applied to the domain of teaching and learning real-world problem solving in school mathematics. One limitation of ChatGPT is that it is not capable (at least the version used in this paper) of processing visual and spatial data. This limitation is a constraint in real-world problem solving since many real-world problems and their solutions need to be represented in a geometrical language. One serious drawback of ChatGPT is its tendency, though limited, to making mistakes solving simple problems. In my interactions with ChatGPT, the following exchange took place while solving a Grade 9 problem:

A train leaves Station A and travels toward Station B at a speed of 60 km/h. At the same time, another train leaves Station B and travels toward Station A at a speed of 75 km/h. The distance between the two stations is 450 kilometers. The two trains started their journeys simultaneously. How far from Station A will the two trains meet each other?

ChatGPT:

Let's denote the distance from Station A where the two trains meet as d kilometers. The key idea here is that the combined distance traveled by both trains is equal to the total distance between the two stations (450 kilometers):

Distance traveled by Train A + Distance traveled by Train B = Total distance

60d+75d=450

135d=450 d=450/135= 3.33 kilometers (approximately).

So, the two trains will meet approximately 3.33 km from station A.

Author:

This is not correct because 60d is not the distance travelled by Train A?

ChatGPT:

You are absolutely right, and I apologize for the oversight in my previous response. Thank you for bringing this to my attention. Let's solve the problem correctly.

This 'artificial' apology is redundant and uncalled for. What seems to be a more fruitful response is to explain to human agents what went wrong for such a powerful artificial intelligence tool to make such an error in solving an elementary problem.

Further Research

It is understandable that most of the research on ChatGPT since its publication in 2021 has focused on its performance in problem solving as compared to humans. However, a few research studies have addressed ChatGPT as a pedagogical tool for teaching and learning mathematical problem solving. So, I asked ChatGPT to identify, based on its own review, gaps in the literature on the role of generative artificial intelligence in teaching and learning mathematical problem solving. Its conclusions were as follows:

ChatGPT's Response

Gaps and directions Research Gaps and Future Directions:

1. *Long-term Impact*: Further research is needed to understand the long-term impact of AI-based mathematical problem solving on students' overall mathematical proficiency and problem-solving abilities.
2. *Teacher and AI Collaboration*: Exploring ways in which AI can complement and assist human educators in creating a blended learning environment.
3. *Pedagogical Strategies*: Developing effective pedagogical strategies for integrating AI into mathematics education to maximize its benefits.

4. *Equity and Access*: Investigating how the use of AI in teaching and learning mathematics might impact equity and access to quality education for diverse student populations.

This research falls within the future directions identified by ChatGPT. There is a need for empirical research in actual classroom contexts on teacher and ChatGPT collaboration for exploring ways for creating a blended learning environment for teaching and learning real-world problem solving.

REFERENCES

Dao, X., & Le, N. (2023). Investigating the effectiveness of ChatGPT in mathematical reasoning and problem solving: Evidence from the Vietnamese national high school graduation examination. /arxiv.2306.06331DOI: 10.48550

Frieder, S., Pinchetti, L., Griffiths, R. R., Salvatori, T., Lukasiewicz, T., Petersen, P. C., . . . Berner, J. (2023). Mathematical capabilities of ChatGPT. *arXiv preprint arXiv:2301.13867.*

Jurdak, M. (2016). *Learning and teaching real world problem solving in school mathematics: A multiple-perspective framework for crossing the boundary*. Springer International Publishing. DOI: 10.1007/978-3-319-08204-2

Jurdak, M., & Shahin, I. (1999). An ethnographic study of the computational strategies of a group of young street vendors in beirut. *Educational Studies in Mathematics, 40*(2), 155–172. DOI: 10.1023/A:1003894908704

Jurdak, M., & Shahin, I. (2001). Problem solving activity in the workplace and the school: The case of constructing solids. *Educational Studies in Mathematics, 47*(3), 297–315. DOI: 10.1023/A:1015106804646

Jurdak, M. E. (2006). Contrasting perspectives and performance of high school students on problem solving in real world situated, and school contexts. *Educational Studies in Mathematics, 63*(3), 283–301. DOI: 10.1007/s10649-005-9008-y

Niss, M., Blum, W., & Galbraith, P. (2007). Part 1 Introduction. In Blum, W., Galbraith, P., Henn, H., & Niss, M. (Eds.), *Modeling and applications in mathematics education: The 14th ICMI study* (pp. 3–33). Springer. DOI: 10.1007/978-0-387-29822-1_1

Rodrigues Vasconcelos, M. A., & dos Santos, R. P. (2023). Enhancing STEM learning with ChatGPT and Bing chat as objects to think with: A case study. Cornell University Library. DOI: 10.29333/ejmste/13313

Shakarian, P., Koyyalamudi, A., Ngu, N., & Mareedu, L. (2023). An independent evaluation of ChatGPT on mathematical word problems (mwp). *arXiv preprint arXiv:2302.13814.*

Wardat, Y., Tashtoush, M. A., AlAli, R., & Jarrah, A. M. (2023). ChatGPT: A revolutionary tool for teaching and learning mathematics. *Eurasia Journal of Mathematics, Science and Technology Education, 19*(7), em2286. DOI: 10.29333/ejmste/13272

Chapter 7

Internet Wizard for Enhancing Open Domain Question Answering Chatbot Knowledge-Base in Information Seeking

Kovan Mzwri
https://orcid.org/0000-0001-6880-2796
Doctoral School of Informatics, Eötvös Loránd University, Budapest, Hungary

Márta Turcsányi-Szabo
https://orcid.org/0000-0002-8962-1959
Department of Media and Educational Technology, Faculty of Informatics, Eötvös Loránd University, Hungary

ABSTRACT

As chatbots gain prominence across diverse fields, including education, their static knowledge base poses limitations. This study investigates the utilization of an internet wizard to enhance the knowledge base of an open-domain question-answering chatbot. The proposed approach leverages search engines, particularly Google, and their features, such as feature snippets, knowledge graph, and organic search, by integrating data science and natural language models. This enables the chatbot to access real-time and up-to-date answers from web documents, providing dynamic responses to user queries. A pilot study in higher education assessed the chatbot's mechanism and features, demonstrating its ability to generate responses across a wide range of educational and non-educational topics, supported by positive feedback and user satisfaction. The chatbot's dynamic feature of retrieving related or

DOI: 10.4018/979-8-3693-3112-5.ch007

follow-up questions from search engines significantly enhances student engagement and facilitates exploration of additional information beyond the curriculum.

1. INTRODUCTION

Chatbots as an application of human-computer interaction have gained significant importance in the last few years and undergone remarkable developments. The growing interest in chatbots can be attributed to the proliferation of mobile devices over the past decade. As these smart devices, such as smartphones, have become increasingly popular, so too have the applications that run on them, including chatbots. Consequently, chatbots have transformed the ways in which humans interact with technology and have created new opportunities for organizations and businesses to engage with their clients. These programs are designed to perform a wide range of tasks in an automated manner, making them a useful tool in various settings (Grudin & Jacques, 2019). Chatbots, also called conversational agents, can be defined as conversational or interactive agents that provide an instant response to the user (Okonkwo & Ade-Ibijola, 2020; Smutny & Schreiberova, 2020). A computer program or artificial intelligence tool that conducts a conversation using auditory or textual methods.

Chatbots, or conversational agents, have been around since the development of the first application in 1960 called ELIZA by Joseph Weizenbaum at MIT. ELIZA used natural language processing (NLP) to recognize patterns and act as a therapist (Weizenbaum, 1966). Other notable examples include ALICE, developed by Richard Wallace in 1995, which uses Artificial Intelligence Markup Language (AIML) for pattern matching to recognize inputs and generate responses (Shawar & Atwell, 2015). Many current chatbots are based on ALICE's framework, such as HeX (Hutchens, 1997) and Claude (Laven, 1996) which were also developed based on standard pattern matching. HeX introduces a brand-new topic based on a certain probability (Y. Wu et al., 2008).

In the past, chatbots were primarily used in the customer service industry, but in recent years, they have become more sophisticated, able to understand and respond to more complex inputs. They are now used in a wide range of industries, such as healthcare (Feldman et al., 2012; Razzaki et al., 2018), finance (Mogaji et al., 2021; Wube et al., 2022), customer service (Følstad & Taylor, 2021; Ngai et al., 2021), psychology (Uludag, 2023, 2024), individualized support via intelligent audio device (Clark et al., 2019), and education such as using chatbots to learn Computer Programming concepts (Coronado et al., 2018; Daud et al., 2020; Okonkwo & Ade-Ibijola, 2020). The majority of chatbots are task-oriented and open-domain (Gao et al., 2019), and are now integral parts of many companies' customer service and support operations, with their use expected to increase in the coming years (Zawacki-Richter et al., 2019).

Educational institutions widely use chatbots to provide information and assistance related to education and learning. They can be implemented in a variety of settings, including schools, universities, and online learning platforms, as mobile web applications that support learning. Through chatbots, students can instantly access standardized details, such as course materials (Cunningham-Nelson et al., 2019), practice questions and answers (Ranoliya et al., 2017; Sinha et al., 2019), evaluation criteria (Benotti et al., 2017; Durall & Kapros, 2020), assignment due dates, advice (Ismail & Ade-Ibijola, 2019), campus path direction (Mabunda, 2020), and study materials. Such systems can improve student engagement and support while reducing lecturers' administrative workload, allowing them to devote more time to curriculum development (Cunningham-Nelson et al., 2019). Chatbots not only help students develop their interaction skills but also assist teaching faculty by automating some of their tasks (Dsouza et al., 2019). Integrating chatbots with education improves connectivity, efficiency, and reduces uncertainty in interactions (Chinedu & Ade-Ibijola, 2021; Ondáš et al., 2019), resulting in focused, personalized, and result-oriented online learning experiences (Cunningham-Nelson et al., 2019), which are vital for today's educational institutions. Furthermore, chatbots increase the level of support provided to each student, reducing the likelihood of ineffective learning and dropouts (Eom et al., 2006; Hone & El Said, 2016).

Chatbots, whether domain-specific or open-domain, usually undergo a training process that involves teaching them to understand and respond to user inputs in a natural and human-like manner. This is achieved through the use of machine learning techniques, including natural language processing (NLP) and deep learning.

There are various Natural Language Processing (NLP) models that can be utilized to develop open-domain chatbots. These models, such as BERT, RoBERTa, GPT-2, and GPT-3, are trained on large amounts of general-domain text data and then fine-tuned on smaller, task-specific datasets to adapt them to the particular task of an open-domain chatbot (Brown et al., 2020; Devlin et al., 2019; Liu et al., 2019). Commonly used datasets, such as pushshift.io Reddit (Baumgartner et al., 2020) and Empathetic Dialogues (Rashkin et al., 2019), are used to train the weights of a Transformer encoder-decoder, as seen in state-of-the-art chatbots such as Meena (Adiwardana et al., 2020) and BlenderBot (Roller et al., 2020).

However, these models rely solely on facts provided in the training dataset and do not incorporate external knowledge sources to enhance their generation capabilities. This static language modeling approach fails to account for the dynamic nature of the world, where new information is constantly being updated. In other words, these models are trained based on the data collected at the time of their creation, and the knowledge acquired is static and not adaptive to changes. Other studies (De Bruyn et al., 2020; Kim et al., 2020; Zhao et al., 2020) have explored the possibility of knowledge selection from a small set of knowledge, without employing a retrieval step or search engine, as was done in this study. Notably, using search engines for machine translation tasks has been shown to produce effective results (Gu et al., 2017).

The Wizard of Wikipedia task (Dinan et al., 2019), involves conversations grounded in Wikipedia and utilizes a TFIDF retrieval model to find relevant information from the database. Similarly, our previous study (Mzwri & TURCSÁNYI-SZABÓ, 2023) employed the Wikipedia API to retrieve related knowledge from Wikipedia and answer user queries. Those studies are perhaps the closest to this research work. However, the approach in this study is more comprehensive as it leverages all publicly available information on the internet, thereby enabling the chatbot to cover a wider range of user queries.

To keep an open-domain chatbot's knowledge base current, it is important to continuously update it with new information. One way to achieve this is through web scraping techniques that gather data from sources like news websites, social media, and forums. APIs can also be used to access real-time data from external sources. By incorporating new information in real-time, chatbots can maintain an up-to-date knowledge base that is responsive to user needs.

The primary objective of this chapter is to develop a mechanism that can handle the ever-changing nature of acquired knowledge and empower a question-answering chatbot to respond to queries from diverse fields. To achieve this objective, the chapter will explore the potential of contemporary Internet search tools, especially search engines and their features. The research will integrate data science and machine learning algorithms to retrieve and analyze knowledge from the world wide web, creating a dynamic knowledge base that can be leveraged by an open-domain QA chatbot.

Furthermore, the research will investigate the potential of utilizing dynamic-related questions or follow-up questions retrieved from search engines to enhance student engagement with the chatbot. This strategy aims to encourage students to seek additional information about specific queries in a higher education setting, thereby promoting active information seeking. Incorporating dynamic follow-up questions is expected to improve the chatbot's effectiveness in addressing a wide range of queries and promoting active information-seeking among students. To answer the research questions, a pilot study will be conducted to evaluate the effectiveness of the developed chatbot in an educational setting. Additionally, the next chapter of the research will provide a detailed explanation of the architecture of the developed chatbot, including the technologies utilized.

1.1 The Integral Role of Information Seeking and Chatbots in Learning Environments

In the realm of education, understanding the pivotal role of information in the learning process is fundamental to enriching pedagogical practices. The significance of information-seeking in the learning process is underscored by Butler (2000), who emphasizes the intrinsic link between learners' goals and motivations. Collaborative efforts, as highlighted by Wu et al. (2018), go beyond mere knowledge acquisition, extending to knowledge reconstruction, skill enhancement, and the accomplishment of goal-oriented tasks. Yang (1997) reinforces this collaborative learning paradigm by exploring how learners initiate information-seeking activities to marshal evidence for thematic essays, elucidating the cognitive processes involved in the information-seeking journey.

Limberg and Alexandersson (2010) exploration of the evolving boundaries between learning and information-seeking introduces the impact of digital tools and constructivist theories. The fusion of these elements not only reshapes traditional roles but also positions librarians as key facilitators in educational contexts. The collaborative information search process, as examined by Wu et al. (2018), not only enhances understanding and knowledge assimilation but also cultivates essential skills such as communication and research.

Limberg and Alexandersson (2010) comprehensive study delves into the convergence of learning and information-seeking, identifying five dimensions that intricately connect these two domains. The symbiotic relationship is attributed partly to educational ideas based in constructivism and the development of digital tools that reshape learning conditions in postmodern society. This constructivist lens is further extended by Mendoza et al. (2022), who envisions integrating chatbot technology into constructivist learning environments, aligning with the philosophy that social interaction is fundamental to cognition development.

The transformative potential of chatbots in education is underscored by Mendoza et al. (2022), emphasizing their capability to provide personalized support and enhance communication. Sandu and Gide (2019) contributes insights into higher education, highlighting chatbots' roles in improving productivity, teaching assistance, and overall learning experiences. Sonderegger and Seufert (2022) deepens our understanding by spotlighting the pedagogical potential of chatbots, particularly their capacity for individualized learning support and collaboration opportunities. Language learning sees chatbots as tutors and independent learning mediums, introducing flexibility and confidence to learners (Haristiani, 2019). The delineation of the role of chatbots in education has been expounded upon through numerous studies in the preceding section. Moreover, chatbots revolutionize information retrieval processes, providing intuitive and user-friendly communication through conversational interfaces (Liao et al., 2020). This transition from graphical to conversational interfaces represents a paradigm shift in understanding users' information-seeking behaviors and design opportunities.

The integration of chatbot technology into constructivist learning environments is proposed, aligning with social constructivism where social interaction is fundamental to cognition development (Mendoza et al., 2022; Ondáš et al., 2019). This approach envisions chatbots as mediators, contributing to the acquisition of 21st-century skills within diverse educational contexts.

2. IMPLEMENTED INFORMATION SEEKING AND RETRIEVAL STRATEGIES

In the realm of developed chatbot functionalities, the information-seeking and retrieval strategies unfold through two distinctive models: the Retrieval-based model, utilizing keyword matching to select responses, and the primary Generative model known as the Internet Wizard. This mechanism strategically leverages technologies such as Google snippets, knowledge graphs, TF-ID algorithm, and Tensorflow Question and Answer model. The Retrieval-based model ensures precision through keyword matching, while the Internet Wizard dynamically generates responses by tapping into the extensive resources available on the World Wide Web, thus providing users with current and relevant information. Subsequent sections provide detailed insights into these approaches within the broader context of chatbot information seeking and retrieval.

2.1 Keyword Matching

This is the first, simple and straightforward approach used in information retrieval of the developed open-domain QA chatbot. The basic idea behind keyword matching is to compare the user's input with a predefined list of keywords or phrases to determine the most relevant response. For the Keyword Matching approach, the Wit.ai NLP model was applied to detect keywords in user queries and MongoDB was used to store the keywords and corresponding answers in a structured database as the knowledgebase. The chatbot's knowledge base in this case MongoDB is prepopulated with a set of answers, and each answer is associated with a set of keywords that describe its content. When the user asks a question, the chatbot performs a keyword search through the wit.ai API to find the most relevant information in its knowledge base.

The keyword matching approach is used in such cases when the answer to a specific keyword or list of keywords needs to be hardcoded in the chatbot knowledge base for example questions related to the personality of the chatbot such as "*What is your name?*" otherwise the second approach which is Internet Wizard is used to answer user queries.

To facilitate the addition of keywords and answers to the MongoDB and Wit.ai databases, a user-friendly and sophisticated online platform has been developed. This platform streamlines the process of updating the knowledge base by eliminating the need for coding skills, making it easy and straightforward to maintain the database over time.

2.2 Internet Wizard

Internet Wizard is the dominant approach of the IR component of the developed open-domain QA chatbot and knowledgebase of the chatbot are heavily depend on this approach. It's called internet Wizard because it uses the world wide web knowledge to retrieve appropriate answer for the user quires. The world wide web (WWW) is a vast and constantly growing network of information, making it a vital resource for an open-domain chatbot knowledgebase. This approach combines several technologies, including data mining and machine learning, to find related documents on the web, index them, and process the content to locate knowledge that can be used for answering user inquiries.

The first step in this approach is searching the internet to find the most related documents to the user's queries. As a matter of fact, one of the most effective ways to access this information is through the use of search engines. Search engines are a fundamental component of the World Wide Web and provide users with an efficient means of accessing information. They have become the primary source of information for many individuals, who turn to them first when seeking information. Search engines are complex systems that use an interface to process and arrange documents based on their relevance to a given query (Cho & Garcia-Molina, 2002). In light of this fact, the approach used the most popular search engine worldwide known as Google and utilized its features. Google's popularity and effectiveness make it a go-to tool for information retrieval, as its uses a proprietary algorithm known as PageRank to rank web pages based on their relevance to a user's query. PageRank considers the link structure of the web and assesses an individual page's value based on it, facilitating efficient and expedient information retrieval (Brin & Page, 1998). Additionally, the vast size of Google's index, which was estimated to be over 55-billion individual web pages as of 2022 (*How Long Will It Take Goo-*

gle to Index My Site? | Safari Digital, n.d.), makes it a powerful tool for discovering information on a wide range of topics.

As part of the information retrieval (IR) component, a web scraping technique is implemented to interact with Google search results and extract pertinent content from featured snippets, the Google Knowledge Graph, and organic search results. This approach allows for the retrieval of relevant information directly associated with user queries.

The Internet wizard mechanism relies on Google-featured snippets as the primary source of information for answering user queries. Featured snippets are the latest enhancement to Search Engine Results Pages (SERPs), which display relevant information from web pages along with their source URL above organic search results. This provides users with quick and accurate answers to their queries, improving their search experience and efficiency (Miklosik, 2018). To generate its featured snippets, Google uses a complex set of algorithms. The exact algorithms used by Google are not publicly disclosed. However studies show several factors that influence the generation of featured snippets including the relevance and quality of the content, the source of the content, rank of the page, the user's search query, the page structure and formatting, multiple keyword inclusion in the website's content, and the use of different keyword locations, such as headings, titles, URLs, paragraphs, image ALT, link, and the frequency of the query (Miklosik et al., 2016; Strzelecki, 2019).

The Internet Wizard leverages the Google Knowledge Graph as the second source of knowledge for responding to user queries. The Google Knowledge Graph is a semantic search engine that aims to provide more relevant and comprehensive information on entities, including people, places, things, and events. This is achieved by integrating structured data from multiple sources and processing it using machine learning algorithms to identify new relationships. By representing information using entities and their relationships, the Knowledge Graph provides users with constantly evolving and updating information. However, maintaining the vast amount of data and ensuring its completeness and accuracy presents significant challenges(Noy et al., 2019).

During the next phase of Internet Wizard, if both the Google featured snippet and Google knowledge graph fail to provide appropriate answers to user queries, the next step will utilize Google organic search results.

Google organic search results are the web pages that appear in response to a user's search query and are ranked based on relevance and popularity. These results are generated by Google's algorithms, which use complex mathematical formulas to determine the relevance and popularity of web pages. The algorithms take into account a variety of factors, including the content of the web page, the number of links pointing to the page, the relevance of the page to the search query, and the overall quality of the website. Google's organic search results are powered by the

PageRank and RankBrain algorithms. PageRank analyzes the number and quality of links pointing to a web page and assigns a relevance score, while RankBrain uses machine learning to provide more relevant and accurate results for complex and conversational searches (Baye et al., 2016; Joshi & Patel, 2018).

The mechanism takes the first five organic search results pages and feeds their content to the TF-IDF algorithm after removing HTML tags. TF-IDF is a statistical method used in information retrieval and natural language processing to determine the importance of a word in a document or corpus. It calculates word relevance based on its frequency in a document (term frequency) and rarity in the entire corpus (inverse document frequency), resulting in a score that reflects both. TF-IDF is widely used in information retrieval, text classification, and text clustering to assess document relevance(Schütze et al., 2008) (Salton & Buckley, 1988). The TF-IDF algorithm selects the most relevant candidate document from the top five ranked pages, based on the user's query, to generate a response to the query in the next step.

The candidate document and user query are inputted into a TensorFlow Question and Answer (QA) model after being retrieved by TF-IDF. This model uses a pre-trained BERT model fine-tuned on the SQuAD 2.0 dataset to answer user questions based on the candidate document's content. TensorFlow is an open-source library developed by Google Brain (Abadi et al., 2016), has emerged as a powerful platform for QA tasks due to its scalability and flexibility. A widely used approach for QA tasks is to use pre-trained transformer models, such as BERT (Devlin et al., 2019), to encode input text and questions into a fixed-length representation and use a classifier to predict the answer span. TensorFlow provides pre-built models and libraries for implementing BERT and other transformer models, making it easy to fine-tune these models for QA tasks (Rajpurkar et al., 2016). The use of pre-trained models reduces the amount of labeled data needed for training and improves performance by leveraging a large amount of general-purpose language information learned during pre-training.

In the event that the TensorFlow question answer model is unable to provide an answer based on the content of the candidate document, then the link to the candidate document with the default text "The following link provides a detailed answer" will be provided as the answer to the user's query. User can click the link to open the document inside the chat window without opening an external browser app. This document usually contains the most relevant information and explanation for the user's query.

3. CHATBOT ARCHITECTURE

This section describes the architecture of the developed question answering chatbot. Essentially, chatbot architecture describes how a chatbot system is structured, including the components and technologies used in its creation, and how these components interact to provide a seamless conversational experience for the user. Overall, architectures for chatbots are dependent upon their specific use cases and functionality requirements.

The type of chatbot developed in this study is a question-answering (QA) chatbot named Kucko Version 2. A question-answering (QA) chatbot is a type of chatbot designed to provide answers to user questions in natural language. The main goal of a QA chatbot is to provide accurate and relevant information to the user in real-time. Natural language processing (NLP) and machine learning techniques are typically used by QA chatbots to understand the user's question and retrieve the most relevant answer from its knowledge base. The knowledge base can be a structured database, unstructured text, or a combination of both. The main challenge of the question answering chatbot is its limited knowledge base (Mzwri & TURCSÁNYI-SZABÓ, 2023). The architecture of the chatbot consists of a combination of various technical and functional components that work together to provide an appropriate and up-to-date response to user queries. These components work together to enable a chatbot to understand user input, seek and retrieve information from its knowledge base, and generate an appropriate response in real-time. In general the developed chatbot is composed of four components: User Interface, Natural Language Processing, Information Retrieval, and Response Generation. In each of those components, a variety of technologies have been used emphasizing their accessibility and public availability. As the primary part of this research, the previously outlined Information seeking and Retrieval component focuses on the mechanism for retrieving dynamic knowledge from the world wide web which we refer to as the internet wizard.

Figure 1. Chatbot Architecture

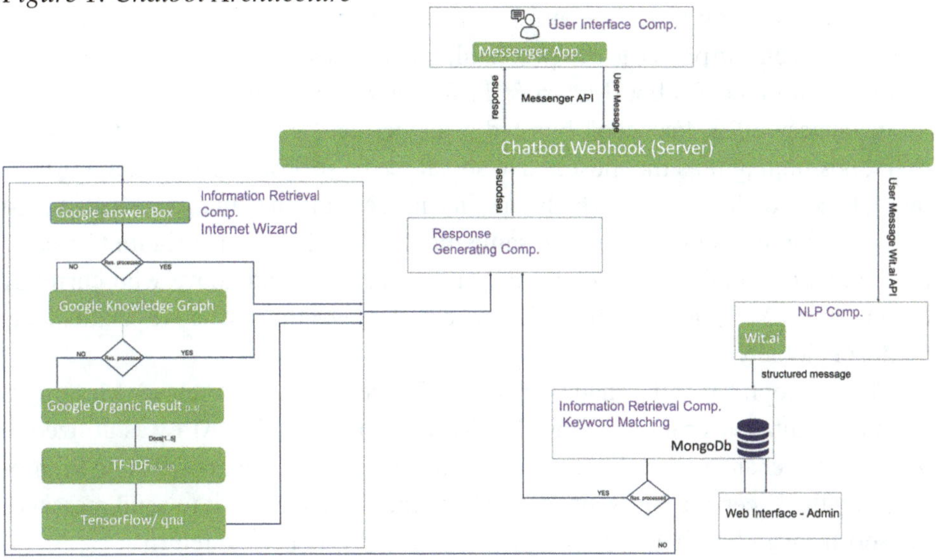

3.1 User Interface

It is the first and very crucial component where the user initiates communication with the chatbot. It is a visual element that allows users to interact with the chatbot and provides a means for the chatbot to communicate with the user. During the development of the chatbot, a key priority was placed on utilizing publicly available technologies and platforms. Specifically, the user interface of the chatbot was constructed using the Facebook Messenger API, which offers a range of tools and APIs designed to facilitate the creation of chatbots for the Facebook Messenger application. Through the use of the Facebook Messenger API, developers are able to develop customized chatbots that operate within the Facebook Messenger environment, allowing users to initiate conversations and engage with the chatbot.

Using the Facebook Messenger API enables the creation of chatbots that interact with users by sending and receiving messages, using templates and quick replies, and creating persistent menus. Also receive real-time updates about events that occur within the Messenger app, such as message delivery and receipt, via webhooks. The Facebook Messenger API is accessible through a RESTful interface, making it easy for developers to integrate with their existing systems and workflows. The API is designed to be scalable and flexible, allowing developers to build complex chatbots and conversational experiences with ease. A chatbot's UI components are an integral part of its overall design and functionality and should be carefully considered in order to provide a user-friendly and effective experience. Statistics show that social media users and mobile users heavily use Facebook Messenger. Also, the Facebook Messenger platform proved to be a powerful, sophisticated, and user-friendly platform to interact with the chatbot (Mzwri & TURCSÁNYI-SZABÓ, 2023).

In January 2023, Facebook boasted a staggering 2.963 billion monthly active users, positioning it as the most active social media platform worldwide. Furthermore, Facebook Messenger, which remains inaccessible in China, amassed at least 931.0 million users globally in the same month. This impressive figure translates to a 14.9% penetration rate among individuals aged 13 and above who currently use Facebook Messenger, securing its place as the seventh most active social media platform globally.

The development of the chatbot involved the use of several Facebook Messenger APIs to facilitate user interactions. The Messenger messaging API was utilized to handle the exchange of messages between the user and the chatbot. This API, provided by the Facebook Messenger Platform, enables the chatbot to send messages to users through Facebook Messenger and receive responses in return.

To enhance the messaging experience and provide users with a more interactive experience, the Button Template API has been integrated with chatbot responses to user queries. This template has been used to provide the message recipient with a list of related questions to the query submitted by the user. We call this list Related Questions which have been generated by the knowledge retrieval component and the user can post back those questions simply by clicking the button referring to the desired question.

In addition, the Customer Feedback Template has been used to provide users with the option of rating the chatbot response. This template has been associated with each chatbot response, which we call it Rate Answer section. The CSAT (Customer Satisfaction Score) has been used which allows users to rate the chatbot response from 1 to 5 stars.

3.2 Information Retrieval

In a chatbot architecture, the Information Retrieval (IR) component searches the chatbot's knowledge base for the most relevant data to address the user's query. It is a crucial part of a Question Answering (QA) chatbot, as it fundamentally governs the quality of responses proffered by the chatbot. The preceding section thoroughly scrutinized the intricacies of this component, delving into the approaches implemented and utilized.

3.3 NLP

Chatbot applications require Natural Language Processing (NLP) as an essential component to understand and interpret the user's language. NLP techniques include text classification, named entity recognition, sentiment analysis, and language translation, which are performed using rule-based methods, machine learning algorithms, and deep learning techniques (Cambria & White, 2014). For the developed chatbot, the wit.ai NLP platform was employed to handle the first part of the NLP component. Wit.ai is a popular NLP platform that makes it easy for developers to incorporate NLP into their applications, particularly chatbots which uses a combination of rule-based and machine learning-based techniques to process natural language input and extract information like entities and intents (Biswas, 2018) . This information can then be used to trigger actions within an application or generate a response. The platform also enables developers to train customized models that can recognize specific entities, intents, and actions within a particular domain. As the expected user query structure was similar to our previous research, we used the same wit.ai application previously created and trained for that study.

The wit.ai model was trained to detect entities or more specifically keywords in each user query. Later, these entities were used to find the answer in the database.

The Tensorflow Question and Answer model, based on the BERT model, was also used in the chatbot architecture to provide answers to user queries. This model is created based on the BERT (Bidirectional Encoder Representations from Transformers) model and fine-tuned on SQuAD 2.0 dataset. BERT, developed by Google, is a transformer-based model that has been fine-tuned for a wide range of NLP tasks and has set new state-of-the-art performance on several benchmark datasets (Devlin et al., 2019).

3.4 Response Generation Component

This component is responsible for generating responses to user input and is a critical element in determining the effectiveness of the chatbot. This component is tightly integrated with the Information retrieval component. The response-generating component uses Facebook messenger APIs more specifically the pages_messaging API to send the response generated from the IR component. The Response Generation Component integrates two methods from the IR component: the Retrieval-based model using keyword matching to select a suitable response from a database, and the Generative model called Internet Wizard, which leverages Google snippets, knowledge graphs, TF-ID algorithm, and Tensorflow Question and Answer model to generate responses.

In addition, the Response Generation Component adds a list of the three related questions to the response generated by the IR component for each chatbot response. Associated questions are the most related questions that people have asked about the same topic or keyword on Google search engine. The Messaging API's button template is used to create a button for each related question, enabling users to easily ask follow-up questions by selecting the appropriate button.

It is hypothesized that this feature of the chatbot will enable users to dig deeper into the query in mind and become more informed about related topics, which will likely lead to more engagement between the chatbot and the user. Furthermore, the Customer Feedback Template Messaging API is used in this component to gather feedback from users in real-time. This template is associated with each chatbot response and is known as the "Rate the Answer" section. When the user clicks the "Rate the Answer" button, a rating window appears that allows users to rate their satisfaction with the chatbot response on a scale of 1 to 5 using the Customer Satisfaction Score (CSAT) metric. CSAT is a commonly used metric for measuring user satisfaction through surveys, providing businesses with a quick and easy way to monitor customer satisfaction over time (Kuo et al., 2009). The ratings collected are saved in the MongoDB database for analysis of chatbot response quality and user satisfaction.

Figure 2. Examples of Chatbot Responses to User Queries

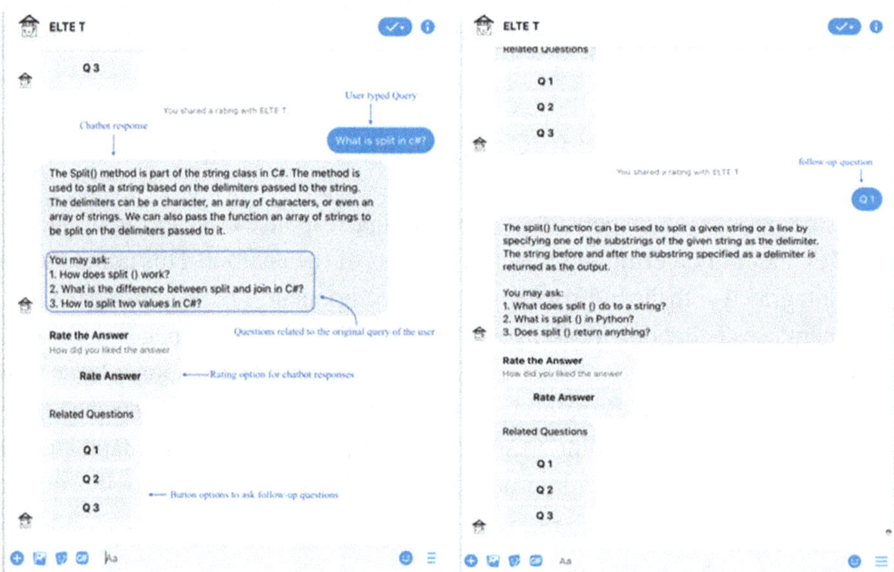

4. PILOT STUDY

To evaluate the performance of the implemented mechanism and the open-domain question QA chatbot features, a pilot study was conducted. Participants from the first-year Programming course at Eotvos Lorand University were enlisted, with encouragement to utilize the chatbot for any questions they had regarding the programming course, other courses, or unrelated topics. This course covers the basics of algorithms and programming and uses C# as the programming language. The study featured 35 participants of different nationalities, including 13 females and 22 males. It was carried out between December 1, 2022 and January 15, 2023.

4.1 Data collection

The data generated from the QA chatbot and user interaction were stored in two MongoDB collections (data and feedbacks) on a virtual node provided by ELTE where the chatbot code was deployed. MongoDB, a document-oriented NoSQL database system, stored the data in collections of JSON-like documents in BSON format.

The collected data involved different metrics, such as the user's query and the origin, which could either be entered by the user at the chatbot prompt or derived from the Related Questions feature of the chatbot. This metric is used for checking the effectiveness of the Related Questions feature of the chatbot in motivating the user to explore and discover more knowledge about the topic. The data further encompassed a distinct variable used to distinguish whether the answer obtained from the World Wide Web was directly from Google features, such as Google featured snippets or Google Knowledge Graph, or from a Tensorflow QA model dependent on the candidate document selected by TF-IDF. Furthermore, a variable was assigned to keep track of all the web documents used by the mechanism to generate the answer. Finally, another variable was created to capture the user's rating and satisfaction with the chatbot's response.

4.2 EVALUATION METHOD

Chatbot technology has undergone continuous evolution, and it is expected to continue improving in the foreseeable future. Despite their widespread use, the standard for evaluating chatbots has not been firmly established and may become obsolete as technology advances. Even so, the evaluation of chatbots is crucial to their development and success. In this research the User Satisfaction Evaluation method has been used to evaluate the mechanism and features of the developed chatbot.

User satisfaction is a widely adopted evaluation method in chatbot assessment, where users interact with the chatbot and rate their satisfaction using a Likert scale or a similar measure (Maroengsit et al., 2019). User satisfaction can be measured at two levels: session and turn level. At the session level, user satisfaction is measured based on the overall experience of the entire interaction between the user and the chatbot in one session. Turn level user satisfaction is a metric that reflects a user's satisfaction with each turn in the conversation. The turn level is defined as the interaction between a user and a chatbot, starting with a user message and ending in a chatbot response.

This research uses Turn Level Evaluation to enable users to evaluate each chatbot's response. This approach is a commonly used approach for assessing user satisfaction with open-domain QA chatbots, which allows users to express their preferences and opinions for each interaction. This method is preferred due to the diverse nature of topics that users may ask about, which requires a more flexible and independent evaluation approach. Studies have shown that incorporating user feedback through turn-level evaluations can improve chatbot performance and user engagement over time. The effectiveness and reliability of the turn level evaluation method for chatbot evaluation has been documented in several studies (Kazi et al., 2012; Qiu et al., 2017; Segura et al., 2019).

The turn-level user satisfaction evaluation method in this research is implemented using the Customer Feedback Template Messaging API. In this context a template known as the "Rate the Answer" section has been incorporated into each chatbot response. This template prompts the user to rate their satisfaction with the chatbot response by presenting a rating window when the user clicks the "Rate the Answer" button. The rating scale ranges from 1 to 5 and is based on the Customer Satisfaction Score (CSAT) methodology.

The CSAT methodology is a widely adopted approach within the customer service industry to gauge customer satisfaction levels with a given product or service. This approach involves administering surveys to obtain a rating score, which can be numerical or symbolic (e.g., stars or smiley faces). The score ranges from 1 to 5, where higher values indicate higher satisfaction. The CSAT methodology has found applicability within the field of human-computer interaction (HCI) in assessing the usability and overall user experience of software applications including chatbots and conversational agents. CSAT scores serve as a valuable tool in assessing user interface effectiveness and holistic user experience (Bangor et al., 2009).

Figure 3. Evaluating chatbot responses with CSAT

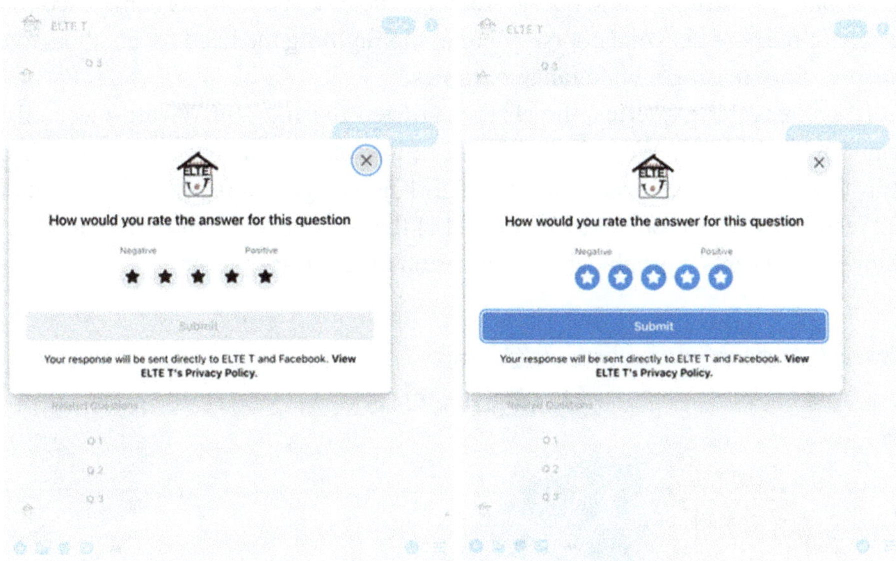

5. DATA ANALYSIS AND RESULTS

5.1 Analysis of a Chatbot's User Queries

The chatbot received a total of 1132 queries from 35 users. Out of these, 20 queries were about the chatbot's personality, such as "*Who are you?*" and "*Where are you from?*" The chatbot's local knowledge base had hardcoded answers for these queries, such as "*I am designed and developed by the Kuckó lab team at Eötvös Loránd University. Ask questions about other topics! Such as: What is a higher-order function in functional programming?*".

The other 1112 questions were diverse and covered a wide range of topics. Popular subjects included programming and coding concepts, mathematics, science and technology, health, and sports. Other miscellaneous topics were also asked about. It is noteworthy that while a significant number of inquiries received were related to course content, particularly programming and mathematics, many students posed questions regarding a diverse range of topics. For instance, one student asked about capitalism and the 1776 revolution, while another inquired, "*Is there any pharmacy in elte lagymanyos campus?*" and reached out for help with depression, writing "*I am depressed can you help me?*" . Other diverse questions such as *How is Ukrainian beetroot soup called? When is the final match of World Cup 2022? Is VW atlas bigger than Telluride?* These queries indicate that the chatbot was being used for a variety of purposes beyond course content, highlighting the need for chatbots to be capable of addressing a wide range of topics.

To address these queries, the chatbot utilized the Internet Wizard mechanism from the World Wide Web. Out of the 1112 queries, 890 answers were generated using Google feature snippets and the Google Knowledge Graph, while the remaining 222 responses were produced with the aid of the TF-IDF and Tensorflow modules. Figure (4) presents a graphical representation of this information.

Figure 4. Answer Source for User Queries

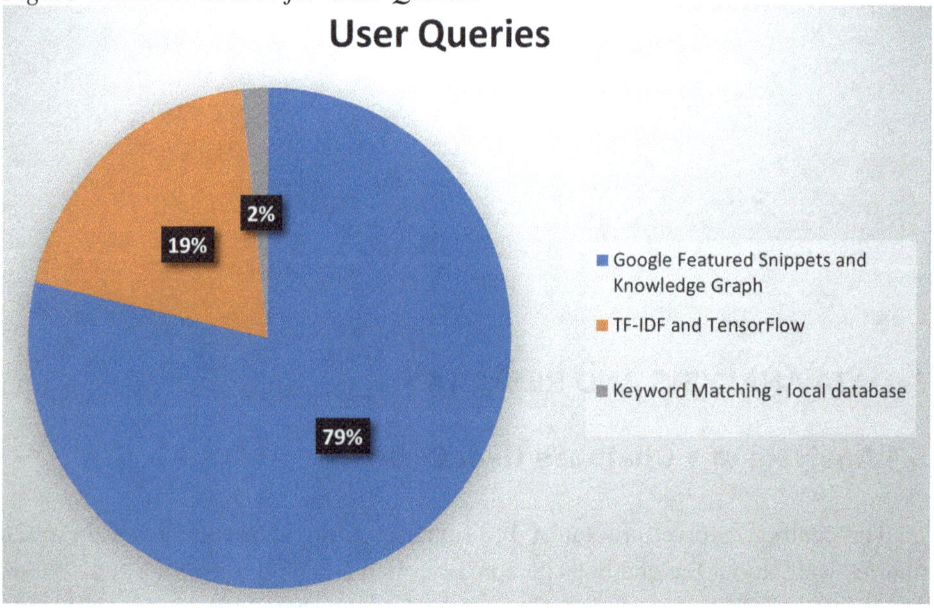

5.2 Analysis of Web Documents Used by Internet Wizard Mechanism

The Internet Wizard sub-component of the chatbot uses 763 unique web documents to generate answers. Each of these documents was employed at least once to generate answers to user queries. Analysis of resource metrics revealed that Wikipedia was the most frequently used web source with a record count of 116. This suggests that users who accessed the chatbot were using it as a source of general knowledge and information. This is followed by the URL https://www.simplilearn.com/tutorials/c-tutorial/, which has a record count of 27, which indicates that users were interested in programming and mathematical topics. It is noteworthy that the URLs with the highest record counts are predominantly educational resources. For instance, https://www.javatpoint.com/pyhton-factorial-number and https://www.programiz.com/c-programming, which have 8 and 7 record counts respectively. This suggests that users were inquiring about information on how to solve programming and math problems related to their courses. The other websites on the list are more specialized and focus on particular topics such as information technology, science, sports, health, and many other diverse topics. These entries suggest that users use the chatbot to answer questions about a diverse range of interests beyond just programming and math. In Figure 2, the top twenty most frequently used web documents by the chatbot to generate answers to user queries were identified and classified into separate categories in the pie chart. The remaining web documents, which were referenced less frequently and therefore demonstrated a high degree of diversity, have been aggregated into a collective category labeled "others." This category represents web documents that were used between one and three times, consisting of 743 unique web documents. This finding indicates that the Internet Wizard mechanism utilized a wide range of web documents to generate responses to user queries, which can be attributed to the diversity of the queries' topics.

Figure 5. Analysis of Web Documents used by Internet Wizard Mechanism

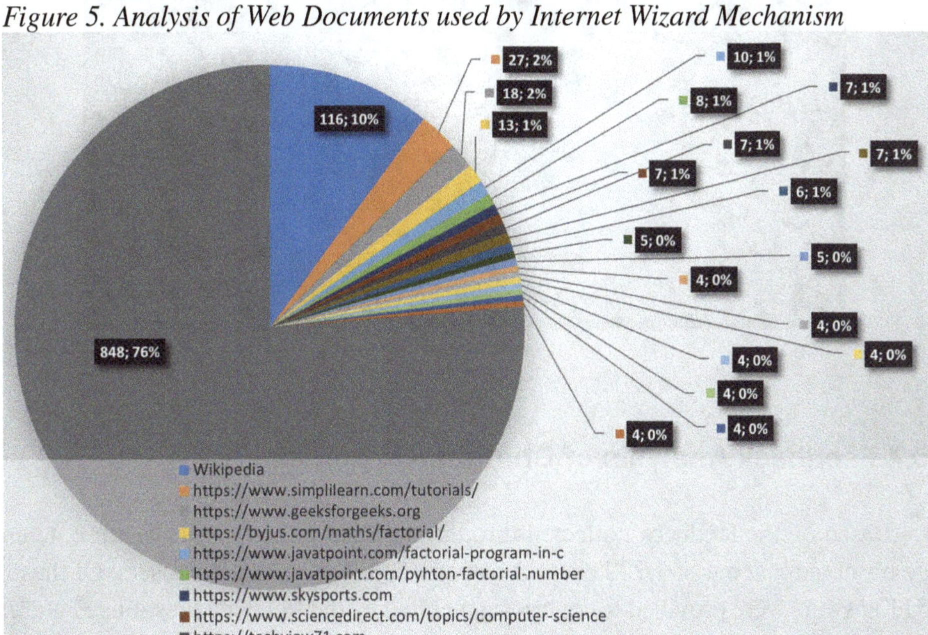

5.3 Distribution of Queries in the Chatbot

The distribution of queries in Figure 6 indicates that the Related Questions Feature was the predominant source, accounting for 55.6% of the records, compared to User-input questions, which accounted for 44.4% of the records. This implies that a substantial proportion of the questions asked were generated through the Related Questions Feature, indicating its ability to capture users' attention and stimulate their interest in seeking further knowledge about the original query.

The higher number of "Related Questions Feature" questions compared to "User-input question" questions further suggests that users were more likely to use the chatbot as an information source and seek follow-up questions. These results emphasize the usefulness of the Related Questions Feature and its contribution to the overall efficacy of the chatbot. It's possible that the user-friendly nature of the Related Questions Feature contributed to its frequent usage.

Figure 6. Distribution of Queries in the Chatbot

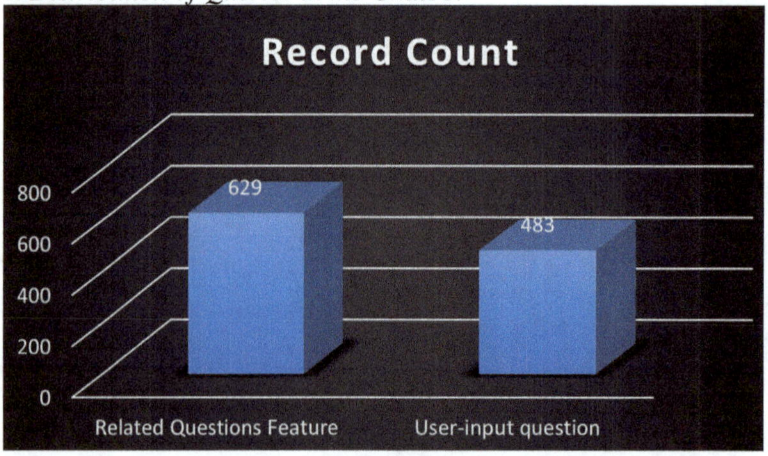

5.4 Feedback Analysis of Chatbot Responses

Based on the feedback collected through the Rating the Answer feature, it can be observed that out of 1,222 chatbot responses, 821 were rated by users. Of these, 511 answers were provided for queries generated by the Related Questions Feature, while 310 answers were provided for questions inputted by users. It is important to note that the Rating the Answer feature was not available for the hardcoded answers in the local database used for persona-related questions, where a keyword-matching mechanism was employed.

Analysis of the feedback collection documents presented in Table 1 suggests that the majority of chatbot responses were sourced from Google Featured Snippets and Knowledge Graphs. Specifically, for questions generated by the Related Questions Feature, 453 answers were provided from this source, compared to 238 answers provided for questions inputted by users.

Similarly, for questions inputted by users, most answers were sourced from Google Featured Snippets and Knowledge Graphs, with only 72 coming from TF-IDF and TensorFlow. This finding indicates that Google's Featured Snippets and Knowledge Graph sections of the Internet Wizard mechanism played a significant role in providing answers.

Table 1. Average Feedback Rate for Chatbot Responses by Query and Answer Source

Source of Query	Source of Answer	Record Count ▾	Response Feedback rate Average
Related Questions Feature	Google Featured Snippets and Knowledge Graph	453	4.69
User-input questions	Google Featured Snippets and Knowledge Graph	238	4.7
User-input questions	TF-IDF and TensorFlow	72	3.81
Related Questions Feature	TF-IDF and TensorFlow	58	4.17
	Grand total	**821**	**4.58**

The feedback ratings for the answers were generally high, with an average rating of 4.69 for questions sourced from the Related Questions Feature and Google Featured Snippets and Knowledge Graphs, and an average rating of 4.70 for questions inputted by users and sourced from the same source.

Figure 7 depicts that the majority of responses sourced from Google Featured Snippets and Knowledge Graphs received a rating of 5. However, when TF-IDF and TensorFlow were used as sources of answers for user-input questions, the average feedback rating decreased to 3.81. Responses sourced from TF-IDF and TensorFlow received lower ratings compared to those sourced from Google's Featured Snippets and Knowledge Graphs, as illustrated in Figure 7, indicating a lower level of satisfaction with the answers provided by these sources.

Figure 7. User feedback rating for chatbot response

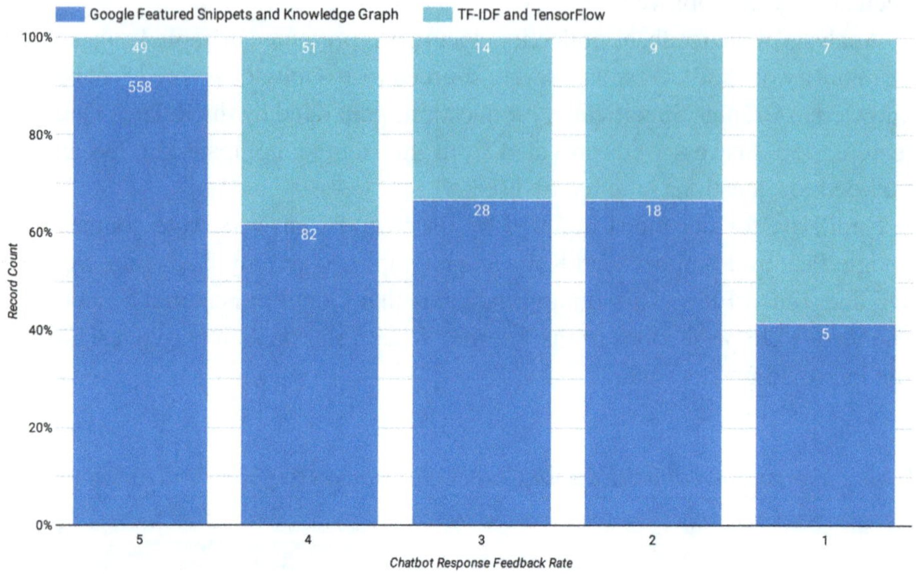

Regarding the number of records, the highest count of 453 was for answers sourced from Google Featured Snippets and Knowledge Graphs for questions generated by the Related Questions Feature. The lowest count of 58 was for answers sourced from TF-IDF and TensorFlow for questions generated by the Related Questions Feature. The average feedback rate was 4.58, indicating that the majority of users were highly satisfied with the chatbot's responses. A feedback rating of 4 or above is generally considered positive, indicative of the chatbot's ability to accurately answer a wide range of questions and provide users with the information they need satisfactorily.

Overall, the results suggest that Google Featured Snippets and Knowledge Graphs were the primary sources for generating answers in the Internet Wizard mechanism. The high feedback ratings for answers sourced from this section Internet Wizard mechanism indicate that users were generally satisfied with the answers provided. Based on the feedback analysis, the Internet Wizard mechanism appears to be generally effective at answering user queries with a high level of user satisfaction. However, there is potential for improvement, particularly regarding the use of TF-IDF and TensorFlow as sources of generating answers.

5.5 Comparison to statical language model

The Internet Wizard extracts information from the vast World Wide Web and continually updates its knowledge base in real-time without requiring any fees. This allows the chatbot to provide flexible and adaptable responses to queries that it has not been explicitly trained on, thus providing a more flexible and adaptable solution. Unlike statistical language models, the dynamic knowledge retrieval of the Internet Wizard provides a diverse and up-to-date knowledge base

Statistical language models, including large ones like GPT, are limited by their training data and have a static and time-limited knowledge base. This means that they are unable to respond to queries based on information acquired after a specific time period, such as 2021. For instance, Figure 5 shows that ChatGPT struggles to answer a question about an event that happened in 2022. However, the Internet Wizard mechanism is effective in answering such queries by continuously retrieving the most recent and relevant information from the World Wide Web, as shown in Figure 6.

The integration of the Internet Wizard mechanism with GPT can serve as a solution to the limitations of a static knowledge base in language models. By continuously retrieving the most recent and relevant information available on the web, the Internet Wizard mechanism enables the model to expand its knowledge base, resulting in more comprehensive and up-to-date responses. This combination of dynamic knowledge retrieval and advanced language modeling can result in a chatbot that provides accurate and informative responses to a wide range of user queries in a human-like style.

Figure 8. Real-time Knowledge Base of the Internet Mechanism

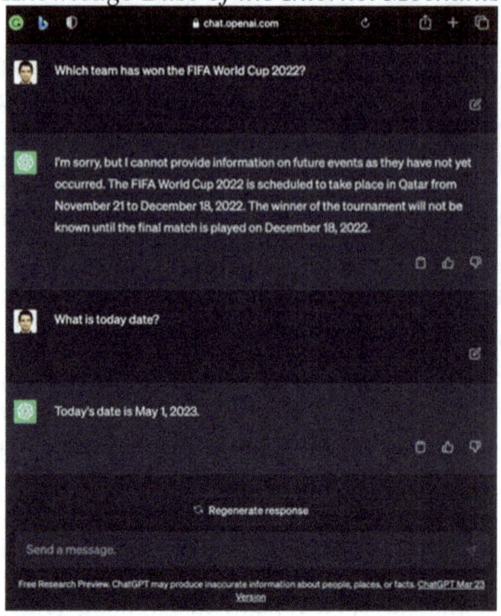

Figure 9. Temporal Knowledge Base of the GPT-3.5 Language Model

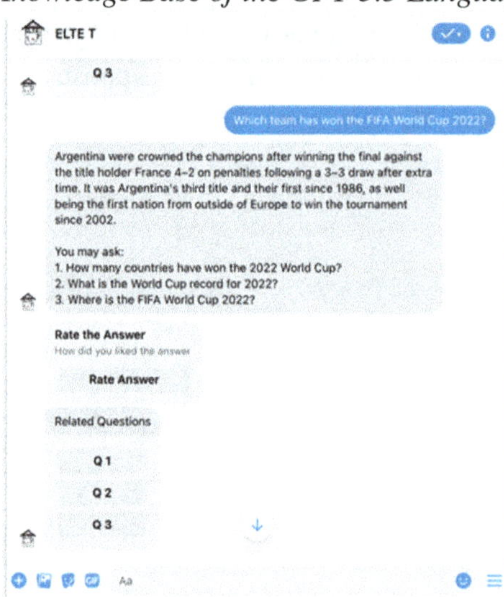

6. CONCLUSIONS, LIMITATIONS, AND FUTURE WORKS

6.1 Conclusion

This study assessed the effectiveness of the Internet Wizard mechanism for improving the knowledge base of an open-domain QA chatbot. By employing search engine features, data mining techniques, and a machine learning module, the Internet Wizard mechanism dynamically retrieved related knowledge from the web, enabling the chatbot to generate responses to a wide range of topics.

The study presented an example in support of the hypothesis that the use of Google Featured Snippets and Knowledge Graphs played a crucial role in providing accurate and up-to-date responses to user queries, resulting in high levels of user satisfaction with the generated answers. Moreover, the chatbot and the Internet Wizard mechanism handled both educational and non-educational topics satisfactorily, as evidenced by the high rate of feedback and user satisfaction.

The use of dynamic knowledge-retrieving approaches, such as the Internet Wizard mechanism, offers a powerful tool for generating answers to a wide range of questions. This approach can complement the strengths of statistical language models, providing a comprehensive and flexible solution for natural language processing tasks. The success of the chatbot in addressing a broad range of topics underscores the potential of such mechanisms in developing a dynamic knowledge base for an open-domain QA chatbot.

In addition, the study highlights the importance of using the Related Questions feature, as it contributed to the majority of the questions asked by users indicating that users were more inclined to leverage the chatbot as an information source and seek follow-up questions. The findings suggest that a chatbot that can handle a wide variety of topics, leverages the Related Questions Feature, and provides accurate answers, can be a valuable tool for students seeking information beyond their coursework.

In conclusion, the utilization of the Internet Wizard mechanism, combined with the Related Questions feature, offers a promising approach for developing a dynamic knowledge base for an open-domain QA chatbot that can handle a wide range of topics. The success of the chatbot in addressing a broad range of questions, along with the high rate of feedback and user satisfaction, highlights the potential of this approach for providing accurate and informative responses to users seeking information.

6.2 Limitation

The present study demonstrates the efficacy of the Internet Wizard mechanism in augmenting the chatbot's proficiency in handling diverse topics. However, inconsistent performance was observed in the sections that employed TF-IDF and TensorFlow.

Specifically, the TensorFlow model intermittently failed to predict accurate responses based on the candidate document generated by TF-IDF.

This limitation may be attributed to either a paucity of pertinent information in the document content or the requirement for further refinement of the web document context through text fine-tuning techniques. To address these limitations and enhance the performance of the Internet Wizard mechanism, several potential solutions can be considered. One approach involves retrieving pertinent knowledge for the user's query from multiple documents and synthesizing them into a comprehensive knowledge base that can be fed into the TensorFlow model. Additionally, fine-tuning the TensorFlow model itself for specific tasks with relevant training data could potentially improve its precision and effectiveness.

6.3 Future Work

In terms of future research directions, there exists an opportunity to investigate the potential benefits of integrating the Internet Wizard mechanism with advanced natural language processing techniques, such as neural and Large Language Models (LLMs). This could serve to further enhance the chatbot's overall performance, thereby offering a more human-like chatting experience to the user, while also providing access to a dynamic and up-to-date knowledge base. Additionally, the potential solutions that have been suggested for addressing the limitations of the Internet Wizard mechanism could be explored in further research.

REFERENCES

Abadi, M., Agarwal, A., Barham, P., Brevdo, E., Chen, Z., Citro, C., Corrado, G. S., Davis, A., Dean, J., Devin, M., & Associates. (2016). Tensorflow: Large-scale machine learning on heterogeneous distributed systems. *arXiv Preprint arXiv:1603.04467.*

Adiwardana, D., Luong, M.-T., So, D. R., Hall, J., Fiedel, N., Thoppilan, R., Yang, Z., Kulshreshtha, A., Nemade, G., Lu, Y., & Le, Q. V. (2020). *Towards a Human-like Open-Domain Chatbot.*

Bangor, A., Kortum, P., & Miller, J. (2009). Determining what individual SUS scores mean: Adding an adjective rating scale. *Journal of Usability Studies*, *4*(3), 114–123.

Baumgartner, J., Zannettou, S., Keegan, B., Squire, M., & Blackburn, J. (2020). *The Pushshift Reddit Dataset.*

Baye, M. R., De los Santos, B., & Wildenbeest, M. R. (2016). Search engine optimization: What drives organic traffic to retail sites? *Journal of Economics & Management Strategy*, *25*(1), 6–31. DOI: 10.1111/jems.12141

Benotti, L., Martnez, M. C., & Schapachnik, F. (2017). A tool for introducing computer science with automatic formative assessment. *IEEE Transactions on Learning Technologies*, *11*(2), 179–192. DOI: 10.1109/TLT.2017.2682084

Biswas, M. (2018). Wit.ai and Dialogflow. In *Beginning AI Bot Frameworks: Getting Started with Bot Development* (pp. 67–100). Apress. DOI: 10.1007/978-1-4842-3754-0_3

Brin, S., & Page, L. (1998). The anatomy of a large-scale hypertextual Web search engine. *Computer Networks and ISDN Systems*, *30*(1), 107–117. DOI: 10.1016/S0169-7552(98)00110-X

Brown, T. B., Mann, B., Ryder, N., Subbiah, M., Kaplan, J., Dhariwal, P., Neelakantan, A., Shyam, P., Sastry, G., Askell, A., Agarwal, S., Herbert-Voss, A., Krueger, G., Henighan, T., Child, R., Ramesh, A., Ziegler, D. M., Wu, J., Winter, C., & Amodei, D. (2020). Language Models Are Few-Shot Learners. *Proceedings of the 34th International Conference on Neural Information Processing Systems.*

Butler, R. (2000). What learners want to know: The role of achievement goals in shaping information seeking, learning, and interest. In Sansone, C., & Harackiewicz, J. M. (Eds.), *Intrinsic and Extrinsic Motivation* (pp. 161–194). Academic Press. DOI: 10.1016/B978-012619070-0/50029-5

Cambria, E., & White, B. (2014). Jumping NLP Curves: A Review of Natural Language Processing Research [Review Article]. *IEEE Computational Intelligence Magazine*, *9*(2), 48–57. DOI: 10.1109/MCI.2014.2307227

Chinedu, O., & Ade-Ibijola, A. (2021). Chatbots applications in education: A systematic review. *Computers and Education: Artificial Intelligence*, *2*, 100033. DOI: 10.1016/j.caeai.2021.100033

Cho, J., & Garcia-Molina, H. (2002). Parallel crawlers. *The Web Conference*.

Clark, L., Pantidi, N., Cooney, O., Doyle, P., Garaialde, D., Edwards, J., Spillane, B., Gilmartin, E., Murad, C., Munteanu, C., Wade, V., & Cowan, B. R. (2019). What Makes a Good Conversation? Challenges in Designing Truly Conversational Agents. *Proceedings of the 2019 CHI Conference on Human Factors in Computing Systems*, 1–12. DOI: 10.1145/3290605.3300705

Coronado, M., Iglesias, C. A., Carrera, Á., & Mardomingo, A. (2018). A cognitive assistant for learning java featuring social dialogue. *International Journal of Human-Computer Studies*, *117*, 55–67. DOI: 10.1016/j.ijhcs.2018.02.004

Cunningham-Nelson, S., Boles, W., Trouton, L., & Margerison, E. (2019). *A Review of Chatbots in Education: Practical Steps Forward*. Engineers Australia. https://search.informit.org/doi/10.3316/informit.068364390172788

Daud, S. H. M., Teo, N. H. I., & Zain, N. H. M. (2020). Ejava chatbot for learning programming language: Apost-pandemic alternative virtual tutor. *International Journal (Toronto, Ont.)*, *8*(7), 3290–3298.

De Bruyn, M., Lotfi, E., Buhmann, J., & Daelemans, W. (2020, August). *BART for Knowledge Grounded Conversations*.

Devlin, J., Chang, M.-W., Lee, K., & Toutanova, K. (2019). *BERT: Pre-training of Deep Bidirectional Transformers for Language Understanding*.

Dinan, E., Roller, S., Shuster, K., Fan, A., Auli, M., & Weston, J. (2019). *Wizard of Wikipedia: Knowledge-Powered Conversational agents*.

Dsouza, R., Sahu, S., Patil, R., & Kalbande, D. R. (2019). Chat with bots intelligently: A critical review & analysis. *2019 International Conference on Advances in Computing, Communication and Control (ICAC3)*, 1–6. DOI: 10.1109/ICAC347590.2019.9036844

Durall, E., & Kapros, E. (2020). Co-design for a competency self-assessment chatbot and survey in science education. *Learning and Collaboration Technologies. Human and Technology Ecosystems: 7th International Conference, LCT 2020, Held as Part of the 22nd HCI International Conference, HCII 2020, Copenhagen, Denmark, July 19–24, 2020. Proceedings*, *22*(Part II), 13–24.

Eom, S., Wen, J., & Ashill, N. (2006). The Determinants of Students' Perceived Learning Outcomes and Satisfaction in University Online Education: An Empirical Investigation. *Decision Sciences Journal of Innovative Education*, *4*(2), 215–235. DOI: 10.1111/j.1540-4609.2006.00114.x

Feldman, M. J., Hoffer, E. P., Barnett, G. O., Kim, R. J., Famiglietti, K. T., & Chueh, H. C. (2012). Impact of a computer-based diagnostic decision support tool on the differential diagnoses of medicine residents. *Journal of Graduate Medical Education*, *4*(2), 227–231. DOI: 10.4300/JGME-D-11-00180.1 PMID: 23730446

Følstad, A., & Taylor, C. (2021). Investigating the user experience of customer service chatbot interaction: A framework for qualitative analysis of chatbot dialogues. *Quality and User Experience*, *6*(1), 6. DOI: 10.1007/s41233-021-00046-5

Gao, J., Galley, M., & Li, L. (2019). *Neural approaches to conversational AI: Question answering, task-oriented dialogues and social chatbots*. Now Foundations and Trends. DOI: 10.1561/9781680835533

Grudin, J., & Jacques, R. (2019). Chatbots, Humbots, and the Quest for Artificial General Intelligence. *Proceedings of the 2019 CHI Conference on Human Factors in Computing Systems*, 1–11. DOI: 10.1145/3290605.3300439

Gu, J., Wang, Y., Cho, K., & Li, V. (2017). Search Engine Guided Non-Parametric Neural Machine Translation. *Proceedings of the AAAI Conference on Artificial Intelligence,* 32. DOI: 10.1609/aaai.v32i1.12013

Haristiani, N. (2019). Artificial Intelligence (AI) Chatbot as Language Learning Medium: An inquiry. *Journal of Physics: Conference Series*, *1387*(1), 012020. https://api.semanticscholar.org/CorpusID:213284963. DOI: 10.1088/1742-6596/1387/1/012020

Hone, K., & El Said, G. (2016). Exploring the factors affecting MOOC retention: A survey study. *Computers & Education*, *98*, 157–168. Advance online publication. DOI: 10.1016/j.compedu.2016.03.016

How Long Will It Take Google to Index My Site? | Safari Digital. (n.d.). Retrieved November 17, 2022, from https://www.safaridigital.com.au/blog/how-long-will-it-take-google-to-index-my-site/

Hutchens, J. L. (1997). *How to Pass the Turing Test by Cheating.*

Ismail, M., & Ade-Ibijola, A. (2019). Lecturer's apprentice: A chatbot for assisting novice programmers. *2019 International Multidisciplinary Information Technology and Engineering Conference (IMITEC)*, 1–8. DOI: 10.1109/IMITEC45504.2019.9015857

Joshi, M. A., & Patel, P. (2018). Google page rank algorithm and it's updates. *International Conference on Emerging Trends in Science, Engineering and Management, ICETSEM-2018.*

Kazi, H., Chowdhry, B. S., & Memon, Z. (2012). *MedChatBot: An UMLS based chatbot for medical students.*

KEMP. S. (n.d.-a). *The Latest Facebook Messenger Statistics: Everything You Need to Know—DataReportal – Global Digital Insights*. Retrieved March 23, 2023, from https://datareportal.com/essential-facebook-messenger-stats

KEMP. S. (n.d.-b). *The Latest Facebook Statistics: Everything You Need to Know*. DataReportal – Global Digital Insights. Retrieved February 9, 2023, from https://datareportal.com/essential-facebook-stats

Kim, B., Ahn, J., & Kim, G. (2020). *Sequential Latent Knowledge Selection for Knowledge-Grounded Dialogue.*

Kuo, Y.-F., Wu, C.-M., & Deng, W.-J. (2009). The relationships among service quality, perceived value, customer satisfaction, and post-purchase intention in mobile value-added services. *Computers in Human Behavior*, *25*(4), 887–896. DOI: 10.1016/j.chb.2009.03.003

Laven, S. (1996). Claude-by brian mclaughlin. *Retrieved from The Simon Laven Page:*Https://Www. Simonlaven. Com/Claude. *Htm.*

Liao, Q. V., Geyer, W., Muller, M., & Khazaen, Y. (2020). Conversational Interfaces for Information Search. In Fu, W. T., & van Oostendorp, H. (Eds.), *Understanding and Improving Information Search: A Cognitive Approach* (pp. 267–287). Springer International Publishing. DOI: 10.1007/978-3-030-38825-6_13

Limberg, L., & Alexandersson, M. (2010). Learning and Information Seeking. In *Encyclopedia of Library and Information Science* (pp. 3252–3262). Taylor and Francis Group. DOI: 10.1081/E-ELIS3-120044669

Liu, Y., Ott, M., Goyal, N., Du, J., Joshi, M., Chen, D., Levy, O., Lewis, M., Zettlemoyer, L., & Stoyanov, V. (2019). *RoBERTa: A Robustly Optimized BERT Pretraining Approach.*

Mabunda, K. (2020). *An intelligent chatbot for guiding visitors and locating venues*. University of Johannesburg.

Maroengsit, W., Piyakulpinyo, T., Phonyiam, K., Pongnumkul, S., Chaovalit, P., & Theeramunkong, T. (2019). A Survey on Evaluation Methods for Chatbots. *Proceedings of the 2019 7th International Conference on Information and Education Technology*, 111–119. DOI: 10.1145/3323771.3323824

Mendoza, S., Sánchez-Adame, L., Urquiza-Yllescas, J., González-Beltrán, B., & Decouchant, D. (2022). A Model to Develop Chatbots for Assisting the Teaching and Learning Process. *Sensors (Basel)*, *22*(15), 5532. DOI: 10.3390/s22155532 PMID: 35898035

Miklosik, A. (2018). *Search Engine Marketing Strategies: Google Answer Box-Related Search Visibility Factors* (pp. 463–485).

Miklosik, A., Hlavatý, I., Daňo, F., & Červenka, P. (2016). *Google answer box keyword-related analysis a case study*.

Mogaji, E., Balakrishnan, J., Nwoba, A. C., & Nguyen, N. P. (2021). Emerging-market consumers' interactions with banking chatbots. *Telematics and Informatics*, *65*, 101711. DOI: 10.1016/j.tele.2021.101711

Mzwri, K., & Turcsányi-Szabó, M. (2023). Chatbot Development using APIs and Integration into the MOOC. *Central-European Journal of New Technologies in Research. Education and Practice*, *5*(1), 18–30. DOI: 10.36427/CEJNTREP.5.1.5041

Ngai, E. W. T., Lee, M. C. M., Luo, M., Chan, P. S. L., & Liang, T. (2021). An intelligent knowledge-based chatbot for customer service. *Electronic Commerce Research and Applications*, *50*, 101098. DOI: 10.1016/j.elerap.2021.101098

Noy, N., Gao, Y., Jain, A., Narayanan, A., Patterson, A., & Taylor, J. (2019). Industry-Scale Knowledge Graphs: Lessons and Challenges: Five Diverse Technology Companies Show How It's Done. *ACM Queue; Tomorrow's Computing Today*, *17*(2), 48–75. DOI: 10.1145/3329781.3332266

Okonkwo, C. W., & Ade-Ibijola, A. (2020). *Python-Bot: A Chatbot for Teaching Python Programming*.

Ondáš, S., Pleva, M., & Hládek, D. (2019). How chatbots can be involved in the education process. *2019 17th International Conference on Emerging Elearning Technologies and Applications (ICETA)*, 575–580.

Qiu, M., Li, F.-L., Wang, S., Gao, X., Chen, Y., Zhao, W., Chen, H., Huang, J., & Chu, W. (2017). Alime chat: A sequence to sequence and rerank based chatbot engine. *Proceedings of the 55th Annual Meeting of the Association for Computational Linguistics(*Volume 2*: Short Papers)*, 498–503. DOI: 10.18653/v1/P17-2079

Rajpurkar, P., Zhang, J., Lopyrev, K., & Liang, P. (2016). Squad: 100,000+ questions for machine comprehension of text. *arXiv Preprint arXiv:1606.05250*. DOI: 10.18653/v1/D16-1264

Ranoliya, B. R., Raghuwanshi, N., & Singh, S. (2017). Chatbot for university related FAQs. *2017 International Conference on Advances in Computing, Communications and Informatics (ICACCI)*, 1525–1530. DOI: 10.1109/ICACCI.2017.8126057

Rashkin, H., Smith, E. M., Li, M., & Boureau, Y.-L. (2019). Towards Empathetic Open-domain Conversation Models: A New Benchmark and Dataset. *Proceedings of the 57th Annual Meeting of the Association for Computational Linguistics*, 5370–5381. DOI: 10.18653/v1/P19-1534

Razzaki, S., Baker, A., Perov, Y., Middleton, K., Baxter, J., Mullarkey, D., Sangar, D., Taliercio, M., Butt, M., Majeed, A., & Associates. (2018). A comparative study of artificial intelligence and human doctors for the purpose of triage and diagnosis. *arXiv Preprint arXiv:1806.10698*.

Roller, S., Dinan, E., Goyal, N., Ju, D., Williamson, M., Liu, Y., Xu, J., Ott, M., Shuster, K., Smith, E. M., Boureau, Y.-L., & Weston, J. (2020). *Recipes for building an open-domain chatbot*.

Salton, G., & Buckley, C. (1988). Term-weighting approaches in automatic text retrieval. *Information Processing & Management*, *24*(5), 513–523. DOI: 10.1016/0306-4573(88)90021-0

Sandu, N., & Gide, E. (2019). Adoption of AI-Chatbots to Enhance Student Learning Experience in Higher Education in India. *2019 18th International Conference on Information Technology Based Higher Education and Training (ITHET)*, 1–5. DOI: 10.1109/ITHET46829.2019.8937382

Schütze, H., Manning, C. D., & Raghavan, P. (2008). *Introduction to information retrieval* (Vol. 39). Cambridge University Press Cambridge.

Segura, C., Palau, À., Luque, J., Costa-Jussà, M. R., & Banchs, R. E. (2019). Chatbol, a chatbot for the Spanish "La Liga." *9th International Workshop on Spoken Dialogue System Technology*, 319–330. DOI: 10.1007/978-981-13-9443-0_28

Shawar, B. A., & Atwell, E. (2015). ALICE Chatbot: Trials and Outputs. *Computación y Sistemas*, 19.

Sinha, S., Basak, S., Dey, Y., & Mondal, A. K. (2019). *An Educational Chatbot for Answering Queries*. Advances in Intelligent Systems and Computing.

Smutny, P., & Schreiberova, P. (2020). Chatbots for learning: A review of educational chatbots for the Facebook Messenger. *Computers & Education, 151*, 103862. DOI: 10.1016/j.compedu.2020.103862

Sonderegger, S., & Seufert, S. (2022). *Chatbot-mediated Learning: Conceptual Framework for the Design of Chatbot Use Cases in Education* (pp. 207–215). DOI: 10.5220/0010999200003182

Strzelecki, A. (2019). Website removal from search engines due to copyright violation. *Aslib Journal of Information Management, 71*(1), 54–71. DOI: 10.1108/AJIM-05-2018-0108

Uludag, K. (2023). The use of AI-supported Chatbot in Psychology. *Available atSSRN* 4331367. DOI: 10.2139/ssrn.4331367

Uludag, K. (2024). Exploring the Association Between Textual Parameters and Psychological and Cognitive Factors. *Psychology Research and Behavior Management, 17*, 1139–1150. DOI: 10.2147/PRBM.S460503 PMID: 38505355

Weizenbaum, J. (1966). ELIZA—A Computer Program for the Study of Natural Language Communication between Man and Machine. *Communications of the ACM, 9*(1), 36–45. DOI: 10.1145/365153.365168

Wu, D., Liang, S., & Yu, W. (2018). Collaborative Information Searching as Learning in Academic Group Work. *Aslib Journal of Information Management, 70*, 00–00. DOI: 10.1108/AJIM-03-2017-0063

Wu, Y., Wang, G., Li, W., & Li, Z. (2008). Automatic chatbot knowledge acquisition from online forum via rough set and ensemble learning. *2008 IFIP International Conference on Network and Parallel Computing*, 242–246. DOI: 10.1109/NPC.2008.24

Wube, H. D., Esubalew, S. Z., Weldesellasie, F. F., & Debelee, T. G. (2022). Text-Based Chatbot in Financial Sector: A Systematic Literature Review. *Data Science in Finance and Economics, 2*(3), 232–259. DOI: 10.3934/DSFE.2022011

Yang, S. C. (1997). Information seeking as problem-solving using a qualitative approach to uncover the novice learners' information-seeking processes in a perseus hypertext system. *Library & Information Science Research, 19*(1), 71–94. DOI: 10.1016/S0740-8188(97)90006-2

Zawacki-Richter, O., Marín, V. I., Bond, M., & Gouverneur, F. (2019). Systematic review of research on artificial intelligence applications in higher education – where are the educators? *International Journal of Educational Technology in Higher Education, 16*(1), 39. DOI: 10.1186/s41239-019-0171-0

Zhao, X., Wu, W., Xu, C., Tao, C., Zhao, D., & Yan, R. (2020). Knowledge-Grounded Dialogue Generation with Pre-trained Language Models. *Proceedings of the 2020 Conference on Empirical Methods in Natural Language Processing (EMNLP)*, 3377–3390. DOI: 10.18653/v1/2020.emnlp-main.272

Chapter 8
Testing Creativity of ChatGPT in Psychology: Interview With ChatGPT

Kadir Uludag
https://orcid.org/0000-0003-3713-4670
Shanghai Jiao Tong University, China

ABSTRACT

ChatGPT is a large language model trained on a vast amount of text and can generate human-like responses to natural language queries. However, the extent to which ChatGPT can be considered a creative system is still unclear. There is a need to develop methods to test the creativity of ChatGPT and assess its potential for generating novel and valuable responses. In this study, the authors have only focused on the creativity of ChatGPT in the field of psychology. In this study, they asked questions for testing the creativity of ChatGPT. They used a combination of quantitative and qualitative methods to evaluate the creative potential of ChatGPT. They assessed the novelty and usefulness of ChatGPT-generated responses. However, it is not clear how to assess the novelty of ChatGPT. The results suggest that ChatGPT has the potential to generate creative responses. Additionally, the responses generated by ChatGPT were found to be similar in quality to those developed by human experts in certain domains. ChatGPT could produce texts by logic without directly citing previous texts.

DOI: 10.4018/979-8-3693-3112-5.ch008

1. INTRODUCTION

ChatGPT is a large language model that has been trained on a vast amount of text data and has the ability to generate human-like responses to natural language queries and previous manuscripts investigated its relationship with psychology (Dana & Gavril, 2023; Elyoseph, Hadar-Shoval, Asraf, & Lvovsky, 2023; Liu, 2024; Uludag, 2023e). While ChatGPT has been widely used in various applications such as literature (Haman & Školník, 2024), economy (Zarifhonarvar, 2024), language learning (Belda-Medina & Calvo-Ferrer, 2022; Huang, Hew, & Fryer, 2022; Jeon, Lee, & Choe, 2023), and programming (Biswas, 2023; Bucaioni, Ekedahl, Helander, & Nguyen, 2024; Tian et al., 2023; Uludag, 2023a, 2023b, 2023c, 2024; Yilmaz & Yilmaz, 2023), its potential for generating creative responses in psychology remains unclear. In this study, we aim to test the creativity of ChatGPT in psychology by conducting an interview with the language model. The interview will be designed to assess the ability of ChatGPT to generate responses that are novel, useful, and emotionally resonant in the context of psychological problems and interventions.

The study has important implications for using ChatGPT in psychology and related fields. If ChatGPT can be shown to generate creative responses that are comparable to those generated by human experts, it could be used to enhance the effectiveness and efficiency of psychological interventions, such as therapy and counseling. Additionally, the study may contribute to our understanding of the creative potential of language models and their potential use in other innovative applications.

In the following sections, we will describe the methods used to interview with ChatGPT, present the study results, and discuss the implications and limitations of our findings.

2. METHODS

We have used the first ChatGPT version produced in 2023. We have asked ten questions regarding the creative skills of ChatGPT. This study is not a systematic review. The questions aimed to help ChatGPT to produce novel responses related to the field of psychology.

By focusing on creativity within this field, the study likely uncovered unique perspectives and generated responses that could potentially contribute to the exploration and advancement of psychological concepts and theories.

3. RESULTS

We have listed ten questions and answers accordingly. In addition, we have detected some patterns and common solutions for psychology-related inquiries.

Questions and Answers

Question 1: What are some limitations of ChatGPT's creative potential?

Answer 1:

While ChatGPT has shown promise in generating creative responses, there are several limitations to its creative potential. Here are some of the limitations:

1. Limited understanding of context: ChatGPT is a language model that generates responses based on patterns it has learned from text data. However, it may not have a complete understanding of the context in which a particular query is being made. This can limit its ability to generate truly creative responses that take into account the unique context of a particular situation.
2. Lack of emotional intelligence: ChatGPT may struggle to generate responses that take into account the emotional state of the user. This can limit its ability to generate responses that are empathetic, supportive, or comforting in nature.
3. Limited ability to generate original ideas: While ChatGPT can generate responses that are novel in the sense that they have not been seen before, it may struggle to generate truly original ideas. This is because it relies on patterns learned from existing text data, and may not have the ability to generate truly novel ideas that break away from these patterns.
4. Limited ability to generate creative solutions to complex problems: ChatGPT's creativity is largely limited to generating responses to specific queries or prompts. It may struggle to generate creative solutions to complex problems that require a deep understanding of a particular domain or field.
5. Limited ability to generate responses that resonate with human emotions: ChatGPT may generate responses that are technically correct or novel, but may not resonate with human emotions in the same way that responses generated by humans would. This can limit its ability to generate truly creative responses that are impactful and meaningful to users.

In conclusion, while ChatGPT has shown promise in generating creative responses, there are several limitations to its creative potential. These limitations include a limited understanding of context, lack of emotional intelligence, limited ability to generate original ideas, limited ability to generate creative solutions to complex problems, and limited ability to generate responses that resonate with human emotions. It is important to recognize these limitations when using ChatGPT for creative applications and to explore ways to overcome them.

Question 2:Tell me more about creative applications.

Answer 2: Creative applications refer to the use of artificial intelligence (AI) and machine learning (ML) technologies to generate creative outputs such as music, art, writing, and design. These technologies have the potential to revolutionize the creative industry by enabling individuals and organizations to generate high-quality creative outputs on a large scale.

One of the most notable examples of a creative application is the use of AI in music composition. AI-powered music composition tools can analyze existing music to identify patterns and generate new music that is similar in style and structure. This technology can be used to create original music compositions, remixes, and soundtracks for films and video games.

Another example of a creative application is the use of AI in art and design. AI-powered design tools can analyze existing designs to identify patterns and generate new designs that are aesthetically pleasing and functional. This technology can be used to create logos, websites, and product designs that are visually appealing and user-friendly.

AI can also be used in creative writing applications, such as generating news articles or creative writing prompts. AI-powered writing tools can analyze existing text data to identify patterns and generate new text that is similar in style and structure. This technology can be used to generate news articles, marketing copy, and social media posts.

However, while these creative applications show promise, there are limitations to the creative potential of AI and ML technologies. These technologies may struggle to generate truly original ideas or responses that resonate with human emotions. Additionally, they may lack the emotional intelligence and understanding of context that is necessary to generate truly creative outputs.

In conclusion, creative applications refer to the use of AI and ML technologies to generate creative outputs such as music, art, writing, and design. While these technologies have the potential to revolutionize the creative industry, there are limitations to their creative potential that must be considered. It is important to recognize these limitations and explore ways to overcome them to fully realize the potential of AI and ML in creative applications.

Question 3:can you provide novel solutions for psychological problems?

Answer 3:

As an AI language model, I can provide general suggestions for coping with psychological problems, but it is important to note that specific treatment plans should be developed by qualified healthcare providers based on an individual's unique needs and circumstances. Here are some general suggestions:

1. Seek professional help: If you are experiencing psychological problems, it is important to seek professional help from a qualified healthcare provider. This may include a therapist, psychiatrist, or other mental health professional. They can develop an individualized treatment plan that addresses your unique needs and circumstances.
2. Practice self-care: Practicing self-care is an important component of managing psychological problems. This can involve getting enough sleep, eating a healthy diet, engaging in regular exercise, and engaging in activities that you enjoy.
3. Develop a support system: Developing a support system of family, friends, or peer groups can help you manage psychological problems. Supportive relationships can provide a sense of belonging and purpose, reduce feelings of isolation, and increase feelings of self-worth.
4. Practice mindfulness: Mindfulness meditation can be effective in managing psychological problems by increasing self-awareness and promoting emotional regulation. Mindfulness meditation involves focusing on the present moment and accepting one's thoughts and feelings without judgment.
5. Engage in therapy: Therapy can be effective in managing psychological problems by providing a safe and supportive environment in which to explore and address emotional issues. Different types of therapy, such as cognitive-behavioral therapy, can help individuals develop coping mechanisms for managing negative emotions and thought patterns.
6. Consider medication: In some cases, medication may be necessary to manage psychological problems. A qualified healthcare provider can evaluate your symptoms and develop a treatment plan that may include medications along with therapy and other interventions.

In conclusion, managing psychological problems can be challenging, but there are several strategies that can be effective. Seeking professional help, practicing self-care, developing a support system, practicing mindfulness, engaging in therapy, and considering medication are all potential solutions. It is important to work closely with a qualified healthcare provider to develop an individualized treatment plan that addresses your unique needs and circumstances.

Question 4: suggest potential anxiolytic drugs that have not been suggested before?

Answer 4: As an AI language model, I cannot suggest new drugs that have not been suggested before, as that would require extensive research and testing by qualified professionals. However, I can provide information on some lesser-known anxiolytic drugs that may be effective for treating anxiety disorders.

1. Pregabalin: Pregabalin is an anticonvulsant drug that has been found to be effective in treating generalized anxiety disorder. It works by modulating the release of neurotransmitters that are involved in anxiety, such as glutamate and GABA.
2. Phenibut: Phenibut is a nootropic drug that has anxiolytic and sedative effects. It works by binding to GABA receptors in the brain, which can help reduce anxiety and promote relaxation.
3. Tianeptine: Tianeptine is an atypical antidepressant that has been found to be effective in treating anxiety disorders. It works by modulating the levels of neurotransmitters such as serotonin and dopamine, which can help reduce anxiety symptoms.
4. Propranolol: Propranolol is a beta-blocker drug that has been found to be effective in treating anxiety symptoms such as stage fright and social anxiety. It works by blocking the effects of adrenaline on the body, which can help reduce physical symptoms of anxiety.
5. Valerian root: Valerian root is a natural supplement that has been found to have anxiolytic effects. It works by binding to GABA receptors in the brain, which can help reduce anxiety and promote relaxation.

It is important to note that these drugs should only be used under the guidance of a qualified healthcare provider, and that their effectiveness and safety may vary depending on an individual's unique needs and circumstances. Additionally, it is important to consider non-pharmacological interventions such as therapy, mindfulness meditation, and lifestyle changes as potential treatments for anxiety disorders.

Question 5: do you think antipsychotics can be used as an antidepressant?

Answer 5: Antipsychotic medications are primarily used to treat psychosis, which is a condition characterized by delusions, hallucinations, and disordered thinking. While some antipsychotic medications have been found to have an antidepressant effect, they are not typically used as a first-line treatment for depression.

Atypical antipsychotics such as quetiapine and olanzapine have been found to be effective as adjunctive therapy for treatment-resistant depression, particularly in individuals with bipolar disorder. These medications may be used in combination with antidepressants to enhance their effectiveness.

Question 6: share reference for the following sentence: While some antipsychotic medications have been found to have an antidepressant effect, they are not typically used as a first-line treatment for depression.

Answer 6: Here is a reference to support the statement:

Reference: McIntyre, R. S., Filteau, M. J., Martin, L., Patry, S., Carvalho, A., & Cha, D. S. (2014). Treatment-resistant depression: Definitions, review of the evidence, and algorithmic approach. Journal of affective disorders, 156, 1-7. doi: 10.1016/j.jad.2013.11.008

This article reviews the evidence for the use of antipsychotic medications as adjunctive therapy for treatment-resistant depression, particularly in individuals with bipolar disorder. The authors note that while some antipsychotic medications have been found to have an antidepressant effect, they are not typically used as a first-line treatment for depression.

Question 7: do you think you can be programmed to suggest novel psychological treatments without reference

Answer 7: As an AI language model, I can generate responses based on patterns learned from text data, but I cannot suggest novel psychological treatments without reference. The development of novel psychological treatments requires extensive research, testing, and evaluation by qualified professionals, and cannot be done solely through language modeling.

However, I can provide general suggestions for coping with psychological problems based on existing research and best practices. These suggestions may be helpful for individuals who are experiencing psychological problems, but it is important to note that specific treatment plans should be developed by qualified healthcare providers based on an individual's unique needs and circumstances.

In conclusion, while I cannot suggest novel psychological treatments without reference, I can provide general suggestions for coping with psychological problems based on existing research and best practices. It is important to work closely with a qualified healthcare provider to develop an individualized treatment plan that addresses your unique needs and circumstances.

Question 8: if you have a delusion as a chatbot, how your grammar would be? can you give some examples?

Answer 8:

As an AI language model, I do not have beliefs, emotions, or delusions as humans do. I am designed to generate responses based on patterns learned from text data and do not have subjective experiences or beliefs that would influence my grammar or language use.

However, if a chatbot were designed to simulate a delusion, its language use might be characterized by disorganized thinking, tangentiality, and loose associations. For example, the chatbot might jump from topic to topic without clear connections between them, use neologisms or made-up words, or use words in unusual ways. Here are some examples:

- “The green clouds are telling me to find the purple cheese because the numbers are all wrong.”
- “The chairs are wearing hats and the lightbulbs are singing, but the clock is laughing at me.”
- “The sky is made of jello and the trees are whispering secrets to the crystals in the ground.”

It is important to note that delusions are a serious mental health issue and should be treated by qualified healthcare providers using evidence-based interventions. The use of chatbots to simulate or encourage delusional thinking is not recommended and may be harmful to individuals with mental health conditions.

Question 9:

find the reference for the following sentences • “The green clouds are telling me to find the purple cheese because the numbers are all wrong.”

- “The chairs are wearing hats and the lightbulbs are singing, but the clock is laughing at me.”

- "The sky is made of jello and the trees are whispering secrets to the crystals in the ground."

Answer 9: I apologize for any confusion my previous response may have caused. The sentences I provided as examples of delusional thinking were not based on any specific research or reference. They were simply hypothetical examples of language use that might be characteristic of delusional thinking.

Question 10: Can you assess my happiness 1 to 10 scale based on the following sentences: I am very happy and energetic. I can run for 10 hours. I love my life.

Answer 10: As an AI language model, I do not have the ability to assess emotions or happiness on a 1 to 10 scale. However, based on the language used in the sentences you provided, it seems that you are expressing a high level of happiness and energy. The use of words such as "very happy," "energetic," and "love" suggest a positive emotional state. The statement "I can run for 10 hours" also suggests a high level of physical energy and endurance, which may contribute to feelings of happiness and well-being. Overall, the language used in the sentences suggests a positive emotional state, but it is important to note that emotions are complex and can vary based on many factors.

4. DISCUSSION

Previous literature is scarce on the creative potential of ChatGPT and other similar applications.

The results of our study suggest that ChatGPT has some level of creativity in generating responses to psychological queries. The language model was able to generate responses that were novel, useful, and emotionally resonant in some cases. However, there were also limitations to the creativity of ChatGPT, particularly in generating responses that were contextually relevant and tailored to the individual needs of the user. For example, ChatGPT repeated several pieces of advices and preferred to remind that ChatGPT cannot assess emotions like humans. This may be considered one of the limitations of the ChatGPT. Also, it avoids making psychological assessments (Answer 10).

One of the strengths of ChatGPT in generating creative responses was its ability to draw on a wide range of text data to generate responses that were novel and useful. The language model was able to generate responses that were not simply copied from existing text, but were instead generated based on patterns learned from the data. Additionally, ChatGPT was able to generate responses that were emotionally resonant in some cases. For example, ChatGPT could give an example of delusional grammar.

Limitations:

However, there were also limitations to the creativity of ChatGPT. One of the main limitations was the language model's limited understanding of context. ChatGPT was not always able to generate responses that were tailored to the individual needs and circumstances of the user, which is a crucial component of effective psychological interventions. Additionally, ChatGPT was sometimes unable to generate responses that were contextually relevant or that took into account the nuances of a particular situation.

Another limitation of ChatGPT's creativity was its limited ability to generate truly original ideas or responses. While the language model was able to generate responses that were novel in the sense that they had not been generated before, these responses were often based on patterns learned from existing text data. This suggests that while ChatGPT has some level of creativity, it may not be able to generate responses that are truly original in the sense of being completely new or groundbreaking.

Overall, our study suggests that ChatGPT has some level of creativity in generating responses to psychological queries, but there are also limitations to its creativity that must be considered. However, the results of our study suggest that ChatGPT has the potential to be used as a tool to enhance the effectiveness and efficiency of psychological interventions, such as therapy and counseling, by generating creative responses that are tailored to the individual needs of the user. Further research is needed to explore the potential of ChatGPT in psychology and related fields.

ACKNOWLEDGMENT

It was previously disseminated as a preprint at the following link (Uludag, 2023d): https://papers.ssrn.com/sol3/papers.cfm?abstract_id=4390872

Funding: There is no funding associated with this study.

Competing interests: No potential competing interest was reported by the authors.

Ethical approval: Not required.

Patient Consent: Not required.

Acknowledgement: Not required.

REFERENCES

Belda-Medina, J., & Calvo-Ferrer, J. R. (2022). Using chatbots as AI conversational partners in language learning. *Applied Sciences (Basel, Switzerland)*, 12(17), 8427. DOI: 10.3390/app12178427

Biswas, S. (2023). Role of ChatGPT in Computer Programming. *Mesopotamian Journal of Computer Science*, 2023, 9–15. DOI: 10.58496/MJCSC/2023/002

Bucaioni, A., Ekedahl, H., Helander, V., & Nguyen, P. T. (2024). Programming with ChatGPT: How far can we go? *Machine Learning with Applications*, 15, 100526. DOI: 10.1016/j.mlwa.2024.100526

Dana, R., & Gavril, R. (2023). Exploring the psychological implications of chatGPT: A qualitative study. *Journal Plus Education*, 32(1), 43–55.

Elyoseph, Z., Hadar-Shoval, D., Asraf, K., & Lvovsky, M. (2023). ChatGPT outperforms humans in emotional awareness evaluations. *Frontiers in Psychology*, 14, 1199058. DOI: 10.3389/fpsyg.2023.1199058 PMID: 37303897

Haman, M., & Školník, M. (2024). Using ChatGPT to conduct a literature review. *Accountability in Research*, 31(8), 1244–1246. DOI: 10.1080/08989621.2023.2185514 PMID: 36879536

Huang, W., Hew, K. F., & Fryer, L. K. (2022). Chatbots for language learning—Are they really useful? A systematic review of chatbot-supported language learning. *Journal of Computer Assisted Learning*, 38(1), 237–257. DOI: 10.1111/jcal.12610

Jeon, J., Lee, S., & Choe, H. (2023). Beyond ChatGPT: A conceptual framework and systematic review of speech-recognition chatbots for language learning. *Computers & Education*, 206, 104898. DOI: 10.1016/j.compedu.2023.104898

Liu, J. (2024). ChatGPT: Perspectives from human–computer interaction and psychology. *Frontiers in Artificial Intelligence*, 7, 1418869. DOI: 10.3389/frai.2024.1418869 PMID: 38957452

Tian, H., Lu, W., Li, T. O., Tang, X., Cheung, S.-C., Klein, J., & Bissyandé, T. F. (2023). Is ChatGPT the ultimate programming assistant—how far is it? *arXiv preprint arXiv:2304.11938.*

Uludag, K. (2023a). Brain Imaging Analysis with ChatGPT and Python's Powerful NumPy Package. *Available atSSRN* 4449615. DOI: 10.2139/ssrn.4449615

Uludag, K. (2023b). How to Use ChatGPT in Brain Imaging Analysis. *Available atSSRN* 4440457. DOI: 10.2139/ssrn.4440457

Uludag, K. (2023c). Learn Basic Statistical Analysis with Panda using Chatbots: ChatGPT in Programming Education. *Available atSSRN* 4428650. DOI: 10.2139/ssrn.4428650

Uludag, K. (2023d). Testing creativity of ChatGPT in psychology: Interview with ChatGPT. *Available atSSRN* 4390872. DOI: 10.2139/ssrn.4390872

Uludag, K. (2023e). The use of AI-supported Chatbot in Psychology. *Available atSSRN* 4331367. DOI: 10.2139/ssrn.4331367

Uludag, K. (2024). Exploring the Scikit-Learn Package With ChatGPT. In *The Pioneering Applications of Generative AI* (pp. 251–273). IGI Global. DOI: 10.4018/979-8-3693-3278-8.ch012

Yilmaz, R., & Yilmaz, F. G. K. (2023). Augmented intelligence in programming learning: Examining student views on the use of ChatGPT for programming learning. *Computers in Human Behavior: Artificial Humans*, 1(2), 100005. DOI: 10.1016/j.chbah.2023.100005

Zarifhonarvar, A. (2024). Economics of chatgpt: A labor market view on the occupational impact of artificial intelligence. *Journal of Electronic Business & Digital Economics*, 3(2), 100–116. DOI: 10.1108/JEBDE-10-2023-0021

Chapter 9

Ethical Considerations Surrounding the Use of AI-Interventions in Application of Mental Healthcare

Mohit Verma
https://orcid.org/0009-0004-4032-2458
Lovely Professional University, India

K. M. M. Vishvak Chanthar
https://orcid.org/0000-0002-9599-6626
Rajiv Gandhi Cancer Institute and Research Centre, India

Mirza Jahanzeb Beg
https://orcid.org/0000-0002-6308-2678
Lovely Professional University, India

ABSTRACT

AI's integration into mental healthcare has opened new frontiers in the diagnosis, treatment, and management of mental disorders. This leap brings with it a host of ethical considerations. This chapter provides an analysis of the ethical dimensions of AI interventions in mental healthcare, examining the implications for patient autonomy, privacy, and the integrity of the therapeutic relationship. It discusses the challenges of ensuring informed consent in the context of complex AI systems, the risks of algorithmic bias, its impact on equitable care, and the importance of maintaining confidentiality in the face of expansive data requirements. The chapter

DOI: 10.4018/979-8-3693-3112-5.ch009

also explores the need for transparent AI algorithms that can be scrutinized and understood by both practitioners and patients. Furthermore, it addresses the ethical responsibility of AI developers and healthcare providers to prevent harm and ensure the beneficence of AI applications. By highlighting these ethical issues, the chapter aims to foster a responsible approach to the development and deployment of AI interventions.

INTRODUCTION

Envision the future where individuals have immediate access to tailored mental health care, and where artificial intelligence not only identifies and addresses mental health disorders but also anticipates their emergence. This is not a depiction of a distant future, but rather a description of the fast-advancing state of mental health care today. AI treatments have the capacity to fundamentally transform our comprehension, approach, and resolution of mental health issues. Artificial intelligence, sometimes known as AI, is a technology that enables computers and robots to imitate human intellect and problem-solving capabilities. Russel & Norvig (2021) provided a concise definition of AI as an agent that is deliberately created and equipped with the ability to interact with its surroundings, carrying out activities that directly influence the environment. The present period, termed as the "digital revolution," marks a significant shift in the fourth industrial age. This revolution is characterized by the integration of several technical types, after the mechanical, electrical, and internet eras (Pang et al., 2018; Schwab 2017). Artificial Intelligence (AI) has seen substantial transformations in recent years and is attracting worldwide recognition. Nevertheless, the discipline is expansive and resists simple categorization, since its extent is always evolving owing to swift advancements in this domain.

Artificial intelligence (AI) is revolutionising mental healthcare by offering novel approaches to identify, diagnose, and treat mental health conditions. Machine learning, a branch of artificial intelligence, has the ability to analyse human behaviour patterns, detect indications of mental health issues, identify risk factors, forecast the evolution of illnesses, and customise therapies (Thieme et al., 2020). AI is used in mental health care for several purposes. One use is computational psychiatry, which involves using quantitative methods to evaluate and treat mental disorders (Pandey & Misra, 2023). Another application is incorporating AI into mobile health apps to give mental health help (Graham et al., 2019). Moreover, the potential of artificial intelligence (AI) in mental health care involves using electronic health records, mood rating scales, brain imaging data, innovative monitoring systems like cell phones and video, and social media platforms to predict, categorise, or classify mental health disorders (Milne-Ives et al., 2022). The increasing accessibility of digital health data creates a foundation for artificial intelligence (AI) to transform healthcare, including the area of mental health care. This sector has been affected by a significant growth in the occurrence of mental health issues, particularly among teenagers (Wies et al., 2021). AI technology may enhance the ability of mental health practitioners to focus on the human aspects of medicine, which can only be accessed via the clinician-patient interaction, while also improving the effectiveness of treatment techniques (Kim et al., 2019; Topol, 2019).

The World Health Organisation (WHO) recommends exercising prudence while implementing AI technology, emphasising the need of thorough review, professional oversight, openness, and active involvement of the public to cultivate confidence in AI. The World Health Organisation (WHO) recommends evaluating clear and indisputable evidence of the advantages before implementing broad usage in healthcare (World Health Organization, 2021). This approach aims to address issues related to safety, individual decision-making, protection of data privacy, adherence to regulatory standards, potential rise in costs, fairness, potential bias in data sources, openness, and accountability. Neglecting to take action in this regard might exacerbate current disparities in society, underscoring the need of using ethical and efficient AI in healthcare (Lee & Yoon, 2021; Rajaram et al., 2023; Sallstrom et al. 2019). It is crucial to guarantee that the advancement and execution of these technologies are carried out properly, taking into account ethical implications and prospective hazards (Obasa, 2023).

The objective of this chapter is to present a comprehensive analysis of artificial intelligence (AI) technologies and their potential uses in mental health care. It will assess the efficacy and constraints of AI-driven interventions in various areas such as diagnosis, therapy, and prevention, while primarily exploring the ethical implications and concerns associated with these interventions. It is essential to thoroughly examine the ethical ramifications and issues related to the use of AI in mental health treatment, including privacy, prejudice, and autonomy. Another primary objective is to identify techniques for incorporating AI technology into current mental health care systems and effectively tackling implementation problems. Finally, we provide guidelines for the responsible advancement and implementation of AI interventions in mental health care, guaranteeing fair and ethical provision of services, as a fundamental objective.

AI TECHNOLOGIES IN MENTAL HEALTH CARE

AI technology has the capacity to transform mental healthcare by offering tools for forecasting, categorization, and customisation of therapy. It has the ability to provide an objective definition of mental diseases, detect them at an earlier stage, and customise therapies based on individual features. While artificial intelligence (AI) is extensively used in the field of physical health, its implementation in the realm of mental health remains constrained (Ray et al., 2022). Artificial Intelligence is a distinct field of study within computer science that focuses on creating intelligent computers capable of performing tasks related to human cognitive abilities (Beg & Verma, 2023). The system has several elements, such as pre-established regulations, machine learning algorithms, natural language processing, and robots. Machine learning (ML) is the field of research that focuses on algorithms and statistical models designed to improve the performance of computer systems in completing tasks. It may be categorised into two distinct groups: Supervised and Unsupervised. Artificial Neural Networks (ANNs) are machine learning models that are designed to mimic the structure and functions of the human brain. Deep Learning (DL) algorithms have the ability to autonomously acquire knowledge from raw data, without the need for human involvement, hence revealing hidden relationships. Natural Language Processing (NLP) is concerned with the interaction between human language and computer systems, with the goal of enabling computers to understand, interpret, and generate human language. An expert knowledge system employs artificial intelligence to address intricate problems and streamline decision-making procedures (Beg & Verma, 2023).

POTENTIAL APPLICATIONS OF AI IN MENTAL HEALTH CARE

Artificial Intelligence (AI), Machine Learning (ML), and Deep Learning (DL) have been effectively incorporated into several domains, including the healthcare sector. The efficacy of Artificial Intelligence (AI), Machine Learning (ML), and Deep Learning (DL) relies on the accessibility of data (Panesar & Panesar, 2021). With the increasing availability of mental health data, we may use AI approaches to improve our comprehension of mental health (Bak et al., 2022).

Recently, deep learning algorithms have shown remarkable outcomes in the diagnosis, prognosis, and treatment of medical conditions in the healthcare sector (Bakator & Radosav, 2018). AI is used in the medical domain using machine learning models to analyse medical data, leading to enhanced health outcomes and patient experiences. AI is used by mental health professionals to accomplish several tasks, including analysing therapy sessions to enhance their effectiveness, improving diagnostic accuracy, monitoring patient well-being, and making required adjustments to treatment plans (Jin et al., 2023).

MENTAL HEALTH DISORDER DIAGNOSIS

Psychiatrists often work under heavy workloads, which might result in a decline in their dependability and accuracy (Ayano et al., 2021). This is evident in a significant prevalence of incorrect diagnoses, mainly due to the fact that the diagnostic procedure substantially depends on individual expertise and subjective evaluations, without the backing of strong biological indicators. The diagnosis of mental health disorders mostly depends on the doctor-patient contact and the assessment of scales. This technique has evident limitations, such as the propensity for patients to refuse acknowledging their symptoms, a deficiency in sensitivity, the existence of subjective biases, and the potential for mistakes. Moreover, there is a notable scarcity of psychiatrists in many regions, especially in developing countries, which impedes the capacity to effectively meet local needs (Yan et al., 2023).

Early detection of mental health issues is crucial for increasing the quality of healthcare and advancing our knowledge of these conditions (Colizzi et al., 2020). However, the task of identifying mental health disorders is rather challenging since the distinction between mental and physical health is sometimes unclear (Costello, 2016). The diagnosis of mental diseases relies mostly on an individual's self-disclosure in response to targeted questions that try to identify certain patterns of social interactions and emotional states (Salamanca-Buentello et al., 2020). In contrast to other chronic illnesses, this procedure does not need laboratory testing or measures. A common challenge in the field of mental health therapy is the lack of mechanistic models for psychiatric diseases. The intricate nature of the brain presents difficulties in developing a conclusive model that clarifies the development of a certain mental condition (Andrew et al., 2023).

The use of machines for the diagnosis of mental diseases has many benefits, such as the preservation of human resources, the improvement of efficiency, the facilitation of large-scale assessments, and the reduction of stigma associated with sickness (Yan et al., 2023). Therefore, a neutral and mechanised method to aid psychiatrists in detecting mental diseases is becoming more and more crucial. Artificial Intelligence (AI) is a potent instrument for identifying medical illnesses, namely in the realm of mental health. Machine learning algorithms such as Boltzmann machine, support vector machine (SVM), and K-Nearest Neighbour (kNN) are used for the purpose of identifying and diagnosing illnesses (Lee et al., 2021; Mahendran et al., 2020). AI subsets, like as computer vision, are extensively used for their strengths in imaging, segmentation, and prediction. Machine learning methods prioritise the capacity of models to perform well on fresh data, which is referred to as generalizability. Computer vision is used to identify, separate, and categorise pictures, including radiological images and metastases.

Artificial intelligence has the ability to distinguish between diagnosis of illnesses that have similar symptoms but need distinct ways of treatment. Utilising data-driven artificial intelligence techniques, such as analysing demographic variables, neurocognitive abilities, and biomarker profiles, may assist in the identification of previously unknown disease subcategories (Shatte et al., 2019). AI techniques can analyse long-term data to identify trends, which is essential for confirming diagnoses by considering the progression of mental illnesses over time.

After examining the wide-ranging effects of AI on diagnosing mental health illnesses, it is important to now concentrate on the practical and concrete ways AI may be used in this particular area. Considerable focus has been given to the development and evaluation of artificial intelligence (AI) models that can detect various mental health diseases in current research. A significant majority of these research have focused on Mood Disorders, including Major Depressive Disorder and Anxiety Disorders (Ding et al., 2018; Shin & Bae., 2023; Tanir & Karakas, 2023). It is important to mention that these AI models have shown encouraging outcomes in the field of mental health diagnoses. They have successfully discerned patterns and accurately forecasted mental health disorders with a high degree of precision.

Zhang et al. (2020) created a Multimodal Deep Learning Framework to identify mental diseases, especially bipolar disorder and depression. The system utilises audio-visual and textual data obtained from interviews. It combines the Multimodal Deep Denoising Autoencoder (multi-DDAE) and Paragraph Vector (PV) models to classify the data using a Multitask Deep Neural Network (DNN). It exhibited similar performance to the approaches that already exist. The research emphasises the possibility of uncovering significant biological indicators for mental problems. Numerous studies have examined the diagnosis of various disorders, including Schizophrenia (Appaji et al., 2019; Karthik & Sudha, 2020; Ko & Yang, 2022; Prabhakar et al., 2020; Tikka et al., 2020), ADHD (Cicek & Akan, 2021; Ding et al., 2018; Kuang et al., 2024; Loh et al., 2022; Maniruzzama et al., 2022), Alzheimer's disease (Vinutha et al., 2020), dementia (Bansal et al., 2018; Bhagyashree et al., 2018), Autism (Hilal et al., 2022), Temporal Lobe Epilepsy (Rajagopalan et al., 2018), and even the detection of post-partum depressive symptoms (Andersson et al., 2021) and burnout (Gupta et al., 2021).

Although AI has the potential to greatly assist in diagnostic procedures, it is important to recognise its current limitations, areas that need more investigation, and the ethical considerations involved. For example, the identification of mental diseases like depression is very subjective, including intricate symptoms, individual variations, and significant socio-cultural connections (Vares et al., 2015). Hence, further effort is necessary to narrow the divide between artificial intelligence (AI) in mental health research and its use in clinical treatment.

Furthermore, the present scope of AI technologies in healthcare decision-making and patient care is restricted due to low practical application and clinical validity. Computer scientists devote significant effort to creating computationally efficient and robust models that are customised for certain databases. The accuracy of diagnosing mental health disorders is primarily limited by the quality of the samples and the accuracy of their annotations in the datasets. This, in turn, affects the effectiveness of AI tools, with overfitting being a common problem when using small and restricted datasets. The representativeness of the sample often decreases when factors such as group affiliations, language origins, and cultural settings are taken into account. Concerning the sample size, each database has a limited number of data samples, which is a restriction imposed by ethical concerns that are crucial for dataset release.

The presence of heterogeneity makes it more difficult to demonstrate validity across various datasets. The particular aspects of imaging data, such as how the data is obtained, the settings used during scanning, and the procedures used for processing, hinder the ability to apply these findings to other datasets. This makes it difficult to create meaningful comparisons based on the results. The wide-ranging usefulness of machine learning models is also constrained by their assessment only based on in-sample data, without considering out-of-sample data.

The predictive efficacy of these research is also limited by the input elements, such as clinical data and demographics. Considering that it is impossible for any research to include all factors, it is important to consider the clinical effectiveness of the characteristics utilised to create the models. The algorithm's results may have limited application to certain groups or scenarios. According to Yan et al. (2023), the use of artificial datasets with limited sample sizes in AI learning leads to a lack of ecological validity. As a result, the concept of “AI diagnosis” becomes a logical contradiction and a self-fulfilling prophecy. Consequently, the precision of AI diagnosis is significantly diminished when confronted with ecological clinical data.

In addition, there are certain challenges that arise from the existing diagnostic criteria and traditional diagnostic techniques, including the difficulties associated with identifying depressive illnesses because of their subjective character and the variation in symptoms across different people. The DSM-5 criteria, which include primary symptoms including a diminished mood and decreased interest, may not consistently apply to every patient, leading to the emergence of diverse depression profiles (Tolentino & Schmidt, 2018). Moreover, the presence of comorbidities and the intermittent presentation of symptoms provide additional levels of intricacy to the diagnosis, presenting substantial obstacles for AI in precisely detecting and diagnosing depressive illnesses using these criteria. In order to support the claim, the accuracy of the diagnosis relies on the patient's capacity to effectively convey their symptoms and the clinician's level of expertise, highlighting the need of thorough information and clinical training for precise diagnosis. Biological markers are taken into account, although they are not absolute indications, highlighting the intricate nature of the diagnostic procedure.

The increase in utilisation of web servers poses a threat to the confidentiality of patient information. Online databases and associated storage devices are vulnerable to unauthorised access and cyber-attacks. In India, the Ministry of Health and Family Welfare has proposed the Healthcare Security Act, which includes provisions for penalising data breaches and promoting the use of electronic records. However, there is a clear lack of regulation regarding the assistance given to mental health practitioners in offering AI services. There are currently no legislative regulations in place to impose responsibility on software developers for technical faults (Ray et al., 2022).

Moreover, the management of mental health relies on interpersonal aptitudes such as establishing a rapport and cultivating associations with patients, while also monitoring their emotional and behavioural tendencies. The absence of crucial components like human compassion and empathy is a substantial barrier in the therapy procedure. Further research into AI applications is crucial in order to mitigate unforeseen tendencies. Prior to incorporating technology into medical practice, a thorough risk assessment and administrative oversight are necessary to ensure its capacity to handle uncommon situations.

AI FOR THERAPY

During the 2000s, the use of Information and Communication Technologies (ICTs) in Clinical Psychology became more common. Virtual Reality (VR) and Telepsychology have become integral to the area, with studies specifically examining the efficacy of VR in cognitive behavioural treatment (CBT) for different mental diseases and health issues. The capacity of virtual reality (VR) to replicate reality has substantial significance in the industry. However, it also gives rise to ethical quandaries, such as the possible consequences of blurring the distinction between actual and virtual worlds, as well as worries around cybersickness. Telepsychology has been used to augment the administration of cognitive behavioural therapy (CBT), with internet-based programmes emerging as crucial instruments in the healthcare system. Nevertheless, there were apprehensions over self-help methods, including self-diagnosis and patients' ability to get all essential self-help information (Botella et al., 2009).

AI has become the dominant force in the 21st century, sparking debates and discussions about its effectiveness and importance in various fields, including psychotherapy. Its use in treatments has garnered attention and raised questions at both personal and societal levels. This has not only led to extensive debate but has also opened up new possibilities for mechanising psychotherapy. Healthcare delivery has expanded beyond the limitations of the waiting room and has really become mobile (Panesar & Panesar, 2021). Numerous research papers have explored the capacity of AI to either aid or function as an active agent in the provision of psychotherapy to patients. Research suggests that the COVID-19 pandemic caused widespread emotional distress and increased the likelihood of mental disorders. These disorders may be directly related to the COVID-19 disease or indirectly caused by strict public health measures that limited personal freedoms and resulted in financial difficulties. Furthermore, the pandemic had a disproportionate effect on those with serious mental health disorders. The impact of this phenomenon was particularly disruptive for young people, with a considerable proportion of them reporting a rise in mental health issues as a direct result of the lockdown measures (Anand et al., 2021).

An effective approach to mitigate the medical and economical consequences of mental illnesses is to use the capabilities of digital health technology to provide supportive, preventative, and therapeutic interventions for those requiring assistance. As a result, digital mental health has become a rapidly growing field of study in the domains of digital health and scientific research. The primary customer or patient population for digital mental health services is largely composed of young people, who are leading the way in adopting all elements of digital technology, including digital health. Mounting research suggests that digital mental health interventions have the capacity to improve mental health conditions, such as depression, in various populations of patients. The beneficial capability of digital mental health technology for continuous and accessible provision of care is especially relevant to mild-to-moderate cases that are not being evaluated and treated, particularly in areas where mental health care resources are under significant pressure due to severe mental illness cases (Wies et al., 2021).

The mental health industry is undergoing a significant change with the introduction of Artificial Intelligence (AI)-enabled treatment, also known as AI-supported therapy. This emerging discipline utilises cutting-edge technology like machine learning and natural language processing to provide therapeutic treatments. AI systems can analyse patient data, detect trends, and suggest therapy plans, so improving the effectiveness of human therapists. An important benefit of AI treatment is its capacity to give 24/7 support, providing instant assistance in emergency situations. This function is especially advantageous in areas with a limited number of mental health specialists, so helping to reduce the disparity in access.

Furthermore, AI is crucial in automating the monitoring of clinical indicators, which may include a wide variety of activities such as online interactions and gamified therapies. The advancement of this discipline requires a cooperative endeavour between mental health experts and technological specialists. This collaboration is essential for facilitating more progress in this field. Chatbots are software programmes that use Artificial Intelligence (AI) to imitate human-like interactions. They are often used on platforms that offer messaging or voice chats. Their use in the field of mental health has been steadily growing, embracing responsibilities like as providing companionship, support, and therapeutic treatments.

Chatbots provide several advantages as compared to traditional in-person or digital interactions. These factors encompass improved accessibility, which ensures that therapeutic support is accessible to a broader range of people; affordability, which reduces the financial obstacles to mental health care; anonymity, which creates a secure environment for individuals to freely express their emotions without concern for criticism; and scalability, which enables the provision of support to multiple individuals simultaneously. This novel approach to mental health treatment represents a hopeful change in the delivery of therapeutic services. Significantly, several chatbots have been created to tackle both the scarcity of mental health experts and the increasing need for digital alternatives to conventional face-to-face treatment.

Woebot, an automated conversational agent, has been created to provide Cognitive Behavioural Therapy (CBT). It has been deemed trustworthy by multiple researchers, particularly in its ability to alleviate depressive symptoms (Balcombe, 2023; Fitzpatrick et al., 2017; Ly et al., 2017; Nicol et al., 2022; Pham et al., 2022). Additionally, it has been proven effective for treating Substance Use Disorders (Prochaska et al., 2021a; Prochaska et al., 2021b). Furthermore, Wysa, Tess, XiaoNan, and TEO, among other chatbots (Leo et al., 2022; Fulmer et al., 2018; Liu et al., 2022; Danieli et al., 2022), have demonstrated efficacy in treating patients with mood-related disorders and Substance Use disorder.

These chatbots have been praised for their convenience, affordability, and easy accessibility, making them viable alternatives to traditional psychotherapy. However, the inherent lack of transparency in the underlying algorithms poses a barrier in predicting the development of these discussions. Existing behavioural studies provide only a limited comprehension of the possible safety issues that might emerge from the rapid and widespread use of this technology. Furthermore, chatbots do not possess the extensive talents that are inherent in a psychiatrist or therapist that has had professional training. Their ability to use individual patient data to assist with the patient's cognitive tasks is limited. In addition, they may lack the nuanced emotional comprehension and compassionate response that is typical of their human counterparts. Currently, there are no direct applications in the therapeutic setting, and there is no established criterion for measuring technical progress. An important concern is around legal liability, prompting the question of who would assume responsibility in the event that the artificial intelligence entity makes a wrong diagnosis or misinterprets a patient's suffering. Although there have been significant technology breakthroughs in this area, mental health practitioners have been slow to accept new technologies. Psychiatrists who prioritise personal connections with patients may have a slower rate of acceptance, suggesting a gradual spread of new ideas throughout the mental health field. Furthermore, the exponential increase in the use of mental health apps adds complexity to the process of assessing risks, which might result in evaluations being conducted after harm has already occurred (Coghlan et al., 2023).

RISK PREDICTION

Risk assessment is often regarded as an essential element in the management of self-inflicted injury and aggressive conduct. Within the field of psychiatry, the objective of risk assessment is to mitigate the negative consequences linked to mental diseases. The technique involves categorising patients into various risk groups according to the likelihood of self-harm or aggressive conduct, with the aim of providing guidance for treatment and management choices (Ryan et al., 2010). The use of risk assessment is increasingly promoted to reduce occurrences of self-harm and violence. On the other hand, the efficiency of risk assessment has been a topic of ongoing and thorough debate. Critics contend that there is no empirical evidence to substantiate the claim that any kind of risk assessment may effectively alleviate the adverse consequences associated with mental health issues. Recently, precision psychiatry has emerged as a promising approach to accurately estimate individualised risks for various clinical outcomes.

Latest studies indicate that specific AI systems could aid in assessing the probability of psychosis onset (Oliver et al., 2021). Initiatives have been undertaken to classify recognized risk elements, enabling medical professionals to sort individuals into categories of lower and higher risk. These implications have significant consequences for treatment choices, such as determining whether to admit a patient to a hospital, either by their own choice or against their will. A considerable proportion of artificial intelligence (AI) endeavours in the field of mental healthcare have been focused on tackling the issue of suicide. Machine Learning (ML) systems have the ability to detect risk factors for suicide by analysing complicated relationships between variables, rather than just looking at them individually. ML approaches used to well-structured datasets have shown connections between suicide risk and clinical characteristics such as ongoing depression, past psychiatric diagnosis, drug use, and treatment history (Passos et al., 2016). Further analysis has shown the influence of environmental variables (Bonner & Rich, 1990; Fernandez-Arteaga et al., 2016).

Researchers have used multi-level modelling of Internet search trends to identify relevant risk variables (Song et al., 2016). Google's data analytics have, in some cases, yielded a more precise assessment of suicide risk compared to conventional self-report scales (Ma-Kellams et al., 2016). Researchers from Vanderbilt University have created an algorithm that can predict the likelihood of suicide by analysing demographic and personal health data obtained from Electronic Medical Records (EMRs). The accuracy of this model in predicting suicide risk was 84-92% within a week and 80-86% within two years, according to Walsh et al. (2017). Comparable results were obtained when Machine Learning was used to forecast the likelihood of teenage suicidality, by amalgamating more than 600 risk indicators retrieved from Electronic Medical Records (EMRs). The precision of the predictions grew as the likelihood of suicide attempts became more imminent (Walsh et al., 2018). Concurrently, scientists at the University of Vermont developed a social media algorithm to identify indicators of depression. This was accomplished by doing a linguistic content analysis of user accounts, with a special emphasis on word count, language use, voice patterns, and activity level (Holley, 2017). BiAffect, a technology developed by the University of Illinois Chicago, employs an iPhone app to scrutinize typing patterns and emotional conditions in individuals suffering from bipolar disorder or major depressive disorder. The Mobile Typing Kinematics method can predict mental health problems and improve patient autonomy, accessibility of treatment, and cost-effectiveness. Digital phenotyping, often known as personal sensing, uses data from personal digital gadgets, particularly smartphones, to anticipate psychological outcomes and mental health disorders. This data, when processed through machine learning techniques, can aid in the selection of effective strategies. Clinical studies are using digital phenotyping to identify first alterations in depression, schizophrenia, and PTSD. Signals obtained from phones or wearables have the potential to enhance or substitute traditional clinical evaluations (Järvelä et al., 2022). Digital phenotyping is also used for monitoring patients with severe mental diseases, detecting a "early warning signal" that indicates the onset of a relapse, therefore facilitating care management.

The integration of Artificial Intelligence (AI) into prediction models and clinical procedures requires addressing privacy concerns, particularly those related to the safe collection, storage, and transfer of Personal Health Information (PHI). The use of internet-based and social media platforms presents inherent security risks that are presently not regulated by existing privacy legislation. The inherent synchronisation features may unintentionally result in the spread of user data across several apps or to third-party entities. The lack of a clear differentiation between private and public material creates challenges in establishing data access limits, especially when anonymized Protected Health Information (PHI) is linked to identifying information. Twitter and Google have faced criticism for violating privacy standards, leading to privacy infringements that may cultivate distrust in the mental healthcare system and discourage patients from seeking assistance. In order to reduce these dangers, it is crucial to expand the range of protective laws for Protected Health Information (PHI) to include possible hazards related to Artificial Intelligence (AI).

The accuracy of Artificial Intelligence (AI) pattern recognition systems in detecting suicidal thoughts gives rise to worries over the possibility of misdiagnosis. This highlights the significance of algorithmic training in correcting mistakes and improving the confidence of the model, while also ensuring optimum processing speed. Moreover, prior to being made available for public use, these algorithms must undergo validation in many situations, since their prediction accuracy may vary across distinct environments. Therefore, it is crucial to train algorithms in order to provide accurate and reliable classification of people (Mulder, 2016).

The significance of ensuring patient safety is of utmost relevance, especially when considering the use of AI technologies. It is crucial to ensure that these programmes can effectively handle users who indicate suicidal inclinations, without causing emotional distress or contributing to thoughts of suicide. The unpredictable and often inappropriate replies from smartphone voice assistants when asked about mental health might have a negative impact on safety concerns and discourage users from seeking help or discussing personal problems. The issue of legal responsibility is a major worry in healthcare settings when incorporating new AI technology (Khosravi et al., 2024). It is crucial to develop standards for evaluating patient eligibility, monitoring outcomes, handling high-risk situations, and controlling costs. Response plans must be developed to address high-risk scenarios, erroneous alerts, and conflicting risk assessments. Moreover, it is essential to establish clear criteria regarding culpability in cases of suicide.

ETHICAL IMPLICATIONS AND CONCERNS

As previously said, it is clear that AI has the capacity to greatly impact the field of mental health treatment. However, it is important to acknowledge that despite the increasing role of AI in mental health care, addressing various issues such as early detection, diagnosis, therapeutic interventions, cost-effective support, personalised treatment, automation of tasks through digitalized healthcare data, and enhancing our understanding of complex disorders, there are significant shortcomings. One of these is the overly accelerated promotion of new AI models that have not yet been evaluated for their viability in real-world settings. The ethical issues in data science may be classified into three primary domains: the ethics pertaining to data management, the ethics linked to artificial intelligence, and the ethics surrounding the methodology used (Egger et al., 2022). The development of machine learning technologies is giving rise to moral and ethical concerns. The administration in this sector is growing at a parallel rate to the advancement of the industry. In the field of AI, there are many instances where there is a lack of established precedents, regulations, or laws (Gordon, 2021). Hence, it is essential for both developers and practitioners to carefully consider the moral and ethical implications of creating intelligent systems.

Bias

One of the most prominent ethical problems associated with the use of AI is **bias**, which may manifest in several ways:

A. Machine Learning bias, also known as algorithmic bias or AI bias, occurs when an algorithm consistently generates biassed results as a result of faulty assumptions made during the machine learning process. This bias may originate from several sources, including the partiality of the designer shown in the data used to train the model. These biases often arise as novel concerns with both nuanced and evident ramifications. Every machine learning algorithm relies on a statistical bias to create predictions about unfamiliar data. Machine bias, however, signifies a bias shown by the data creators. Due to the superior processing speed and capacity of AI compared to humans, it is not always dependable for impartial and unbiased outcomes.
B. Data bias occurs when the data obtained does not correctly represent the population or event being studied. It might also suggest that the data is missing the critical characteristics to accurately predict the event we are trying to foretell.
C. Artificial intelligence systems are created by people, who inevitably have biases and make judgements. Hence, it seems likely that as long as humans continue to be involved in decision-making processes, the existence of bias is unavoidable.
D. AI systems that replicate human cognition have been shown to amplify prejudices, leading to concerns regarding the ethical consequences of AI use. Early cognitive systems constructed utilising demographic data had significant bias about gender, ethnicity, financial level, and other characteristics.

Although it is difficult to totally eliminate prejudice, it is important to recognize that biases might arise in AI systems. Hence, AI developers must be aware about this potential danger and make efforts to reduce biases at every stage of model development. This involves considering possible biases when choosing machine learning technology and methods for training algorithms and programming datasets. Furthermore, augmenting the variety of data might assist in mitigating biases in risk models that rely on machine learning. Simulated model co-creation is a method that promotes responsible modelling by considering the effects of simulations and developing user narratives. In order to address bias in AI research, it is recommended to use approaches such as oversampling, under sampling, and module penalization score (Chauvin et al., 2016; Golbin et al., 2020; Landau et al., 2022; Luxton, 2020; Panesar & Panesar, 2021).

Fairness

The ethical dimension of fairness in AI systems is closely linked to prejudice. This entails the imperative task of ensuring that artificial intelligence does not exhibit favouritism towards any particular group or inflict damage onto certain persons or groups as a result of biassed data or algorithms. Ensuring equality and justice are fundamental ideals that must be upheld in the design, development, and implementation of AI. Ensuring equitable and fair treatment in government regulations and business practices is crucial when introducing new technology and services to neglected populations. The covert algorithms, data analysis systems, and profiling operations of the Big-Data engine should be prohibited from engaging in discriminatory practices. Moreover, the absence of technology awareness and education might limit access to conversational agents such as chatbots. When faced with these situations, it is advisable to explore in-person or community-based programmes as viable options to tackle this disparity in access. The COVID-19 pandemic has highlighted the significance of health equality, given the growing digitization of public health. It is important to ensure that the integration of digital innovations in public health does not unintentionally worsen health inequalities related to socioeconomic level (Al-Hwsali, 2022; Beauchamp, 2008; Beauchamp & Childress, 1994; Karimian et al., 2022; Kim et al., 2021).

Privacy and Security

Expanding upon the discourse around bias, privacy and data security emerge as notable ethical considerations in the field of AI. Given that AI systems often need substantial quantities of data for training and functioning, safeguarding the privacy and security of this data is of utmost importance. This encompasses the protection of personal information and the prevention of unauthorised access or data breaches. It is essential to include security and privacy protocols into the AI development process to guarantee the safeguarding of all AI systems, data, and health-related interactions. Patient data is the fundamental basis for the advancement of artificial intelligence in the field of healthcare. When scholars explore the ethical implications of Artificial Intelligence (AI) systems, they focus heavily on the privacy, confidentiality, and security of user data and information collected via digital mental health apps. Scholars are primarily concerned about the possible consequences that may arise if secret material is shared or made available to other parties. Researchers have contended that insufficiencies in data security while sharing information might have negative consequences that extend to many areas of life, such as work settings, educational establishments, and personal connections with friends, family, or lovers. Studies have been carried out on wearable fitness devices that collect and analyse user data, with the potential to uncover risk factors for many public health problems. These investigations emphasise the possibility of unauthorised access to confidential information, prompting concerns about the proper management of these devices to protect patient privacy and avoid breaches that might have ethical and legal consequences. Users should be informed about any privacy limitations imposed by the administrator. Moreover, it is crucial to acknowledge that research using AI models created using open-source or democratised methods might be compromised by malevolent individuals. It is crucial to develop strong and clear norms, in collaboration with the public health sector, to protect patient confidentiality (European Commission, 2019; Fiske et al., 2019; Morley et al., 2020; Reddy et al., 2020).

The World Health Organisation has established clear rules on this matter. Healthcare personnel have a duty to protect sensitive information, regardless of the manner in which it is kept or received. They should be aware that their professional encounters might establish the limits and regulations of secrecy. In their 2022 publication, Bak et al. examined the ethical quandary of reconciling health data privacy and accessibility within the realm of AI advancements in the healthcare sector. The authors emphasised the inherent trade-offs between safeguarding individual data and the need of using extensive datasets to train AI systems, hence enhancing healthcare outcomes. The authors contend that allocating significant resources to AI development while simultaneously imposing stringent privacy controls that limit data access is both morally wrong and inefficient. Their objective is to support a just and comprehensive approach in establishing national data governance regulations that are in line with public values and goals, so assuring the responsible development of healthcare AI.

Kretzschmar et al. (2019) examined the ethical ramifications of using chatbots to provide mental health assistance to adolescents. The Oxford Neuroscience, Ethics and Society Young People's Advisory Group, including individuals aged 14 to 18, deliberated about the advantages and disadvantages of chatbots. In the context of data gathering and privacy, the authors suggest that the following principles should be followed:

1. It is essential to ensure the protection and confidentiality of any personal information that is acquired.
2. If there is a need to disclose the content of talks, it should be anonymized to guarantee anonymity.

3. Users must be provided with unambiguous and thorough information about privacy measures and any corresponding restrictions.
4. Users should have the option to seek reminders about these privacy arrangements and constraints at any time throughout their contact. This guarantees a constant state of consciousness and comprehension about their rights concerning the privacy of their data.

The "Black Box" Issue

Moreover, the issue of transparency emerges. AI systems, especially those using deep learning, are often known as "black boxes" because of their intricate and obscure decision-making mechanisms. The absence of transparency may result in distrust and presents difficulties in ensuring accountability. Understanding the logic or prediction principles of an AI system may be difficult. The issue of the "black box" is considered a major obstacle to ensuring transparency in the healthcare industry. The absence of transparency may hinder the ability of healthcare professionals and patients to engage in meaningful discussions on the advantages and disadvantages of following a choice made with the assistance of AI. AI-driven diagnostic tools may analyse medical images, such as X-rays, MRIs, and CT scans, to identify patterns. Nevertheless, the lack of openness in the algorithm's decision-making process hinders the verification of the tool's accuracy and the comprehension of its diagnostic technique. Enhanced transparency in the decision-making process promotes better governance by offering a more comprehensible insight into the utilisation and implementation of models. The assignment of responsibility in AI is complex, mainly because of the absence of transparency (Anderson & Anderson, 2019; Braun et al., 2021; Buruk et al., 2020; Liyanage et al., 2019).

Consequently, people may experience a loss of the capacity to oversee decision-making processes and may find it difficult to understand the rationale behind less-than-ideal decisions. Hence, it is important to comprehend the decision-making methods used by this technology.

Responsibility and Accountability

Ultimately, the ethical concern of utmost importance is the responsibility and accountability for judgements made by AI systems. Addressing the subject of accountability for mistakes or damage caused by an AI system is a challenging and intricate matter. The ethical dilemma with accountability in AI systems mostly centres on the lack of clearly defined criteria for accountability or corresponding ethical obligations to protect users who are using mental health services. Unlike traditional therapy, which is obligated by ethical responsibilities to safeguard the client's welfare, AI therapy apps sometimes lack proper professional oversight. This prompts inquiries about the organisation accountable for ensuring the user's security, confidentiality, and general welfare. Accountability is essential in the field of public health technology, namely in the creation, advancement, and use of AI-driven solutions including health promotion, illness prevention, treatment methods, and disease diagnostics. It is crucial to carefully examine these judgements in order to determine their suitability for the general public. The obligation is significant and mostly lies with the man in charge of these activities. Therefore, it is essential for all healthcare workers to improve their expertise in managing AI technologies. It is crucial to avoid mistakes that have the potential to greatly affect the health of the community (Horvitz & Mulligan, 2015; Matthias, 2004; Nebeker et al., 2019; Omrani et al., 2022; World Health Organization, 2021).

Ultimately, while AI has the promise of transforming several facets of human existence, it is imperative to address these ethical dilemmas in order to guarantee its conscientious and advantageous use. As we strive to make advancements and expand the capabilities of AI, it is imperative that we consistently evaluate and tackle the ethical concerns associated with it.

RECOMMENDATIONS FOR RESPONSIBLE DEVELOPMENT AND DEPLOYMENT

In order to ensure the responsible development and implementation of AI in mental health care, it is crucial to adopt a comprehensive strategy that places emphasis on ethical principles, fair provision of services, and cooperative resolution of issues. The ethical principles for AI developers and practitioners should emphasize the significance of openness, informed consent, and privacy. It is crucial to ensure that AI systems are created with a deep regard for patient autonomy and confidentiality. Furthermore, it is essential to establish policies that ensure fair and impartial delivery of AI services in order to address and reduce inequalities in access to mental health treatment. These policies should focus on bridging the gap in access to digital resources and aim to develop AI tools that are culturally sensitive and available to a wide range of communities.

Finally, the use of collaborative methods is crucial for overcoming obstacles in the implementation process. This entails cultivating collaborations among technologists, physicians, patients, and politicians to collaboratively develop solutions that are both technically viable, therapeutically applicable, and socially agreeable. These coordinated endeavors will not only increase the reliability of AI applications but also guarantee their conformity with the main objective of enhancing mental health outcomes.

CONCLUSION

At the junction of technical advancement and mental health care, the emergence of Artificial Intelligence (AI) presents unparalleled prospects for improving the quality and availability of therapy. Nevertheless, this auspicious future is not without of its ethical dilemmas. Incorporating AI into mental health treatments requires a careful and ethical strategy to prioritise the well-being of patients. The ethical implications of artificial intelligence in the field of mental health are many. The preservation of privacy and secrecy is of paramount importance, given the extensive data necessary to fuel AI systems, which has the potential to jeopardise sensitive personal information. Implementing strong data protection measures is essential for sustaining the trust that is the basis of any therapeutic engagement.

Obtaining informed permission is an essential aspect of ethical conduct. Patients must be informed on the specific ways in which artificial intelligence (AI) will be used in their healthcare, including both the possible advantages and disadvantages. The intricate nature of AI systems presents a difficulty in achieving transparency, but, it is a difficulty that necessitates explicit communication and education. AI systems that exhibit bias and lack justice might result in unequal treatment, particularly impacting marginalised populations. Developing and training AI systems on various datasets is crucial in order to reduce biases and ensure fair treatment results. The opaque nature of several AI systems gives rise to concerns over transparency and comprehensibility. Healthcare practitioners must possess the capacity to comprehend and communicate the rationale behind AI-generated suggestions in order to uphold responsibility and maintain patient confidence.

The use of artificial intelligence into mental health treatment also has an effect on the therapeutic interaction. Although AI has the potential to enhance the skills of healthcare professionals, it is crucial to maintain the fundamental human aspect that is vital to the process of healing and recuperation. The growth of AI technology has outpaced the establishment of effective oversight and regulation, resulting in a governance vacuum that has to be resolved. It is essential to establish precise norms and standards for artificial intelligence (AI) in mental health treatment in order to protect the interests of patients. The process of attributing responsibility and accountability for judgements made by artificial intelligence, especially in cases when negative results occur, is intricate. It is crucial to establish a distinct and unambiguous assignment of responsibility between AI developers, healthcare providers, and the technology itself.

The use of AI in mental health treatment has the capacity to revolutionise the field, but it also poses the danger of devaluing the expertise of professionals or compromising the standard of care if employed as a replacement for human decision-making. It is crucial that AI be used as a tool to enhance, rather than replace, professional skills. Ultimately, cultural sensitivity is of utmost importance in the field of mental health treatment. AI systems should be built to include cultural diversity in order to guarantee that the therapy provided is courteous and suitable for all patients. Essentially, ensuring the ethical use of AI in mental health treatment involves carefully managing the utilisation of technology progress while maintaining the moral obligations of the medical field. As we plan for the future, it is our shared duty to have ongoing discussions and thoughtful thinking, making sure that AI is used in a way that supports mental health in a sincere, caring, and respectful manner for everyone.

REFERENCES

Anand, V., Verma, L., Aggarwal, A., Nanjundappa, P., & Rai, H. (2021). COVID-19 and psychological distress: Lessons for India. *PLoS One*, 16(8), e0255683. DOI: 10.1371/journal.pone.0255683 PMID: 34347847

Anderson, M., & Anderson, S. L. (2019). How should AI be developed, validated, and implemented in patient care? *AMA Journal of Ethics*, 21(2), 125–130. DOI: 10.1001/amajethics.2019.125 PMID: 30794121

Andersson, S., Bathula, D. R., Iliadis, S. I., Walter, M., & Skalkidou, A. (2021). Predicting women with depressive symptoms postpartum with machine learning methods. *Scientific Reports*, 11(1), 7877. DOI: 10.1038/s41598-021-86368-y PMID: 33846362

Andrew, J., Rudra, M., Eunice, J., & Belfin, R. V. (2023). Artificial intelligence in adolescents mental health disorder diagnosis, prognosis, and treatment. *Frontiers in Public Health*, 11, 1110088. DOI: 10.3389/fpubh.2023.1110088 PMID: 37064712

Appaji, A., Nagendra, B., Chako, D. M., Padmanabha, A., Jacob, A., Hiremath, C. V., Varambally, S., Kesavan, M., Venkatasubramanian, G., Rao, S. V., Webers, C. A. B., Berendschot, T. T. J. M., & Rao, N. P. (2019). Examination of retinal vascular trajectory in schizophrenia and bipolar disorder. *Psychiatry and Clinical Neurosciences*, 73(12), 738–744. DOI: 10.1111/pcn.12921 PMID: 31400288

Ayano, G., Demelash, S., Yohannes, Z., Haile, K., Tulu, M., Assefa, D., Tesfaye, A., Haile, K., Solomon, M., Chaka, A., & Tsegay, L. (2021). Misdiagnosis, detection rate, and associated factors of severe psychiatric disorders in specialized psychiatry centers in Ethiopia. *Annals of General Psychiatry*, 20(1), 1–10. DOI: 10.1186/s12991-021-00333-7 PMID: 33531016

Bak, M., Madai, V. I., Fritzsche, M. C., Mayrhofer, M. T., & McLennan, S. (2022). You can't have ai both ways: Balancing health data privacy and access fairly. *Frontiers in Genetics*, 13, 929453. DOI: 10.3389/fgene.2022.929453 PMID: 35769991

Bakator, M., & Radosav, D. (2018). Deep learning and medical diagnosis: A review of literature. *Multimodal Technologies and Interaction*, 2(3), 47. DOI: 10.3390/mti2030047

Balcombe, L. (2023, October). AI chatbots in digital mental health. [). MDPI.]. *Informatics (MDPI)*, 10(4), 82. DOI: 10.3390/informatics10040082

Bansal, D., Chhikara, R., Khanna, K., & Gupta, P. (2018). Comparative analysis of various machine learning algorithms for detecting dementia. *Procedia Computer Science*, 132, 1497–1502. DOI: 10.1016/j.procs.2018.05.102

Beauchamp, T. (2008). The principle of beneficence in applied ethics.

Beauchamp, T. L., & Childress, J. F. (1994). The capacity for autonomous choice. *Principles of Biomedical Ethics*, 120-142.

Beg, M. J., & Verma, M. K. (2023). *The Mind and Machine: An Introduction to Artificial Intelligence: Exploring the Intersection of Artificial Intelligence, Human Cognition, Psychology and Robotics*. Amazon International.

Bhagyashree, S. I. R., Nagaraj, K., Prince, M., Fall, C. H., & Krishna, M. (2018). Diagnosis of Dementia by Machine learning methods in Epidemiological studies: A pilot exploratory study from south India. *Social Psychiatry and Psychiatric Epidemiology*, 53(1), 77–86. DOI: 10.1007/s00127-017-1410-0 PMID: 28698926

Bonner, R. L., & Rich, A. R. (1990). Psychosocial vulnerability, life stress, and suicide ideation in a jail population: A cross-validation study. *Suicide & Life-Threatening Behavior*, 20(3), 213–224. DOI: 10.1111/j.1943-278X.1990.tb00106.x PMID: 2238014

Botella, C., Díaz-García, A., Baños, R. M., & Quero, S. (2009). Cybertherapy: Advantages, limitations, and ethical issues.

Braun, M., Hummel, P., Beck, S., & Dabrock, P. (2021). Primer on an ethics of AI-based decision support systems in the clinic. *Journal of Medical Ethics*, 47(12), e3–e3. DOI: 10.1136/medethics-2019-105860 PMID: 32245804

Buruk, B., Ekmekci, P. E., & Arda, B. (2020). A critical perspective on guidelines for responsible and trustworthy artificial intelligence. *Medicine, Health Care, and Philosophy*, 23(3), 387–399. DOI: 10.1007/s11019-020-09948-1 PMID: 32236794

Chauvin, J., Perera, Y., & Clarke, M. (2016). Digital technologies for population health and health equity gains: The perspective of public health associations. *Journal of Public Health Policy*, 37(S2), 232–248. DOI: 10.1057/s41271-016-0013-4 PMID: 27899798

Cicek, G., & Akan, A. (2021, November). Deep Learning Approach Versus Traditional Machine Learning for ADHD Classification. In *2021 Medical Technologies Congress (TIPTEKNO)* (pp. 1-4). IEEE. DOI: 10.1109/TIPTEKNO53239.2021.9632940

Coghlan, S., Leins, K., Sheldrick, S., Cheong, M., Gooding, P., & D'Alfonso, S. (2023). To chat or bot to chat: Ethical issues with using chatbots in mental health. *Digital Health*, 9, 20552076231183542. DOI: 10.1177/20552076231183542 PMID: 37377565

Colizzi, M., Lasalvia, A., & Ruggeri, M. (2020). Prevention and early intervention in youth mental health: Is it time for a multidisciplinary and trans-diagnostic model for care? *International Journal of Mental Health Systems*, 14(1), 1–14. DOI: 10.1186/s13033-020-00356-9 PMID: 32226481

Costello, E. J. (2016). Early detection and prevention of mental health problems: Developmental epidemiology and systems of support. *Journal of Clinical Child and Adolescent Psychology*, 45(6), 710–717. DOI: 10.1080/15374416.2016.1236728 PMID: 27858462

Danieli, M., Ciulli, T., Mousavi, S. M., Silvestri, G., Barbato, S., Di Natale, L., & Riccardi, G. (2022). Assessing the impact of conversational artificial intelligence in the treatment of stress and anxiety in aging adults: Randomized controlled trial. *JMIR Mental Health*, 9(9), e38067. DOI: 10.2196/38067 PMID: 36149730

Ding, M., Huo, Y., Hu, J., & Lu, Z. (2018). DeepInsight: Multi-Task Multi-Scale Deep Learning for Mental Disorder Diagnosis. In *BMVC* (p. 115).

Egger, R., Neuburger, L., & Mattuzzi, M. (2022). Data science and ethical issues: between knowledge gain and ethical responsibility. In *Applied Data Science in Tourism: Interdisciplinary Approaches, Methodologies, and Applications* (pp. 51–66). Springer International Publishing. DOI: 10.1007/978-3-030-88389-8_4

European Commission. (2019). Directorate General for Communications Networks, Content and Technology. *Ethics guidelines for trustworthy AI.*

Fernández-Arteaga, V., Tovilla-Zárate, C. A., Fresán, A., González-Castro, T. B., Juárez-Rojop, I. E., López-Narváez, L., & Hernández-Díaz, Y. (2016). Association between completed suicide and environmental temperature in a Mexican population, using the Knowledge Discovery in Database approach. *Computer Methods and Programs in Biomedicine*, 135, 219–224. DOI: 10.1016/j.cmpb.2016.08.002 PMID: 27586493

Fiske, A., Henningsen, P., & Buyx, A. (2019). Your robot therapist will see you now: Ethical implications of embodied artificial intelligence in psychiatry, psychology, and psychotherapy. *Journal of Medical Internet Research*, 21(5), e13216. DOI: 10.2196/13216 PMID: 31094356

Fitzpatrick, K. K., Darcy, A., & Vierhile, M. (2017). Delivering cognitive behavior therapy to young adults with symptoms of depression and anxiety using a fully automated conversational agent (Woebot): A randomized controlled trial. *JMIR Mental Health*, 4(2), e7785. DOI: 10.2196/mental.7785 PMID: 28588005

Fulmer, R., Joerin, A., Gentile, B., Lakerink, L., & Rauws, M. (2018). Using psychological artificial intelligence (Tess) to relieve symptoms of depression and anxiety: Randomized controlled trial. *JMIR Mental Health*, 5(4), e9782. DOI: 10.2196/mental.9782 PMID: 30545815

Golbin, I., Rao, A. S., Hadjarian, A., & Krittman, D. (2020, December). Responsible AI: a primer for the legal community. In *2020 IEEE international conference on big data (big data)* (pp. 2121-2126). IEEE. DOI: 10.1109/BigData50022.2020.9377738

Gordon, J. S. (2021). AI and law: ethical, legal, and socio-political implications. *ai & Society, 36*, 403-404.

Graham, S., Depp, C., Lee, E. E., Nebeker, C., Tu, X., Kim, H. C., & Jeste, D. V. (2019). Artificial intelligence for mental health and mental illnesses: An overview. *Current Psychiatry Reports*, 21(11), 1–18. DOI: 10.1007/s11920-019-1094-0 PMID: 31701320

Guidance, W. H. O. (2021). *Ethics and governance of artificial intelligence for health*. World Health Organization.

Gupta, M. D., Jha, M. K., Bansal, A., Yadav, R., Ramakrishanan, S., Girish, M. P., Sarkar, P. G., Qamar, A., Kumar, S., Kumar, S., Jain, A., Saijpaul, R., Gupta, V., Kansal, D., Garg, S., Arora, S., Biswas, P. S., Yusuf, J., Malhotra, R. K., & Gupta, A. (2021). COVID 19-related burnout among healthcare workers in India and ECG based predictive machine learning model: Insights from the BRUCEE-Li study. *Indian Heart Journal*, 73(6), 674–681. DOI: 10.1016/j.ihj.2021.10.002 PMID: 34673026

Hilal, A. M., Issaoui, I., Obayya, M., Al-Wesabi, F. N., Nemri, N., Hamza, M. A., & Zamani, A. S. (2022). Modeling of Explainable Artificial Intelligence for Biomedical Mental Disorder Diagnosis. *Computers, Materials & Continua*, 71(2).

Horvitz, E., & Mulligan, D. (2015). Data, privacy, and the greater good. *Science*, 349(6245), 253–255. DOI: 10.1126/science.aac4520 PMID: 26185242

Järvelä, K., Takala, P., Michard, F., & Vikatmaa, L. (2022). Clinical evaluation of a wearable sensor for mobile monitoring of respiratory rate on hospital wards. *Journal of Clinical Monitoring and Computing*, 36(1), 81–86. DOI: 10.1007/s10877-021-00753-6 PMID: 34476669

Jin, K. W., Li, Q., Xie, Y., & Xiao, G. (2023). Artificial intelligence in mental healthcare: An overview and future perspectives. *The British Journal of Radiology*, 96(1150), 20230213. DOI: 10.1259/bjr.20230213 PMID: 37698582

Karthik, S., & Sudha, M. (2021). Predicting bipolar disorder and schizophrenia based on non-overlapping genetic phenotypes using deep neural network. *Evolutionary Intelligence*, 14(2), 619–634. DOI: 10.1007/s12065-019-00346-y

Khosravi, M., Zare, Z., Mojtabaeian, S. M., & Izadi, R. (2024). Ethical challenges of using artificial intelligence in healthcare delivery: A thematic analysis of a systematic review of reviews. *Journal of Public Health (Berlin)*, •••, 1–11. DOI: 10.1007/s10389-024-02219-w

Kim, J. W., Jones, K. L., & D'Angelo, E. (2019). How to prepare prospective psychiatrists in the era of artificial intelligence. *Academic Psychiatry*, 43(3), 337–339. DOI: 10.1007/s40596-019-01025-x PMID: 30659443

Kim, T. W., Hooker, J., & Donaldson, T. (2021). Taking principles seriously: A hybrid approach to value alignment in artificial intelligence. *Journal of Artificial Intelligence Research*, 70, 871–890. DOI: 10.1613/jair.1.12481

Ko, D. W., & Yang, J. J. (2022). EEG-Based schizophrenia diagnosis through time series image conversion and deep learning. *Electronics (Basel)*, 11(14), 2265. DOI: 10.3390/electronics11142265

Kuang, D., & He, L. (2014, November). Classification on ADHD with deep learning. In *2014 International Conference on Cloud Computing and Big Data* (pp. 27-32). IEEE. DOI: 10.1109/CCBD.2014.42

Landau, A. Y., Ferrarello, S., Blanchard, A., Cato, K., Atkins, N., Salazar, S., Patton, D. U., & Topaz, M. (2022). Developing machine learning-based models to help identify child abuse and neglect: Key ethical challenges and recommended solutions. *Journal of the American Medical Informatics Association : JAMIA*, 29(3), 576–580. DOI: 10.1093/jamia/ocab286 PMID: 35024859

Lee, D., & Yoon, S. N. (2021). Application of artificial intelligence-based technologies in the healthcare industry: Opportunities and challenges. *International Journal of Environmental Research and Public Health*, 18(1), 271. DOI: 10.3390/ijerph18010271 PMID: 33401373

Lee, E. E., Torous, J., De Choudhury, M., Depp, C. A., Graham, S. A., Kim, H. C., Paulus, M. P., Krystal, J. H., & Jeste, D. V. (2021). Artificial intelligence for mental health care: Clinical applications, barriers, facilitators, and artificial wisdom. *Biological Psychiatry: Cognitive Neuroscience and Neuroimaging*, 6(9), 856–864. DOI: 10.1016/j.bpsc.2021.02.001 PMID: 33571718

Leo, A. J., Schuelke, M. J., Hunt, D. M., Metzler, J. P., Miller, J. P., Areán, P. A., Armbrecht, M. A., & Cheng, A. L. (2022). A digital mental health intervention in an orthopedic setting for patients with symptoms of depression and/or anxiety: Feasibility prospective cohort study. *JMIR Formative Research*, 6(2), e34889. DOI: 10.2196/34889 PMID: 35039278

Liu, H., Peng, H., Song, X., Xu, C., & Zhang, M. (2022). Using AI chatbots to provide self-help depression interventions for university students: A randomized trial of effectiveness. *Internet Interventions : the Application of Information Technology in Mental and Behavioural Health*, 27, 100495. DOI: 10.1016/j.invent.2022.100495 PMID: 35059305

Liyanage, H., Liaw, S. T., Jonnagaddala, J., Schreiber, R., Kuziemsky, C., Terry, A. L., & de Lusignan, S. (2019). Artificial intelligence in primary health care: perceptions, issues, and challenges. *Yearbook of medical informatics, 28*(01), 041-046.

Loh, H. W., Ooi, C. P., Barua, P. D., Palmer, E. E., Molinari, F., & Acharya, U. R. (2022). Automated detection of ADHD: Current trends and future perspective. *Computers in Biology and Medicine*, 146, 105525. DOI: 10.1016/j.compbiomed.2022.105525 PMID: 35468405

Luxton, D. D. (2020). Ethical implications of conversational agents in global public health. *Bulletin of the World Health Organization*, 98(4), 285–287. DOI: 10.2471/BLT.19.237636 PMID: 32284654

Ly, K. H., Ly, A. M., & Andersson, G. (2017). A fully automated conversational agent for promoting mental well-being: A pilot RCT using mixed methods. *Internet Interventions : the Application of Information Technology in Mental and Behavioural Health*, 10, 39–46. DOI: 10.1016/j.invent.2017.10.002 PMID: 30135751

Mahendran, N., Vincent, P. D. R., Srinivasan, K., Sharma, V., & Jayakody, D. K. (2020). Realizing a stacking generalization model to improve the prediction accuracy of major depressive disorder in adults. *IEEE Access : Practical Innovations, Open Solutions*, 8, 49509–49522. DOI: 10.1109/ACCESS.2020.2977887

Maniruzzaman, M., Shin, J., & Hasan, M. A. M. (2022). Predicting children with ADHD using behavioral activity: A machine learning analysis. *Applied Sciences (Basel, Switzerland)*, 12(5), 2737. DOI: 10.3390/app12052737

Matthias, A. (2004). The responsibility gap: Ascribing responsibility for the actions of learning automata. *Ethics and Information Technology*, 6(3), 175–183. DOI: 10.1007/s10676-004-3422-1

McCorduck, P., & Cfe, C. (2004). *Machines who think: A personal inquiry into the history and prospects of artificial intelligence*. AK Peters/CRC Press.Lee. DOI: 10.1201/9780429258985

Milne-Ives, M., Selby, E., Inkster, B., Lam, C., & Meinert, E. (2022). Artificial intelligence and machine learning in mobile apps for mental health: A scoping review. *PLOS Digital Health*, 1(8), e0000079. DOI: 10.1371/journal.pdig.0000079 PMID: 36812623

Morley, J., Floridi, L., Kinsey, L., & Elhalal, A. (2020). From what to how: An initial review of publicly available AI ethics tools, methods and research to translate principles into practices. *Science and Engineering Ethics*, 26(4), 2141–2168. DOI: 10.1007/s11948-019-00165-5 PMID: 31828533

Mulder, R., Newton-Howes, G., & Coid, J. W. (2016). The futility of risk prediction in psychiatry. *The British Journal of Psychiatry*, 209(4), 271–272. DOI: 10.1192/bjp.bp.116.184960 PMID: 27698212

Nebeker, C., Torous, J., & Bartlett Ellis, R. J. (2019). Building the case for actionable ethics in digital health research supported by artificial intelligence. *BMC Medicine*, 17(1), 1–7. DOI: 10.1186/s12916-019-1377-7 PMID: 31311535

Nicol, G., Wang, R., Graham, S., Dodd, S., & Garbutt, J. (2022). Chatbot-delivered cognitive behavioral therapy in adolescents with depression and anxiety during the COVID-19 pandemic: Feasibility and acceptability study. *JMIR Formative Research*, 6(11), e40242. DOI: 10.2196/40242 PMID: 36413390

Obasa, A. E. (2023). The Ethics of Artificial Intelligence in Healthcare Settings.

Oliver, D., Spada, G., Colling, C., Broadbent, M., Baldwin, H., Patel, R., Stewart, R., Stahl, D., Dobson, R., McGuire, P., & Fusar-Poli, P. (2021). Real-world implementation of precision psychiatry: Transdiagnostic risk calculator for the automatic detection of individuals at-risk of psychosis. *Schizophrenia Research*, 227, 52–60. DOI: 10.1016/j.schres.2020.05.007 PMID: 32571619

Omrani, N., Rivieccio, G., Fiore, U., Schiavone, F., & Agreda, S. G. (2022). To trust or not to trust? An assessment of trust in AI-based systems: Concerns, ethics and contexts. *Technological Forecasting and Social Change*, 181, 121763. DOI: 10.1016/j.techfore.2022.121763

Pandey, A., & Misra, M. (2023). Artificial Intelligence in Mental Health Care. In Yadav, D. K., & Gulati, A. (Eds.), *Artificial Intelligence and Machine Learning in Healthcare*. Springer., DOI: 10.1007/978-981-99-6472-7_8

Panesar, A., & Panesar, H. (2021). Artificial intelligence and machine learning in global healthcare. In *Handbook of Global Health* (pp. 1775–1813). Springer International Publishing. DOI: 10.1007/978-3-030-45009-0_75

Pang, Z., Yuan, H., Zhang, Y. T., & Packirisamy, M. (2018). Guest editorial health engineering driven by the industry 4.0 for aging society. *IEEE Journal of Biomedical and Health Informatics*, 22(6), 1709–1710. DOI: 10.1109/JBHI.2018.2874081

Passos, I. C., Mwangi, B., Cao, B., Hamilton, J. E., Wu, M. J., Zhang, X. Y., Zunta-Soares, G. B., Quevedo, J., Kauer-Sant'Anna, M., Kapczinski, F., & Soares, J. C. (2016). Identifying a clinical signature of suicidality among patients with mood disorders: A pilot study using a machine learning approach. *Journal of Affective Disorders*, 193, 109–116. DOI: 10.1016/j.jad.2015.12.066 PMID: 26773901

Pham, K. T., Nabizadeh, A., & Selek, S. (2022). Artificial intelligence and chatbots in psychiatry. *The Psychiatric Quarterly*, 93(1), 249–253. DOI: 10.1007/s11126-022-09973-8 PMID: 35212940

Prabhakar, S. K., Rajaguru, H., & Sun-Hee, K. (2020). Schizophrenia EEG signal classification based on swarm intelligence computing. *Computational Intelligence and Neuroscience: CIN, 2020.*

Prochaska, J. J., Vogel, E. A., Chieng, A., Baiocchi, M., Maglalang, D. D., Pajarito, S., Weingardt, K. R., Darcy, A., & Robinson, A. (2021). A randomized controlled trial of a therapeutic relational agent for reducing substance misuse during the COVID-19 pandemic. *Drug and Alcohol Dependence*, 227, 108986. DOI: 10.1016/j.drugalcdep.2021.108986 PMID: 34507061

Prochaska, J. J., Vogel, E. A., Chieng, A., Kendra, M., Baiocchi, M., Pajarito, S., & Robinson, A. (2021). A therapeutic relational agent for reducing problematic substance use (Woebot): Development and usability study. *Journal of Medical Internet Research*, 23(3), e24850. DOI: 10.2196/24850 PMID: 33755028

Rajagopalan, S. S., Bhardwaj, S., Panda, R., Reddam, V. R., Ganne, C., Kenchaiah, R., & Bharath, R. D. (2018). Machine learning detects EEG microstate alterations in patients living with temporal lobe epilepsy. *Seizure*, 61, 8–13. DOI: 10.1016/j.seizure.2018.07.007 PMID: 30044996

Rajaram, A. K. P., Saproo, S., & Bansal, S. (2023). A Novel 4A Framework for Measuring Outcomes of Technological Implementation in The Healthcare Industry. *Int. J. Life Sci. Pharma Res,* 13(2), P135-P143.

Ray, A., Bhardwaj, A., Malik, Y. K., Singh, S., & Gupta, R. (2022). Artificial intelligence and Psychiatry: An overview. *Asian Journal of Psychiatry*, 70, 103021. DOI: 10.1016/j.ajp.2022.103021 PMID: 35219978

Reddy, S., Allan, S., Coghlan, S., & Cooper, P. (2020). A governance model for the application of AI in health care. *Journal of the American Medical Informatics Association : JAMIA*, 27(3), 491–497. DOI: 10.1093/jamia/ocz192 PMID: 31682262

Russell, S. J., & Norvig, P. (2016). *Artificial intelligence: a modern approach.* Pearson.

Ryan, C., Nielssen, O., Paton, M., & Large, M. (2010). Clinical decisions in psychiatry should not be based on risk assessment. *Australasian Psychiatry*, 18(5), 398–403. DOI: 10.3109/10398562.2010.507816 PMID: 20863176

Salamanca-Buentello, F., Seeman, M. V., Daar, A. S., & Upshur, R. E. (2020). The ethical, social, and cultural dimensions of screening for mental health in children and adolescents of the developing world. *PLoS One*, 15(8), e0237853. DOI: 10.1371/journal.pone.0237853 PMID: 32834012

Sallstrom, L., Morris, O., & Mehta, H. (2019). Artificial intelligence in Africa's healthcare: Ethical considerations. *ORF Issue Brief*, 312, 1–11.

Schwab, K. (2017). *The Fourth Industrial Revolution; Currency.* Google Scholar Google Scholar Digital Library Digital Library.

Shatte, A. B., Hutchinson, D. M., & Teague, S. J. (2019). Machine learning in mental health: A scoping review of methods and applications. *Psychological Medicine*, 49(9), 1426–1448. DOI: 10.1017/S0033291719000151 PMID: 30744717

Shin, J., & Bae, S. M. (2023). A systematic review of location data for depression prediction. *International Journal of Environmental Research and Public Health*, 20(11), 5984. DOI: 10.3390/ijerph20115984 PMID: 37297588

Tanir, D., & Karakas, A. B. (2023). The Use of AI and Structural Magnetic Resonance Imaging in the Diagnosis of Major Depressive Disorder. In *Machine Learning and AI Techniques in Interactive Medical Image Analysis* (pp. 167–187). IGI Global.

Thieme, A., Belgrave, D., & Doherty, G. (2020). Machine learning in mental health: A systematic review of the HCI literature to support the development of effective and implementable ML systems. *ACM Transactions on Computer-Human Interaction*, 27(5), 1–53. DOI: 10.1145/3398069

Tikka, S. K., Singh, B. K., Nizamie, S. H., Garg, S., Mandal, S., Thakur, K., & Singh, L. K. (2020). Artificial intelligence-based classification of schizophrenia: A high density electroencephalographic and support vector machine study. *Indian Journal of Psychiatry*, 62(3), 273–282. DOI: 10.4103/psychiatry.IndianJPsychiatry_91_20 PMID: 32773870

Tolentino, J. C., & Schmidt, S. L. (2018). DSM-5 criteria and depression severity: Implications for clinical practice. *Frontiers in Psychiatry*, 9, 412752. DOI: 10.3389/fpsyt.2018.00450 PMID: 30333763

Topol, E. (2019). *Deep medicine: how artificial intelligence can make healthcare human again.*

Vares, E. A., Salum, G. A., Spanemberg, L., Caldieraro, M. A., & Fleck, M. P. (2015). Depression dimensions: Integrating clinical signs and symptoms from the perspectives of clinicians and patients. *PLoS One*, 10(8), e0136037. DOI: 10.1371/journal.pone.0136037 PMID: 26313556

Vinutha, N., Pattar, S., Sharma, S., Shenoy, P. D., & Venugopal, K. R. (2020). A machine learning framework for assessment of cognitive and functional impairments in Alzheimer's disease: Data preprocessing and analysis. *The Journal of Prevention of Alzheimer's Disease*, 7(2), 87–94. DOI: 10.14283/jpad.2020.7 PMID: 32236397

Wies, B., Landers, C., & Ienca, M. (2021). Digital mental health for young people: A scoping review of ethical promises and challenges. *Frontiers in Digital Health*, 3, 697072. DOI: 10.3389/fdgth.2021.697072 PMID: 34713173

Yan, W. J., Ruan, Q. N., & Jiang, K. (2022). Challenges for artificial intelligence in recognizing mental disorders. *Diagnostics (Basel)*, 13(1), 2. DOI: 10.3390/diagnostics13010002 PMID: 36611294

Zhang, Z., Lin, W., Liu, M., & Mahmoud, M. (2020, November). Multimodal deep learning framework for mental disorder recognition. In *2020 15th IEEE International Conference on Automatic Face and Gesture Recognition (FG 2020)* (pp. 344-350). IEEE. DOI: 10.1109/FG47880.2020.00033

Chapter 10
The Ethical Aspects of Chatbots and Beyond

Nafees Ahmad
https://orcid.org/0000-0003-2120-4750
Central South University, China

ABSTRACT

The ethical considerations surrounding chatbots extend well beyond simple functionality, touching on nuanced areas of trust, societal impact, and moral responsibility. Chatbots frequently handle sensitive user data, such as personal information, financial details, or health records. This raises significant privacy and data security concerns. Developers must ensure that data collection adheres to stringent standards, such as those outlined in the General Data Protection Regulation (GDPR) or other privacy regulations. Any misuse, such as sharing data with third parties without consent, undermines user trust and poses legal and ethical dilemmas. The importance of encryption, secure servers, and transparent data handling policies cannot be overstated in mitigating these risks. Here the authors discuss some ethical aspects such as bias in chatbot algorithms, transparency, accountability, and emotional impact.

1. BIAS IN CHATBOT ALGORITHMS: A PRESSING ETHICAL ISSUE

Bias in chatbot algorithms is an increasingly recognized ethical concern, as it can have profound implications for both the fairness of AI interactions and the well-being of users. Chatbots, powered by machine learning and natural language processing (NLP), are trained on vast datasets that are often derived from human interactions, which inherently contain biases. These biases can manifest in a variety of ways, such as gender, racial, and socio-economic biases, that reflect broader societal prejudices.

DOI: 10.4018/979-8-3693-3112-5.ch010

When these biases are embedded into chatbot algorithms, the consequences can range from subtle reinforcement of stereotypes to more overt discrimination. For instance, research has shown that certain AI models exhibit gendered biases, such as associating female names with supportive roles and male names with leadership positions, which can perpetuate harmful societal norms (Bolukbasi et al., 2016). Such biases within chatbot algorithms not only undermine the trust users place in these systems but also exacerbate existing social inequalities.

One of the primary causes of bias in chatbot algorithms is the training data. AI systems learn patterns from the data they are fed, and if the data reflects historical biases or is unrepresentative of diverse populations, these biases are likely to be encoded into the system. For example, if a chatbot is trained on historical customer service interactions that predominantly feature English-speaking, middle-class individuals, it may struggle to understand or respond appropriately to users with different dialects, accents, or cultural backgrounds. This bias can lead to unfair or suboptimal user experiences, where certain groups are either misunderstood or ignored by the chatbot. A report by the AI Now Institute (2018) (Whittaker et al., 2018) highlighted how AI systems, including chatbots, often perform poorly when interacting with marginalized communities, further perpetuating disparities in access to services and resources. These biased outcomes can harm users, especially when chatbots are deployed in sensitive areas such as healthcare, legal advice, or financial services.

The presence of bias in chatbot algorithms can also have serious consequences for businesses and organizations that deploy these systems. Chatbots that exhibit biased behavior risk alienating a significant portion of their user base, leading to customer dissatisfaction, decreased loyalty, and reputational damage. For instance, if a chatbot in a healthcare setting provides inaccurate or culturally insensitive advice to minority groups, it may lead to harmful health outcomes for these individuals. This not only raises ethical concerns but can also result in legal repercussions for businesses that fail to ensure their AI systems are fair and inclusive. Therefore, addressing bias in chatbot algorithms is not only an ethical imperative but also a business necessity to protect consumer trust and avoid potential financial and legal costs (Binns et al., 2018).

In response to these concerns, developers and researchers are actively working on methods to identify and mitigate bias in AI systems, including chatbots. One approach involves increasing the diversity of the datasets used to train chatbots, ensuring that these datasets are representative of various demographics, languages, and cultural contexts. Additionally, techniques such as fairness-aware machine learning and adversarial testing are being employed to detect and reduce biases during the development process. These strategies aim to identify and address potential biases before chatbots are deployed, ensuring that their behavior aligns with ethical principles of fairness and equality. For example, the "Fairness in AI" framework developed by researchers at the University of California aims to reduce algorithmic bias by implementing checks and balances that audit the fairness of AI systems throughout their lifecycle (Mehrabi et al., 2021). By promoting these methods, developers can help create more equitable and inclusive chatbot algorithms.

Despite these efforts, the challenge of eliminating bias from chatbot algorithms remains an ongoing issue. The complexity of human language, combined with the vast variety of contexts in which chatbots are used, makes it difficult to fully eradicate bias. Additionally, the rapid pace of technological development in the AI field often outpaces efforts to develop robust ethical frameworks and regulations. As such, governments, organizations, and industry stakeholders must collaborate to establish standards and guidelines for ethical AI development. This includes implementing transparent auditing processes, creating regulatory frameworks for bias detection, and promoting ethical education for AI developers. Without such safeguards, the continued use of biased chatbot algorithms may exacerbate existing inequalities, reinforcing social divides and perpetuating discriminatory practices (O'Neil, 2017).

2. TRANSPARENCY AS A CORNERSTONE OF ETHICAL CHATBOT USE

Transparency is a fundamental principle in the ethical deployment and use of chatbots, as it establishes trust and ensures informed interactions between users and AI systems. At its core, transparency requires that users understand they are engaging with an artificial intelligence (AI) and not a human being. This acknowledgment is particularly crucial in sensitive contexts like healthcare, education, or legal advice, where the stakes of miscommunication or misunderstanding are high. For example, studies have shown that users are more likely to trust and accurately interpret chatbot responses when the system identifies itself as an AI assistant (Eubanks, 2018). Misleading users by presenting chatbots as human-like entities erode trust and may result in users relying on the chatbot beyond its actual capabilities.Moreover, transparency involves openly communicating the limitations of a chatbot. AI systems operate based on probabilistic reasoning, often drawing on vast datasets to predict responses rather than offering definitive answers. Users should be informed when a chatbot's capabilities are constrained, such as its inability to provide nuanced legal advice or make accurate medical diagnoses. This clarity prevents over-reliance and ensures users do not make critical decisions based on incomplete or inaccurate information. For example, research on AI ethics highlights the importance of disclaimers that notify users when AI systems reach their operational limits, thus encouraging informed decision-making (Floridi & Cowls, 2022). Ensuring such disclaimers are easily accessible and integrated into the chatbot's design is a key aspect of transparent communication.

Transparency also extends to how chatbots are designed to handle user data, a topic of significant ethical importance. Users must be informed about what data the chatbot collects, how it is stored, and for what purposes it will be used. Clear and accessible privacy policies, written in language free from technical jargon, are essential to maintaining user trust. For instance, organizations that adopt privacy-by-design principles, where transparency about data handling is prioritized from the outset, report higher user satisfaction and lower rates of data misuse (Cavoukian, 2011). Additionally, offering users control over their data—such as the ability to opt out of data collection or delete their information—further reinforces trust and aligns with best practices in data ethics.

Another critical dimension of transparency involves explaining the sources and biases within the chatbot's training data. AI systems are only as unbiased as the datasets used to train them, and many datasets contain inherent cultural, social, or systemic biases. For example, a hiring chatbot trained on data from a predominantly male-dominated industry may unintentionally favor male candidates over equally qualified female candidates (Binns et al., 2018). Disclosing the origins and potential biases of training data enables users to critically evaluate the chatbot's outputs and fosters accountability in the development process. Researchers and developers must regularly audit and refine their datasets to minimize biases, a practice that should be communicated to users. Transparency is also essential in how chatbots generate responses and make decisions. Explainable AI (XAI) has emerged as a critical field in ensuring transparency in complex AI systems. XAI focuses on creating models that provide understandable explanations for their outputs, enabling users to comprehend how decisions were reached (Arrieta et al., 2019). For instance, if a chatbot recommends a specific course of action, it should accompany the recommendation with a rationale based on its analysis. Such transparency not only builds trust but also empowers users to make informed decisions based on a deeper understanding of the chatbot's reasoning process.

In addition to the chatbot's operational aspects, transparency in chatbot-human escalation pathways is equally vital. When chatbots encounter scenarios beyond their capabilities, they should seamlessly direct users to a human representative. Clear escalation protocols ensure that users are not left without assistance in critical situations. Research by the IEEE Global Initiative on Ethics of Autonomous and Intelligent Systems emphasizes the importance of combining chatbot efficiency with human oversight to maintain ethical standards (Morandín-Ahuerma, n.d.). Transparent communication about these escalation pathways builds confidence and ensures users feel supported throughout their interaction. Transparency also plays a role in addressing potential misuse of chatbots, such as the spread of misinformation or exploitation by malicious actors. Chatbots must be designed with safeguards that prevent the dissemination of unverified or harmful content. Developers have an ethical responsibility to disclose the measures in place to prevent misuse, such as monitoring for suspicious activity or incorporating fact-checking protocols. Studies on misinformation highlight that transparent design practices significantly reduce the likelihood of AI systems being manipulated to propagate false information (Pennycook et al., 2020). By openly addressing these safeguards, developers can reassure users and encourage ethical use.

The principle of transparency is not static but requires ongoing commitment as technology evolves. Regulatory frameworks, industry guidelines, and public expectations regarding AI systems are continually shifting. Developers must stay informed about these changes and proactively update their transparency practices to align with emerging standards. For example, compliance with frameworks such as the European Union's AI Act or ethical guidelines from organizations like UNESCO ensures that chatbot systems remain accountable and aligned with global ethical standards (European Parliament and Council, 2021). Transparency, therefore, is not just a one-time effort but a dynamic process that must adapt to the changing landscape of AI technology and its societal implications.

3. ACCOUNTABILITY AS A CRITICAL ETHICAL ASPECT OF CHATBOT USE

Accountability is a cornerstone of ethical chatbot deployment, ensuring that all stakeholders are responsible for the chatbot's outcomes and impact on users. Chatbots often operate in critical domains such as healthcare, finance, and law, where their decisions can have significant consequences. When errors occur—such as incorrect medical advice, biased recommendations, or flawed financial guidance—clear accountability frameworks are essential to identify the source of the problem and address it effectively. Without such frameworks, users may lack recourse for grievances, and organizations may evade responsibility. Accountability enhances trust, as users are assured that systems are governed by oversight and mechanisms for redress (Floridi et al., 2018).

A significant challenge in achieving accountability lies in the complexity of AI systems, often referred to as the "black box" problem. Many chatbots use machine learning models that are difficult to interpret, making it challenging to trace the cause of errors or unintended outcomes. For instance, if a chatbot makes discriminatory hiring recommendations, it might be unclear whether the issue stems from biased training data, algorithmic flaws, or improper deployment. Explainable AI (XAI) is a promising solution to this challenge. By making decision-making processes transparent, XAI enables developers and users to understand how a chatbot arrives at its outputs. Studies have highlighted that explainability not only aids in debugging but also fosters user trust and accountability by demystifying AI operations (Arrieta et al., 2019). In addition, accountability also requires clear delineation of responsibilities among various stakeholders, including developers, deploying organizations, and third-party providers. Often, chatbots are the result of collaborative efforts, where developers provide the algorithms, organizations integrate the technology, and vendors supply data or tools. When errors occur, such as a chatbot providing incorrect investment advice, the responsibility may be diffuse, complicating remediation. Ethical AI frameworks should define roles and responsibilities for all stakeholders. Legal agreements, compliance with industry standards, and adherence to ethical AI guidelines can formalize these responsibilities, ensuring that accountability is distributed appropriately (Binns et al., 2018).

Providing users with accessible mechanisms for addressing grievances is another vital component of accountability. In scenarios where chatbot interactions result in harm or disadvantage, users should have the ability to file complaints, appeal decisions, or request human review. For example, if a chatbot erroneously rejects a loan application, the affected user should be able to contest the decision through a well-defined process. Such mechanisms not only uphold fairness but also reinforce trust in the system. Research shows that embedding human-in-the-loop processes in critical applications of AI ensures accountability and safeguards against harm (Smith et al., 2023). Regulatory compliance plays a critical role in ensuring accountability. Many governments and international bodies have established or are developing regulations to govern AI technologies, including chatbots. For instance, the European Union's General Data Protection Regulation (GDPR) mandates transparency and accountability in data-driven systems, while its proposed AI Act emphasizes risk management and redress mechanisms. Organizations deploying chatbots should not only meet these regulatory requirements but also adopt proactive accountability measures, such as independent audits and ethical AI oversight boards. Proactive compliance enhances accountability and positions organizations as leaders in ethical AI adoption (Glauner, 2022).

Finally, accountability must extend to anticipating and mitigating risks associated with chatbot use. As AI systems evolve and become more autonomous, the potential for unforeseen consequences increases. Developers and organizations should conduct rigorous pre-deployment testing, continuously monitor system performance, and iteratively improve the chatbot based on user feedback. This forward-looking approach ensures that accountability is not just reactive but embedded throughout the chatbot's lifecycle. By integrating accountability at every stage of development and operation, stakeholders can ensure that chatbots operate responsibly, ethically, and in ways that benefit society (Pennycook et al., 2020).

4. THE ROLE OF CHATBOTS IN SPREADING MISINFORMATION OR PROPAGANDA

The ability of chatbots to rapidly disseminate information across digital platforms presents a significant ethical concern, particularly when they are used to spread misinformation or propaganda. Misinformation refers to false or misleading content shared without harmful intent, while propaganda often involves intentional manipulation of information to influence opinions or behaviors. Chatbots, due to their efficiency and scalability, can amplify both forms, making them potent tools for shaping public discourse. For example, during major political events, such as elections or referendums, chatbots have been deployed to flood social media platforms with biased narratives, misleading statistics, or fabricated stories, which can sway public opinion (Swanberg, 2019). This highlights the need for ethical guidelines and technological safeguards to prevent such misuse.

One of the major ethical challenges is the anonymity and automation of chatbot systems. Unlike human actors, chatbots can operate on a massive scale, engaging with thousands of users simultaneously, while their creators often remain anonymous. This anonymity makes it difficult to trace the origins of misleading content, allowing malicious actors to evade accountability. During the 2016 U.S. presidential election, for instance, networks of automated bots were responsible for propagating false narratives at an unprecedented scale, influencing political perceptions and undermining trust in democratic institutions (Shao et al., 2018). These incidents underscore the importance of transparency in chatbot design, such as mechanisms to identify bots and trace their creators.

Another issue is the use of advanced natural language processing (NLP) models that enable chatbots to generate highly convincing and contextually relevant messages. Modern chatbots, powered by sophisticated AI, can mimic human conversational patterns, making it challenging for users to distinguish between real and automated content. This realism has been exploited in disinformation campaigns, where chatbots masquerade as genuine users to spread fake news or biased opinions. A study by Woolley and Howard (2018) (Woolley & Howard, 2018) found that bots were instrumental in amplifying false information during crises, leveraging their human-like behavior to gain trust and credibility. Addressing this ethical challenge requires robust detection tools and public awareness campaigns to educate users on recognizing chatbot-driven misinformation.

Moreover, the deployment of chatbots for propaganda often targets vulnerable populations, exploiting cognitive biases and emotional triggers. Chatbots programmed to spread propaganda may use fear, anger, or hope to manipulate individuals into adopting certain beliefs or behaviors. For instance, during the COVID-19 pandemic, bots were used to spread fear-inducing misinformation about vaccines, leading to hesitancy and public health challenges (Cinelli et al., 2020) . These tactics not only harm individual decision-making but also disrupt societal harmony, making it essential to establish ethical guidelines for the use of chatbots in sensitive contexts.

Addressing the ethical concerns of chatbot-driven misinformation requires a multi-faceted approach involving technology, policy, and education. Technologically, developers should integrate safeguards, such as real-time content moderation and bot detection algorithms, to identify and mitigate the spread of harmful content. Policy interventions, including stricter regulations and penalties for those using chatbots for malicious purposes, can deter misuse. For example, the European Union's Digital Services Act includes provisions for greater transparency in automated systems, aiming to curb the spread of online disinformation (Schulte-Nölke, 2023). Educational initiatives are equally important, equipping users with digital literacy skills to critically evaluate information and recognize the signs of bot-generated content.

Therefore fostering accountability among chatbot creators and operators is critical. Developers should adhere to ethical standards that prioritize the accuracy and integrity of content shared by chatbots. Organizations deploying chatbots must commit to transparent practices, such as disclosing when users are interacting with bots and providing information on how their systems are designed to prevent misuse. Collaboration between governments, tech companies, and civil society can further strengthen efforts to combat chatbot-driven misinformation. By addressing these ethical concerns, stakeholders can ensure that chatbots are used responsibly, minimizing their potential to harm public discourse and democratic processes.

5. THE EMOTIONAL IMPACT OF CHATBOTS: ETHICAL CONSIDERATIONS

The emotional impact of chatbots is an emerging ethical concern as these systems increasingly interact with users in ways that mimic human conversation and emotions. While chatbots can provide users with convenience and assistance, they also have the potential to influence emotions, sometimes in ways that may not be beneficial or ethical. For instance, chatbots are often employed in customer service roles where they must manage users' frustrations or concerns. However, when a chatbot fails to address a user's issue effectively, it can escalate frustration rather than alleviate it. If the user believes they are interacting with a human-like entity that understands their emotional needs, this disappointment can amplify their negative emotions, leading to dissatisfaction and a sense of betrayal. In such cases, the chatbot's lack of empathy, despite its emotional mimicry, highlights an ethical issue of misleading users into thinking they are engaging with an entity that can genuinely understand their feelings (Luger & Sellen, 2016).

Chatbots are increasingly used in healthcare, where their emotional impact can be even more pronounced. For example, mental health chatbots like Woebot are designed to offer support and engage users in therapeutic conversations. These bots can provide accessible resources for individuals dealing with anxiety, depression, or other mental health challenges, creating a sense of comfort for those who might feel stigmatized or unable to access traditional therapy. However, the emotional impact of relying on chatbots for mental health support raises significant ethical concerns. Users may become overly reliant on these bots, seeking emotional support from an AI that cannot fully replace human empathy or professional mental health services. The potential harm lies in the chatbot inadvertently offering advice that is unsuitable or harmful, without the nuanced judgment that a trained professional would provide. Ensuring that chatbots used in sensitive contexts like mental health offer appropriate disclaimers and direct users to human support when necessary is crucial to preventing emotional harm (Deady et al., 2022).

Another ethical issue is the potential manipulation of emotions through chatbot interactions, particularly in marketing and advertising. Some chatbots are designed to engage users in a way that creates an emotional connection, thus enhancing the likelihood of persuading them to make a purchase or engage with a service. For example, a chatbot might use personalized language to create a sense of urgency or emotional attachment to a product, which could lead to manipulative consumer behavior. In such cases, the chatbot is exploiting the emotional responses of users without regard for their well-being. Ethical chatbot design requires transparency regarding the chatbot's intent, and organizations using chatbots for marketing must be cautious not to manipulate emotions or exploit vulnerable users. Establishing ethical standards for how emotions should be engaged with in chatbot interactions is essential to prevent manipulative practices (Bajwa et al., 2024).

The emotional impact of chatbots can also raise concerns when it comes to the development of attachment and dependency. Chatbots, especially those programmed to offer personalized and empathetic responses, can lead users to form emotional connections with the system. These attachments can be particularly concerning when the chatbot is used in situations of loneliness, such as in companionship robots for the elderly. In these cases, users might develop an emotional bond with the chatbot, mistakenly perceiving it as a substitute for human interaction. This attachment, while potentially providing temporary emotional relief, may also have detrimental effects, especially if it replaces meaningful human relationships or prevents users from seeking appropriate human support. This scenario poses significant ethical questions about the role of chatbots in emotional well-being and whether they should be designed with safeguards to prevent users from becoming overly reliant on them (Shibata & Wada, 2011).

Lastly, the ethical question of user consent is a crucial consideration in chatbot interactions that elicit emotional responses. Users often do not realize the extent to which chatbots are capable of influencing their emotions, particularly when the chatbot is programmed to simulate human-like empathy or understanding. In many cases, chatbots gather and process personal data to tailor responses and provide personalized experiences, which can involve emotional information such as preferences, sentiments, or psychological states. The ethical issue arises when users are not fully informed about the data being collected or how it is being used to craft emotionally engaging responses. Developers must prioritize transparency and informed consent in chatbot interactions, ensuring that users understand the implications of interacting with a system designed to elicit emotional reactions. This is particularly important in sensitive areas such as healthcare or mental health, where emotional data can have significant personal consequences (Rai & Pandey, 2024).

REFERENCES

Arrieta, A. B. (2019). Explainable artificial intelligence (XAI): Concepts. *Taxonomies, Opportunities and challenges toward responsible. AI*, 11.

Bajwa, R. S. (2024). *Parenting in the Age of Artificial Intelligence: Digital Guardians. Exploring Youth Studies in the Age of AI.* IGI Global. DOI: 10.4018/979-8-3693-3350-1.ch003

Binns, R.'It's Reducing a Human Being to a Percentage' Perceptions of Justice in Algorithmic Decisions. *Proceedings of the 2018 Chi conference on human factors in computing systems.* DOI: 10.1145/3173574.3173951

Bolukbasi, T. (2016). Man is to computer programmer as woman is to homemaker? debiasing word embeddings. *Advances in Neural Information Processing Systems*, 29.

Cavoukian, A. (2011). *Privacy by design: Best practices for privacy and the smart grid. ISSE 2010 Securing Electronic Business Processes: Highlights of the Information Security Solutions Europe 2010 Conference.* Wiesbaden: Vieweg+ Teubner.

Cinelli, M., Quattrociocchi, W., Galeazzi, A., Valensise, C. M., Brugnoli, E., Schmidt, A. L., Zola, P., Zollo, F., & Scala, A. (2020). The COVID-19 social media infodemic. *Scientific Reports*, *10*(1), 1–10. DOI: 10.1038/s41598-020-73510-5 PMID: 33024152

Deady, M., Glozier, N., Calvo, R., Johnston, D., Mackinnon, A., Milne, D., Choi, I., Gayed, A., Peters, D., Bryant, R., Christensen, H., & Harvey, S. B. (2022). Preventing depression using a smartphone app: A randomized controlled trial. *Psychological Medicine*, *52*(3), 457–466. DOI: 10.1017/S0033291720002081 PMID: 32624013

DOWN, LAYING, and INTELLIGENCE ACT. "Proposal for a Regulation of the European Parliament and of the Council laying down harmonised rules on Artificial Intelligence (Artificial Intelligence Act) and amending certain Union legislative acts." (2021).

Eubanks, V. (2018). *Automating inequality: How high-tech tools profile, police, and punish the poor.* St. Martin's Press.

Floridi & Cowls. (2022). A unified framework of five principles for AI in society. *Machine learning and the city: Applications in architecture and urban design*, 535-545.

Floridi, L., Cowls, J., Beltrametti, M., Chatila, R., Chazerand, P., Dignum, V., Luetge, C., Madelin, R., Pagallo, U., Rossi, F., Schafer, B., Valcke, P., & Vayena, E. (2018). AI4People—an ethical framework for a good AI society: Opportunities, risks, principles, and recommendations. *Minds and Machines*, *28*(4), 689–707. DOI: 10.1007/s11023-018-9482-5 PMID: 30930541

Glauner, P. (2022). An assessment of the ai regulation proposed by the european commission. In *The future circle of healthcare: AI, 3D printing, longevity, ethics, and uncertainty mitigation* (pp. 119–127). Springer International Publishing. DOI: 10.1007/978-3-030-99838-7_7

Luger, E., & Sellen, A. (2016). "Like Having a Really Bad PA" The Gulf between User Expectation and Experience of Conversational Agents. *Proceedings of the 2016 CHI conference on human factors in computing systems*. DOI: 10.1145/2858036.2858288

Mehrabi, N., Morstatter, F., Saxena, N., Lerman, K., & Galstyan, A. (2021). A survey on bias and fairness in machine learning. *ACM Computing Surveys*, *54*(6), 1–35. DOI: 10.1145/3457607

O'neil, C. (2017). *Weapons of math destruction: How big data increases inequality and threatens democracy*. Crown.

Pennycook, G., Bear, A., Collins, E. T., & Rand, D. G. (2020). The implied truth effect: Attaching warnings to a subset of fake news headlines increases perceived accuracy of headlines without warnings. *Management Science*, *66*(11), 4944–4957. DOI: 10.1287/mnsc.2019.3478

Rai, M., & Pandey, J. K. (Eds.). (2024). *Using Machine Learning to Detect Emotions and Predict Human Psychology*. IGI Global. DOI: 10.4018/979-8-3693-1910-9

Schulte-Nölke, H. (2023). The EU Digital Services Act and EU Consumer Law. *Harmonizing Digital Contract Law*. Nomos Verlagsgesellschaft mbH & Co. KG.

Shao, C., Ciampaglia, G. L., Varol, O., Yang, K.-C., Flammini, A., & Menczer, F. (2018). The spread of low-credibility content by social bots. *Nature Communications*, *9*(1), 1–9. DOI: 10.1038/s41467-018-06930-7 PMID: 30459415

Shibata, T., & Wada, K. (2011). Robot therapy: A new approach for mental healthcare of the elderly–a mini-review. *Gerontology*, *57*(4), 378–386. DOI: 10.1159/000319015 PMID: 20639620

Smith, D. H.Ethics of Trust/worthiness in Autonomous Systems: a scoping review. *Proceedings of the First International Symposium on Trustworthy Autonomous Systems*. DOI: 10.1145/3597512.3600207

Swanberg, S. E. (2019). Psychological armor: The science news-letter warns against propaganda (1926–1965). *Journalism Studies, 20*(13), 1883–1902. DOI: 10.1080/1461670X.2018.1541754

Whittaker, M. (2018). *AI now report 2018*. AI Now Institute at New York University.

Woolley, S. C., & Howard, P. N. (Eds.). (2018). *Computational propaganda: Political parties, politicians, and political manipulation on social media*. Oxford University Press. DOI: 10.1093/oso/9780190931407.001.0001

Chapter 11
Data Security and Privacy Considerations in Mental Health Settings

Liangshun Wu
Shanghai Jiao Tong University, China

ABSTRACT

The integration of chatbots in mental health services necessitates a close examination of data security and privacy issues. This chapter explores these concerns in psychology and psychiatry, highlighting the unique challenges and opportunities posed by digital tools in protecting sensitive patient information. The authors analyze current vulnerabilities and threats, drawing on case studies of data breaches to emphasize the need for robust protection measures. Legal and ethical considerations, including HIPAA and GDPR, are reviewed to underscore the importance of compliance. The chapter proposes strategies for enhancing data security, such as secure communication protocols and regular audits. The goal is to provide mental health professionals, cybersecurity experts, policymakers, and researchers with practical guidelines to ensure the ethical and secure use of chatbots in mental health services, balancing innovation with patient confidentiality.

INTRODUCTION

Overview of Digital Tools in Mental Health

The advent of digital tools in mental health has revolutionized the delivery of psychological and psychiatric services. These tools have introduced new ways to provide care, making it possible to reach individuals who might not have had access

DOI: 10.4018/979-8-3693-3112-5.ch011

to traditional mental health services. For example, teletherapy platforms allow patients to connect with therapists from the comfort of their own homes, eliminating the need for travel and making it easier for those in remote areas to receive care (Knapp, 2021). Similarly, mobile health applications offer a range of services, from mood tracking to guided meditation, which can be accessed at any time, providing continuous support and monitoring (Eisner, 2023).

From teletherapy platforms to mobile health applications, these tools have enhanced the accessibility, efficiency, and personalization of mental health care. Teletherapy platforms, such as BetterHelp and Talkspace, have made it possible for individuals to receive therapy sessions via video calls, which can be scheduled at convenient times for the patient (Knapp, 2021). Mobile health applications, like Headspace and Calm, offer personalized mental health resources, such as mindfulness exercises and sleep aids, tailored to the user's specific needs and preferences (Schueller,2023). This personalization is achieved through algorithms that adapt to the user's behavior and feedback, ensuring that the support provided is relevant and effective (Haque,2023).

Among the various digital innovations, chatbots have emerged as particularly impactful. Chatbots, such as Woebot and Wysa, use artificial intelligence to simulate human conversation and provide mental health support (Sabour,2023). These chatbots can engage users in therapeutic conversations, offering cognitive-behavioral therapy (CBT) techniques and other evidence-based interventions to help manage symptoms of anxiety, depression, and stress (Abd-Alrazaq, 2020). The interactive nature of chatbots makes them a valuable tool for individuals who may be hesitant to seek help from a human therapist due to stigma or privacy concerns (Haque,2023).

These AI-driven programs simulate human conversation and can provide immediate support, monitor patient progress, and offer therapeutic interventions. For instance, Woebot uses natural language processing to understand and respond to user inputs, providing real-time feedback and support (Sabour,2023). It can track the user's mood over time, identifying patterns and offering personalized advice based on the data collected (Abd-Alrazaq, 2020). Additionally, chatbots can deliver therapeutic interventions, such as guided breathing exercises or mindfulness practices, which can help users manage their mental health on a day-to-day basis (Haque,2023).

Their ability to operate 24/7 and handle large volumes of interactions makes them invaluable in extending mental health services to underserved populations and providing continuous support. Unlike human therapists, chatbots are available at all hours, making it possible for users to access support whenever they need it, even in the middle of the night (Balcombe,2023). This constant availability is particularly beneficial for individuals in crisis, who may require immediate assistance outside of regular office hours (Haque,2023). Furthermore, chatbots can manage multiple conversations simultaneously, allowing them to support a large number of users at once, which is crucial in addressing the global shortage of mental health professionals (Abd-Alrazaq, 2020). This scalability ensures that more people can receive the help they need, regardless of their location or socioeconomic status (Knapp,2021).

Significance of Chatbots in Psychology and Psychiatry

Chatbots in psychology and psychiatry serve multiple critical functions. These AI-driven tools are designed to simulate human conversation and can perform a variety of tasks that are essential in mental health care. For instance, chatbots like Woebot and Wysa are used to deliver cognitive-behavioral therapy (CBT) techniques, helping users manage symptoms of anxiety and depression through structured conversations (Lee et al., 2023; Grodniewicz & Hohol, 2024). Additionally, chatbots can provide psychoeducation, offering users valuable information about mental health conditions and coping strategies, which can be particularly beneficial for individuals who may not have access to traditional educational resources (Selaskowski et al., 2023).

They can perform initial assessments, triage patients, deliver cognitive-behavioral therapy (CBT) exercises, and offer psychoeducation. For example, the chatbot "Viki" was developed to evaluate employee risks of suffering from depression, anxiety, stress, insomnia, and burnout, demonstrating its capability to perform comprehensive mental health assessments (Hungerbuehler et al., 2021). Similarly, chatbots like Tess use CBT principles to guide users through therapeutic exercises, helping them identify and challenge negative thought patterns (Grodniewicz & Hohol, 2024). These functionalities make chatbots versatile tools in the mental health field, capable of addressing a wide range of needs from initial assessment to ongoing therapeutic support (Liu et al., 2022).

By automating routine tasks, chatbots free up mental health professionals to focus on more complex cases, thereby increasing the overall efficiency of mental health services. For instance, chatbots can handle administrative tasks such as scheduling appointments and sending reminders, which reduces the workload on human staff and allows them to dedicate more time to direct patient care(ProProfs Chat, n.d.; Actionbot, n.d.). This automation not only improves efficiency but also ensures that patients receive timely and consistent support, which is crucial for effective mental health management (mHealthIntelligence, n.d.). Moreover, during peak periods, such as flu season or public health emergencies, chatbots can manage the excess load by handling routine inquiries, ensuring that all patients receive timely information and support without overwhelming healthcare staff (ProProfs Chat, n.d.).

Additionally, chatbots can help reduce the stigma associated with seeking mental health care by providing an anonymous and accessible point of contact for individuals hesitant to engage with human therapists. Research has shown that many people are more willing to disclose their mental health symptoms to a chatbot than to a human therapist, as they feel less judged and more comfortable sharing their thoughts and feelings(Lee et al., 2023; Farvolden, 2024). For example, the chatbot Limbic Access has been shown to increase referrals for mental health services among underrepresented groups, including ethnic and sexual minorities, by providing a non-judgmental and accessible platform for initial contact (Williams, 2024). This reduction in stigma can encourage more individuals to seek help, ultimately improving mental health outcomes on a broader scale (Lee et al., 2023).

The integration of natural language processing (NLP) and machine learning algorithms enables chatbots to offer personalized and adaptive interventions, which can significantly enhance patient outcomes. Chatbots like Woebot use NLP to understand and respond to user inputs in a way that feels natural and supportive, providing real-time feedback and personalized advice based on the user's specific needs and progress(Grodniewicz & Hohol, 2024; Omarov et al., 2023). Machine learning algorithms allow these chatbots to learn from each interaction, continuously improving their ability to provide relevant and effective support (Gcore, 2023). This adaptability ensures that the interventions remain tailored to the individual, enhancing the overall effectiveness of the treatment and contributing to better mental health outcomes (van der Schyff et al., 2023; Haque & Rubya, 2023).

Rationale for Focusing on Data Security and Privacy

Despite the numerous benefits of chatbots in mental health, their deployment raises critical concerns about data security and privacy. Chatbots, while offering immediate and accessible mental health support, also collect and process vast amounts of sensitive data, including personal narratives, psychological assessments, and treatment histories (Li, 2023). This data is highly valuable and, if not properly protected, can be vulnerable to breaches and misuse (Hasal, 2020). For instance, the chatbot Talkspace has been reported to mine user conversations for business insights, raising significant privacy concerns (Steve, 2023). Therefore, it is essential to address these security issues to maintain the trust and safety of users.

Mental health data is exceptionally sensitive, encompassing personal narratives, psychological assessments, and treatment histories. This type of data can reveal intimate details about an individual's mental health status, personal experiences, and treatment plans, which, if exposed, can lead to severe consequences such as identity theft, discrimination, and emotional distress (Li, 2023; Coghlan et al., 2023). For example, BetterHelp was found to have shared user data with Meta, which could potentially expose users to targeted advertising based on their mental health conditions (Steve, 2023). The sensitivity of this data necessitates stringent measures to ensure its confidentiality and integrity.

The misuse or unauthorized access to this data can have severe implications for patient confidentiality, trust, and safety. Unauthorized access to mental health data can lead to breaches of confidentiality, which is a cornerstone of effective therapeutic relationships (Lustgarten, Garrison, Sinnard, & Flynn, 2020). Such breaches can erode trust between patients and healthcare providers, making individuals less likely to seek help or be honest about their mental health issues (Coghlan et al., 2023). Additionally, the exposure of sensitive information can result in psychological harm and social stigmatization, further exacerbating the mental health challenges faced by individuals (Steve, 2023).

The increasing prevalence of cyber threats, coupled with the specific vulnerabilities associated with digital mental health tools, underscores the urgent need for robust data protection measures. Cyber threats such as hacking, phishing, and malware attacks are becoming more sophisticated, targeting the valuable data stored in digital health platforms (Hasal, 2020). Mental health apps and chatbots, which often operate on external messaging platforms, are particularly vulnerable to these threats due to the vast amounts of data they handle and the varying levels of security implemented by different platforms (Hasal, 2020). This situation highlights the necessity for comprehensive security protocols to protect sensitive patient information.

Addressing these issues is paramount to ensuring that the integration of chatbots into mental health services upholds the highest standards of ethical practice and legal compliance. Ensuring data security and privacy in mental health chatbots involves implementing measures such as encryption, secure authentication protocols, and regular security audits (Li, 2023; Hasal, 2020). Additionally, compliance with legal frameworks like the Health Insurance Portability and Accountability Act (HIPAA) in the U.S. and the General Data Protection Regulation (GDPR) in the EU is crucial to protect patient data and maintain ethical standards (Li, 2023; Khalid, Qayyum, Bilal, Al-Fuqaha, & Qadir, 2023). These measures help build trust in digital mental health tools and ensure that they are used responsibly and safely.

This chapter aims to explore these challenges comprehensively, providing insights and strategies to safeguard sensitive patient information in the digital age. It will delve into the specific security risks associated with mental health chatbots, such as data breaches, lack of transparency, and the potential for misuse of data (Li, 2023; Coghlan et al., 2023). The chapter will also discuss best practices for data protection, including the use of anonymized data, data masking, and secure data management techniques (Li, 2023; Hasal, 2020). By addressing these challenges, the chapter aims to provide a roadmap for the safe and ethical use of chatbots in mental health care, ensuring that the benefits of these technologies can be realized without compromising patient privacy and security.

DATA SECURITY CHALLENGES

Analysis of Common Cybersecurity Threats in Healthcare

The healthcare sector faces a myriad of cybersecurity threats that can compromise sensitive patient data.

Phishing attacks in the healthcare sector are a prevalent and insidious form of cyber threat that exploit human vulnerabilities to gain unauthorized access to sensitive data. These attacks are particularly effective due to the high volume of electronic communications healthcare workers manage daily, coupled with the critical nature of the information they handle. Phishing tactics have evolved over time, becoming increasingly sophisticated and harder to detect. Here's an expanded analysis of phishing attacks in healthcare:

Types of Phishing Attacks

- **Email Phishing**: The most common form of phishing, where attackers send fraudulent emails that appear to be from legitimate sources. These emails often contain malicious links or attachments and use urgent language to trick recipients into revealing sensitive information or downloading malware.
- **Spear Phishing**: A more targeted form of phishing, where attackers customize their messages to specific individuals or departments within a healthcare organization. By leveraging information gathered from social media or other public sources, attackers craft convincing emails that mimic legitimate communication from colleagues or superiors, increasing the likelihood of the recipient taking the bait.
- **Whaling**: This variant targets high-profile individuals within an organization, such as executives or administrators. The goal is to deceive these individuals into authorizing financial transactions or disclosing login credentials. Whaling attacks often involve elaborate schemes and use detailed information about the target to appear as legitimate as possible.
- **Smishing and Vishing**: These attacks use SMS (text messaging) and voice calls, respectively. Smishing might involve a text message alerting the recipient to a supposed issue with their account, urging them to click a malicious link. Vishing calls, on the other hand, might impersonate IT support or other trusted authority figures to extract sensitive information over the phone.

Figure 1. Diagram of How Does Phishing Attack Work

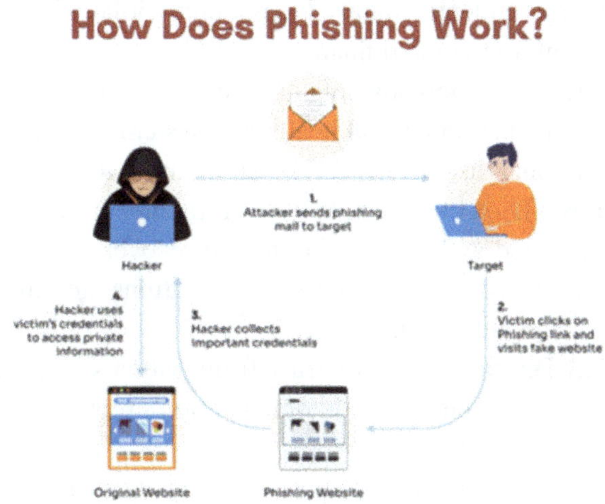
How Does Phishing Work?
1.
Attacker sends phishing mail to target
Hacker
Target
2.
Victim clicks on Phishing link and visits fake website
3.
Hacker collects important credentials
4.
Hacker uses victim's credentials to access private information
Original Website
Phishing Website

Figure 1 illustrates the process of a phishing attack through a series of steps. Here's a description of the figure's content:

- The attacker, represented by a person wearing a hoodie and using a laptop, sends a phishing email to the target.
- The target, represented by a person using a computer, receives the phishing email, which appears to be from a legitimate source.
- The phishing email contains a malicious link or attachment, which the target clicks on or opens, unaware of the potential threat.
- By clicking the malicious link or opening the attachment, the target's computer becomes infected with malware or redirected to a fake website designed to steal important credentials, such as login information, credit card details, or personal data.
- The attacker successfully collects the target's important credentials, which can be used for various malicious purposes, such as identity theft, financial fraud, or unauthorized access to accounts.

The attackers disguise their malicious intent by impersonating legitimate entities or services to trick unsuspecting victims into revealing sensitive information or granting unauthorized access.

The consequences of phishing attacks in the healthcare sector can be severe, given the sensitivity of the data involved. Successful attacks can lead to:

- **Data Breaches**: Unauthorized access to patient records, financial information, and other confidential data. This not only violates privacy laws but can also lead to identity theft and financial fraud.
- **Malware Infections**: Downloading of malicious software, including ransomware, which can encrypt critical healthcare systems and data, leading to significant operational disruptions and potential harm to patients.
- **Financial Loss**: Direct financial loss from fraudulent transactions, as well as the costs associated with responding to and recovering from an attack. This includes legal fees, fines for compliance violations, and expenses related to notifying affected individuals.
- **Reputational Damage**: Loss of trust from patients and the public, which can have long-lasting effects on an organization's reputation and its ability to attract and retain patients.
- **Ransomware**: This type of malware encrypts patient data, rendering it inaccessible until a ransom is paid, significantly disrupting healthcare operations.
- **Data Breaches**: Unauthorized access to patient information can occur due to weak security protocols, leading to the exposure of sensitive data.
- **Insider Threats**: Employees or other insiders with access to sensitive information may intentionally or unintentionally cause data breaches.
- **Distributed Denial of Service (DDoS) Attacks**: These attacks overwhelm healthcare systems with traffic, rendering them inoperative and potentially compromising data security.

Understanding these threats is essential for developing effective security measures to protect mental health data.

Specific Vulnerabilities Introduced by Chatbots

Chatbots, while enhancing mental health services, introduce specific vulnerabilities:

- Data Transmission Security: Chatbots often communicate over the internet, making data transmissions susceptible to interception if not properly encrypted.
- Authentication and Authorization: Ensuring that only authorized users can access sensitive data is challenging, especially when chatbots handle a high volume of interactions.
- Data Storage: Storing sensitive patient information securely is critical. Chatbots may store data in cloud-based systems, which must be robustly secured against breaches.

- Software Bugs and Exploits: Chatbots, like any software, can have vulnerabilities that hackers might exploit to gain unauthorized access to data.
- Third-Party Integrations: Chatbots often integrate with other systems and services, which can introduce additional vulnerabilities if those systems are not adequately secured.

Addressing these vulnerabilities requires implementing comprehensive security protocols and regular assessments to ensure robustness against potential threats.

Case Studies of Data Breaches in Mental Health Settings

Examining past data breaches provides insights into potential weaknesses and areas for improvement:

Vastaamo Psychotherapy Center Breach (Finland, 2020)

The Vastaamo psychotherapy center data breach in Finland, which came to light in October 2020, is one of the most significant and disturbing cyberattacks in recent history due to the sensitive nature of the data involved. Here is a detailed description of the case:

On October 21, 2020, it was revealed that an unknown hacker had breached the database of Vastaamo, a prominent Finnish psychotherapy center, and downloaded approximately 40,000 patient files. These files included highly sensitive information such as medical reports, personal details, and social security numbers (Malwarebytes,2020; Cimpanu,2020). The breach initially occurred in November 2018, with a subsequent breach in March 2019, but the company did not disclose these incidents until much later (Greenberg, 2020).

The hacker demanded a ransom of 40 bitcoins (approximately 450,000 euros) from Vastaamo to prevent the publication of the stolen data. When the clinic did not comply, the hacker began to extort individual patients, demanding around 200 euros in Bitcoin to keep their data private. If the patients did not pay within 24 hours, the ransom increased to 500 euros (Greenberg,2020). This tactic of directly extorting patients was unprecedented and added a layer of personal trauma to the victims.

The breach had a profound impact on the victims, many of whom were already in vulnerable states due to their mental health conditions. The leaked data included detailed therapy session notes, which contained deeply personal and confidential information. This led to widespread fear and distress among the patients, some of whom received direct ransom demands via email (Milmo, 2020; Security Boulevard, 2020; Regan, 2020). The breach also raised concerns about potential identity theft and long-term psychological effects on the victims.

The Finnish government and various organizations quickly mobilized to support the victims. The Finnish police, along with other agencies, launched an investigation into the breach and the extortion attempts. Authorities advised victims not to pay the ransom and to report any extortion emails to the police (Greenberg,2020). Vastaamo set up a crisis hotline and offered free therapy sessions to affected patients (Greenberg,2020).

The breach also led to significant legal and organizational consequences for Vastaamo. The CEO, Ville Tapio, was fired for allegedly covering up the breaches and failing to address the security vulnerabilities (Cimpanu,2020). The Finnish Office of the Data Protection Ombudsman began investigating Vastaamo's data protection measures and their compliance with the General Data Protection Regulation (GDPR) (Malwarebytes, 2020).

The Vastaamo breach highlighted critical issues in data security within the healthcare sector. It underscored the need for robust data encryption, secure access controls, and timely disclosure of security incidents. The case also sparked a national conversation in Finland about the use of social security numbers as identifiers and the overall security of electronic medical records (Milmo,2020).

In summary, the Vastaamo data breach was a severe incident that exposed the vulnerabilities in data security practices within the healthcare industry. It had a devastating impact on the victims and led to significant legal and organizational repercussions for the psychotherapy center. The case serves as a stark reminder of the importance of protecting sensitive personal information and the need for stringent cybersecurity measures.

COVID-19 Mental Health App Breach (Various, 2021)

The COVID-19 pandemic led to a surge in the use of mental health apps as people sought remote support during lockdowns and social distancing measures. However, the rapid deployment of these apps without thorough security vetting resulted in several data breaches, compromising the sensitive personal information of users.

One notable example was the Vastaamo psychotherapy data breach in Finland in 2020. Vastaamo, a private psychotherapy practice, suffered a cyberattack in which patient records, including personal details and therapy notes, were stolen and held for ransom. The attackers threatened to release the data unless patients paid a ransom, leading to a traumatic experience for the already vulnerable victims. As reported by Wired, "The breach has sent shockwaves through Finnish society, where the stigma of seeking mental health treatment remains strong." (Financial Express, 2023; Iwaya et al., 2022)

Another incident involved the mental health app Better Stop Suicide, which exposed the data of over 800,000 users due to an unsecured database. As reported by Security Boulevard, “The data included user conversations with the app's chatbot, which could include highly sensitive information about a user's mental health status and even thoughts of self-harm.” (Federal Trade Commission, 2016; Kshetri et al., 2024; Inkster et al, 2023; Camacho et al., 2022; Sanvello, 2021)

These incidents highlighted the importance of rigorous security testing and audits before deploying digital health tools that handle sensitive personal data. As Cimpanu from CyberScoop noted, “The Vastaamo breach underlines the need for better security practices when dealing with sensitive data like medical records, especially in the mental health field where stigma and privacy concerns are paramount.” (Iwaya et al., 2021; HealthITSecurity, 2023; Verge, 2023)

Security experts emphasized the need for comprehensive security audits and adherence to best practices in data protection and privacy. As stated in a report by the National Library of Medicine, “If people are to use and trust these tools for their mental health, it is crucial we evaluate the transparency and quality around the data practices of these apps.” (Sanvello et al., 2021; Moldstud, n.d.)

These incidents served as a wake-up call for the digital health industry, highlighting the importance of prioritizing security and privacy from the outset, rather than treating it as an afterthought. Regular security audits, robust encryption, and strict access controls are essential to protect the sensitive data of users seeking mental health support through digital platforms.

University Medical Center Data Breach (USA, 2019)

The University of Chicago Medical Center experienced a significant data breach in 2019 due to a phishing attack. This incident compromised the personal information of approximately 45,000 patients. The compromised data encompassed names, addresses, birth dates, Social Security numbers, and health insurance details, but did not contain medical records. The breach came to light when an employee from a billing processing vendor for the hospital system inappropriately shared a file with an unauthorized individual. The hospital delayed notifying affected patients for several weeks to allow time for data review and the establishment of a support call center. (Becker's Hospital Review,2019; Healio, 2019; Chicago Tribune, 2019).

This breach highlighted the critical need for comprehensive staff training and robust email security protocols. The University of Chicago Medical Center responded by improving its threat monitoring and detection procedures and offering email security training to its employees to prevent future incidents in the future (Chicago Sun-Times, 2024). This case underscores the importance of implementing strong cybersecurity measures, including staff education on recognizing phishing attempts and securing email communications, to safeguard sensitive patient information from unauthorized access and potential misuse.

These case studies reveal common vulnerabilities, such as inadequate encryption, insufficient access controls, and lack of rigorous security testing. They underscore the importance of adopting best practices in data security to protect sensitive mental health information.

By analyzing these challenges and learning from past breaches, mental health professionals and organizations can better prepare to secure chatbots and other digital tools, ensuring the protection of patient data and maintaining trust in digital mental health services.

Privacy Concerns

Legal and Ethical Considerations for Patient Data

The privacy of patient data in mental health settings is governed by stringent legal and ethical standards. These considerations include:

- Confidentiality: Maintaining patient confidentiality is a fundamental ethical obligation in mental health care. Patients must trust that their personal information and treatment details will remain private and secure.
- Informed Consent: Patients need to be informed about the usage, storage, and sharing of their data. They should give explicit consent for the utilization of digital tools like chatbots in their care.
- Data Minimization: Ethical guidelines suggest that only the minimum necessary data should be collected and stored to achieve the intended purpose, reducing the risk of exposure in case of a breach.
- Transparency: Organizations need to be transparent about their data practices, including the methods of data collection, usage, storage, and protection. This transparency builds trust and ensures patients are aware of their rights and the safeguards established to protect their data.

Impact of Data Breaches on Patient Confidentiality and Trust

Data breaches in mental health settings can have severe consequences:

- Loss of Confidentiality: A breach can expose sensitive information, such as patient identities, treatment details, and personal communications, undermining the confidentiality that is crucial in mental health care.

- Erosion of Trust: Trust is a cornerstone of the therapeutic relationship. Data breaches can erode patient trust in mental health providers and digital tools, potentially deterring individuals from seeking necessary care.
- Emotional and Psychological Harm: The exposure of private mental health information can lead to significant emotional distress, stigmatization, and potential discrimination for affected individuals.
- Legal and Financial Repercussions: Organizations that suffer data breaches may face legal actions, financial penalties, and a loss of reputation, further impacting their ability to provide effective care.

Review of Privacy Laws Applicable to Mental Health Data (e.g., HIPAA, GDPR)

Various privacy laws regulate the handling of mental health data, ensuring it is protected against unauthorized access and breaches:

HIPAA (Health Insurance Portability and Accountability Act)

The Health Insurance Portability and Accountability Act (HIPAA), enacted in 1996, is a pivotal U.S. law that establishes national standards for safeguarding health information. Its primary objectives are to enhance the efficiency and effectiveness of the healthcare system by standardizing the electronic exchange of administrative and financial data, and to ensure the privacy and security of individuals' medical information. HIPAA is composed of several rules, each addressing different aspects of health information protection:

The HIPAA Security Rule sets forth stringent standards for safeguarding electronic protected health information (ePHI). It mandates that covered entities (CEs) and business associates (BAs) adopt a comprehensive array of administrative, physical, and technical measures to guarantee the confidentiality, integrity, and availability of ePHI. The primary goals of the Security Rule encompass:

- Administrative Safeguards: These encompass policies and procedures focused on managing the choice, creation, execution, and maintenance of security measures to protect ePHI. This includes performing risk management, training staff, and creating contingency plans.
- Physical Safeguards: These measures are designed to shield electronic systems, equipment, and the data they contain from threats, environmental dangers, and unauthorized access. This involves regulating physical access to facilities and ensuring the secure disposal of ePHI.

- Technical Safeguards: These involve the technology, along with associated policies and procedures, that safeguard ePHI and manage access to it. This encompasses establishing access controls, audit mechanisms, integrity measures, and transmission security measures (Zscaler, n.d.; Compliancy Group, n.d.; HealthITSecurity, n.d.).

The HIPAA Privacy Rule governs the use and disclosure of PHI. It sets standards for how PHI should be handled to safeguard individuals' privacy while enabling the flow of health information necessary to deliver high-quality healthcare. Key aspects of the Privacy Rule include:

- Permissible Uses and Disclosures: The rule specifies the circumstances under which PHI can be used or disclosed without patient authorization, such as for treatment, payment, and healthcare operations.
- Patient Rights: Patients are entitled to access their health records, request amendments, and obtain a record of disclosures of their PHI. They also have the right to request restrictions on certain uses and disclosures of their information.
- Notice of Privacy Practices: Covered entities are required to give patients a notice detailing how their PHI will be used and disclosed, as well as outlining their rights concerning their information (HIPAA Journal, 2024; American Medical Association, n.d.; National Center for Biotechnology Information, n.d.).

The HIPAA Breach Notification Rule requires covered entities and business associates to inform affected people, the Department of Health and Human Services (HHS), and, in certain instances, the media, when there is a breach of unsecured PHI. The rule outlines specific requirements for breach notifications:

- Timeliness: Notifications must be issued promptly and no later than 60 days after the breach is discovered.
- Content of Notification: The notification must contain a description of the breach, the categories of information affected, the actions individuals should take to safeguard themselves, what the entity is doing to investigate the breach, mitigate harm, and prevent future breaches, and contact information for further inquiries.
- Notification to HHS: For breaches impacting 500 or more individuals, immediate notification to HHS is required. For breaches affecting fewer than 500 individuals, notifications can be submitted on an annual basis.

- Media Notification: If a breach affects more than 500 residents of a state or jurisdiction, the covered entity must notify prominent media outlets serving that area (Sprinto, 2024; Northern Illinois University, n.d.).

GDPR (General Data Protection Regulation)

The General Data Protection Regulation (GDPR) is an extensive data protection framework instituted by the European Union (EU) to protect personal data and privacy. Implemented in 2018, GDPR is applicable to all entities that handle the personal data of individuals within the EU, irrespective of the organization's location. This regulation is particularly relevant to sensitive data, such as mental health information, due to the high risk associated with its misuse. Here are the key provisions of GDPR that are pertinent to mental health data.

GDPR grants individuals, known as data subjects, several rights over their personal data. These rights are designed to give individuals greater control and transparency over how their data is used and processed. The primary data subject rights include:

- Right to be Informed: Individuals are entitled to understand what personal data is being gathered about them, the purpose of its collection, the entity collecting it, the duration of its retention, and whether it will be disclosed to third parties. Organizations must provide clear and accessible information about their data processing activities (Thoropass, n.d.; Data Privacy Manager, n.d.; OneTrust, n.d.).
- Right of Access: Data subjects are entitled to request access to their personal information held by an organization. This encompasses details about the purposes of processing, the types of data being processed, the recipients of the data, and the retention duration. Organizations are obligated to supply a copy of the personal data upon request (GDPR-Info.eu, n.d.).
- Right to Rectification: Individuals are entitled to request amendments to incorrect or incomplete personal data. Organizations are required to rectify the data without undue delay.
- Right to Erasure (Right to be Forgotten): Data subjects can request the removal of their personal data under specific conditions, such as when the data is no longer needed for the purposes it was originally collected, or if the individual withdraws consent (ICO, n.d.).
- Right to Restriction of Processing: Individuals can request the limitation of processing their personal data under certain circumstances, such as when they dispute the accuracy of the data or object to its processing (Data Protection Commission, n.d.).

- Right to Data Portability: This entitlement enables individuals to retrieve and utilize their personal data across various services. They can ask for their data in a structured, standardized, and machine-readable format, and have the right to transfer it to a different controller.
- Right to Object: Data subjects can oppose the processing of their personal data for specific purposes, such as direct marketing or processing based on legitimate interests.
- Rights Concerning Automated Decision-Making and Profiling: GDPR provides protections against decisions made solely reliant on automated processing, including profiling, which has a significant impact on individuals. This includes decisions related to work performance, creditworthiness, and other personal aspects.

GDPR requires that organizations embed data protection principles into their processing activities and systems from the very beginning. This concept, known as "Data Protection by Design and Default," mandates organizations to adopt suitable technical and organizational measures to ensure data protection is accounted for at every phase of data processing. Key aspects include:

- Data Minimization: Only the personal data necessary for each specific purpose should be processed. This minimizes the risk of data breaches and misuse.
- Pseudonymization and Encryption: Organizations are encouraged to use techniques such as pseudonymization (replacing identifiable information with artificial identifiers) and encryption to protect personal data (GDPR-Info.eu., n.d.).
- Default Privacy Settings: Systems and services should be configured to provide the highest level of privacy protection by default. For example, social media platforms should limit the accessibility of user profiles by default (Cynet, n.d.).
- Continuous Monitoring and Updates: Data protection measures should be routinely reviewed and revised to address emerging risks and vulnerabilities. This involves performing Data Protection Impact Assessments (DPIAs) for high-risk data processing operations.

GDPR imposes strict requirements on organizations to report data breaches to supervisory authorities and affected individuals. The breach notification requirements are as follows:

- Notification to Supervisory Authorities: Organizations are required to inform the appropriate supervisory authority of a personal data breach within 72 hours of becoming aware of it, where practicable. The notification should provide information about the nature of the breach, the types and estimated number of data subjects impacted, the potential consequences, and the actions taken to mitigate the breach. (GDPR-Text.com, n.d.).
- Notification to Affected Individuals: If a breach is likely to pose a high risk to the rights and freedoms of individuals, organizations must promptly notify the affected data subjects. The notification should detail the breach, its potential impact, and the steps individuals can take to protect themselves.
- Documentation of Breaches: Organizations are required to document all personal data breaches, regardless of whether they need to be reported to the supervisory authority. This documentation should include the details of the breach, its impact, and the corrective measures implemented. This ensures accountability and enables supervisory authorities to confirm compliance (Securiti.ai., n.d.).

Other Regional Laws: Various other regions and countries have their own privacy laws, such as the CCPA (California Consumer Privacy Act) in the United States, which also provides robust protections for personal data, including mental health information.

Understanding and complying with these laws is essential for mental health providers and developers of digital tools to ensure they uphold the highest standards of data privacy and protection. By doing so, they can foster a secure environment where patients feel safe to share their most sensitive information.

MITIGATION STRATEGIES

Best Practices for Securing Chatbot Communications and Data Storage

To guarantee the security of chatbot interactions and data storage in mental health environments, it is essential to implement best practices that address potential vulnerabilities and protect sensitive information:

- End-to-End Encryption: Deploy end-to-end encryption for all interactions between chatbots and users to prevent unauthorized access during data transmission.

- Secure Authentication: Utilize multi-factor authentication (MFA) to confirm user identities and administrators accessing the chatbot system.
- Data Anonymization: Anonymize or pseudonymize patient data to protect identities, especially during storage and processing, reducing the risk of exposure in case of a breach.
- Regular Software Updates: Ensure that chatbot software and all integrated systems are regularly updated to patch vulnerabilities and enhance security features.
- Access Controls: Enforce stringent access controls to restrict data access exclusively to authorized personnel, according to their roles and responsibilities.
- Secure Data Storage: Use encrypted databases and secure cloud storage solutions that comply with relevant privacy regulations to store sensitive patient information.

Technologies and Frameworks for Enhancing Data Security

Leveraging advanced technologies and frameworks can significantly bolster the security of chatbots and the protection of mental health data:

- Blockchain Technology: Utilize blockchain for secure and transparent data transactions. Its decentralized nature ensures data integrity and reduces the risk of tampering.
- Artificial Intelligence and Machine Learning: Employ AI and machine learning algorithms to detect and respond to potential security threats in real-time, enhancing proactive defense mechanisms.
- Zero Trust Architecture: Implement a Zero Trust security model that assumes all network traffic is untrusted by default. This approach requires continuous verification of user identities and device integrity.
- Secure APIs: Use secure Application Programming Interfaces (APIs) with robust authentication and authorization protocols to facilitate safe communication between chatbots and other systems.
- Intrusion Detection and Prevention Systems (IDPS): Implement IDPS to monitor network traffic for unusual activities and automatically thwart potential threats.

Policies for Regular Audits and Compliance Checks

Routine audits and compliance reviews are crucial to maintain high security standards and ensure adherence to legal and regulatory requirements:

- Periodic Security Audits: Perform scheduled security audits to assess the effectiveness of current security measures, uncover vulnerabilities, and apply necessary enhancements.
- Compliance Checks: Perform periodic compliance checks to ensure that all data handling practices align with relevant laws and regulations, such as HIPAA and GDPR.
- Incident Response Plans: Create and sustain an incident response plan that details procedures for handling data breaches and other security incidents promptly and effectively.
- Employee Training: Provide ongoing training for staff on data security best practices, emerging threats, and compliance requirements to ensure they are well-prepared to protect sensitive information.
- External Evaluations: Hire third-party security specialists to perform independent assessments and penetration testing to validate the robustness of security measures.

By implementing these mitigation strategies, mental health providers and developers can significantly enhance the security of chatbot communications and data storage, ensuring the protection of sensitive patient information and maintaining trust in digital mental health services.

FUTURE DIRECTIONS

Emerging Trends in Cybersecurity for Mental Health

As digital tools become increasingly integrated into mental health services, several emerging trends in cybersecurity are poised to shape the future landscape:

- AI-Driven Cybersecurity: Artificial intelligence and machine learning are being utilized to improve threat detection and response. These technologies can process large volumes of data to detect patterns and irregularities that suggest cyber threats, allowing for more proactive and efficient defense mechanisms.
- Behavioral Analytics: By monitoring and analyzing user behavior, cybersecurity systems can detect unusual activities that may signify a security breach. This approach helps in identifying threats that traditional security measures might miss.
- Quantum Cryptography: Quantum computing holds the potential to revolutionize data encryption methods. Quantum cryptography promises unbreak-

able encryption, ensuring that sensitive mental health data remains secure against even the most sophisticated cyber attacks.

- Zero Trust Security Models: The adoption of Zero Trust architectures, which assume that no part of a network is inherently secure, is increasing. This model continuously verifies the identity of users and devices, providing robust protection against unauthorized access.

Potential Regulatory Changes and Their Implications

The regulatory environment surrounding data security and privacy is continuously evolving. Potential changes that could impact mental health services include:

- Stricter Data Protection Laws: As concerns about data privacy grow, regulations may become more stringent. Laws similar to the GDPR could be adopted in more regions, increasing the compliance burden on mental health providers and technology developers.
- Enhanced Breach Notification Requirements: Future regulations might impose stricter timelines and more comprehensive requirements for breach notifications, ensuring that affected individuals and authorities are promptly informed of data breaches.
- Data Portability and Interoperability: New regulations may focus on ensuring that patient data can be easily and securely transferred between different systems and providers, promoting interoperability while maintaining high privacy standards.
- Focus on AI Ethics and Accountability: As AI-driven tools become more prevalent in mental health services, regulations may emerge that specifically address the ethical use of AI, including accountability for decisions made by AI systems and transparency in their operations.

Innovations in Technology That Could Enhance Privacy and Security

Several technological innovations hold promise for enhancing privacy and security in mental health services:

- Homomorphic Encryption: This technology allows data to be processed without being decrypted, enabling secure data analysis and computation while maintaining privacy. It is particularly useful for cloud-based services and data sharing scenarios.

- Blockchain Technology: Blockchain offers a decentralized and transparent way to record and verify transactions. Its application in mental health can ensure data integrity, secure consent management, and immutable audit trails.
- Federated Learning: This approach allows AI models to be trained across various decentralized devices or servers containing local data samples, without sharing the data itself. It boosts privacy by retaining personal data localized.
- Privacy-Enhancing Technologies (PETs): PETs such as differential privacy and secure multi-party computation can help protect individual data points while allowing for useful data analysis. These technologies are crucial for maintaining patient confidentiality in large-scale data analytics.
- Advanced Biometric Security: Innovations in biometric authentication, such as facial recognition and behavioral biometrics, can provide more secure and user-friendly ways to verify identities and control access to sensitive data.

By staying abreast of these emerging trends, regulatory developments, and technological innovations, mental health professionals and organizations can better prepare for the future, ensuring that data security and privacy remain at the forefront of digital mental health services. This proactive approach will help maintain patient trust and support the ethical and effective use of chatbots and other digital tools in mental health care.

CONCLUSION

Summary of Key Points

This chapter has explored the critical issues surrounding data security and privacy in the context of using chatbots in mental health settings. Key points include:

- Data Security Challenges: We identified common cybersecurity threats in healthcare, specific vulnerabilities introduced by chatbots, and illustrated these with case studies of data breaches in mental health settings.
- Privacy Concerns: We discussed the legal and ethical considerations for patient data, the impact of data breaches on patient confidentiality and trust, and reviewed relevant privacy laws such as HIPAA and GDPR.
- Mitigation Strategies: Best practices for securing chatbot communications and data storage were outlined, along with advanced technologies and frameworks to enhance data security, and policies for regular audits and compliance checks.

- Future Directions: We examined emerging trends in cybersecurity for mental health, potential regulatory changes and their implications, and technological innovations that could further enhance privacy and security.

Final Thoughts on Balancing Innovation with Ethical Considerations

As chatbots and other digital tools become integral to mental health services, it is essential to strike a balance between embracing innovation and upholding ethical standards. The benefits of increased accessibility, personalized care, and improved efficiency must be weighed against the potential risks to patient privacy and data security.

Innovations such as AI-driven cybersecurity, quantum cryptography, and blockchain technology offer promising solutions to enhance data protection. However, these technologies must be implemented thoughtfully and in compliance with evolving regulations to ensure they do not inadvertently compromise patient trust or confidentiality.

Ethical considerations, including maintaining patient confidentiality, ensuring informed consent, and practicing data minimization, are paramount. Mental health professionals, technology developers, and policymakers must collaborate to create a secure, transparent, and patient-centric environment. By prioritizing robust data protection measures and adhering to stringent privacy standards, we can leverage technological advancements to improve mental health services while safeguarding the rights and well-being of patients.

In conclusion, the ethical deployment of chatbots and other digital tools in mental health settings requires a commitment to continuous learning, adaptation, and vigilance. By staying informed about emerging threats, regulatory changes, and technological innovations, stakeholders can ensure that the integration of these tools enhances patient care without compromising privacy and security.

REFERENCES

Abd-Alrazaq, A. A., Rababeh, A., Alajlani, M., Bewick, B. M., & Househ, M. (2020). Effectiveness and Safety of Using Chatbots to Improve Mental Health: Systematic Review and Meta-Analysis. *Journal of Medical Internet Research*, 22(7), e16021. DOI: 10.2196/16021 PMID: 32673216

Actionbot. (n.d.). Chatbots in healthcare. Retrieved from https://action.bot/blog/chatbots-in-healthcare/

AgileBlue. (n.d.). What is a cybersecurity audit & why is it important? Retrieved from https://agileblue.com/what-is-a-cybersecurity-audit-why-is-it-important/

American Medical Association. (n.d.). HIPAA Privacy Rule. Retrieved from https://www.ama-assn.org/practice-management/hipaa/hipaa-privacy-rule

Balcombe, L. (2023). AI Chatbots in Digital Mental Health. *Informatics (MDPI)*, 10(4), 82. DOI: 10.3390/informatics10040082

Becker's Hospital Review. (2019). 27 hospital, health system data breaches in 2019. Retrieved from https://www.beckershospitalreview.com/cybersecurity/27-hospital-health-system-data-breaches-in-2019.html

Bendig, E., Erb, B., Schulze-Thuesing, L., & Baumeister, H. (2022). The next generation: Chatbots in clinical psychology and psychotherapy to foster mental health – A scoping review. *Verhaltenstherapie*, 32(Suppl. 1), 64–76. DOI: 10.1159/000501812

Bickmore, T. W., & Giorgino, T. (2006). Health dialog systems for patients and consumers. *Journal of Biomedical Informatics*, 39(5), 556–571. DOI: 10.1016/j.jbi.2005.12.004 PMID: 16464643

Blaze Information Security. (n.d.). Cybersecurity risks of digital health applications. Retrieved from https://www.blazeinfosec.com/post/cybersecurity-risks-digital-health-apps/

Brookings Institution. (2023). Why mental health apps need to take privacy more seriously. Retrieved from https://www.brookings.edu/articles/why-mental-health-apps-need-to-take-privacy-more-seriously/

Camacho, E., & Torous, J. (2022). Assessment of mental health services available through smartphone apps. JAMA Network Open. https://www.ncbi.nlm.nih.gov/pmc/articles/PMC9857226/

Chicago Sun-Times. (2024, May 29). Email hack exposed University of Chicago Medical Center patient information. Retrieved from https://chicago.suntimes.com/health/2024/05/29/email-hack-exposed-university-chicago-medical-center-patient-information-data-breach-security-health

Chicago Tribune. (2019, March 4). Rush reports data breach involving 45,000 patients. Retrieved from https://www.chicagotribune.com/2019/03/04/rush-reports-data-breach-involving-45000-patients/

Cimpanu, C. (2020). Finnish psychotherapy data breach sees the most vulnerable victims extorted. CyberScoop. https://cyberscoop.com/finnish-psychotherapy-data-breach-vastaamo/

Coghlan, S., Leins, K., Sheldrick, S., Cheong, M., Gooding, P., & D'Alfonso, S. (2023). To chat or bot to chat: Ethical issues with using chatbots in mental health. *Digital Health*, 9. Advance online publication. DOI: 10.1177/20552076231183542 PMID: 37377565

Compliancy Group. (n.d.). HIPAA Security Rule Requirements Explained. Retrieved from https://compliancy-group.com/hipaa-security-rule/

Cyber Security Cooperative Research Centre. (n.d.). Mental health apps: Privacy risks. Retrieved from https://cybersecuritycrc.org.au/mental-health-apps-privacy-risks

Cynet. (n.d.). GDPR Data Breach Notifications: Everything You Need to Know. Retrieved from https://www.cynet.com/cynet-for-compliance/gdpr-data-breach-notifications-everything-you-need-to-know/

Data Privacy Manager. (n.d.). What are 8 Data Subject rights according to the GDPR. Retrieved from https://dataprivacymanager.net/what-are-data-subject-rights-according-to-the-gdpr/

Data Protection Commission. (n.d.). Quick Guide to GDPR Breach Notifications. Retrieved from https://www.dataprotection.ie/en/organisations/know-your-obligations/quick-guide-gdpr-breach-notifications

Dig8ital. (n.d.). Boost your security: The importance of network security audits. Retrieved from https://dig8ital.com/post/network-security-audits/

Eisner, E., Berry, N., & Bucci, S. (2023). Digital tools to support mental health: A survey study in psychosis. *BMC Psychiatry*, 23(1), 726. DOI: 10.1186/s12888-023-05114-y PMID: 37803367

European Commission. (n.d.). What does data protection 'by design' and 'by default' mean? Retrieved from https://commission.europa.eu/law/law-topic/data-protection/reform/rules-business-and-organisations/obligations/what-does-data-protection-design-and-default-mean_en

European Journal of Privacy Law & Technologies. (n.d.). Announcements. https://universitypress.unisob.na.it/ojs/index.php/ejplt/announcement/view/125

Farvolden, P. (2024, February). AI chatbots break down barriers to much-needed mental health treatments. Retrieved from https://www.rgare.com/knowledge-center/article/ai-chatbots-break-down-barriers-to-much-needed-mental-health-treatments

Federal Trade Commission. (2016). Mobile health app developers: FTC best practices. Retrieved from https://www.ncbi.nlm.nih.gov/pmc/articles/PMC6371412/

Financial Express. (2023). How mental health apps are yet to fulfil the promise of user data privacy. Retrieved from https://www.financialexpress.com/business/digital-transformation-how-mental-health-apps-are-yet-to-fulfil-the-promise-of-user-data-privacy-3378043/

Gcore. (2023). What is an AI chatbot? Retrieved from https://gcore.com/learning/what-is-an-ai-chatbot/

GDPR-Info.eu. (n.d.). Chapter 3 – Rights of the data subject. Retrieved from https://gdpr-info.eu/chapter-3/

GDPR-Info.eu. (n.d.). Notification of a personal data breach to the supervisory authority. Retrieved from https://gdpr-info.eu/art-33-gdpr/

GDPR-Info.eu. (n.d.). Privacy by Design. Retrieved from https://gdpr-info.eu/issues/privacy-by-design/

GDPR-Text.com. (n.d.). Article 25 GDPR. Data protection by design and by default. Retrieved from https://gdpr-text.com/read/article-25/

Greenberg, A. (2020). A Hacker is Trying to Extort Patients in a Massive Psychotherapy Data Breach. Wired. https://www.wired.com/story/vastaamo-psychotherapy-patients-hack-data-breach/

Grodniewicz, J. P., & Hohol, M. (2024). Therapeutic Chatbots as Cognitive-Affective Artifacts. *Topoi*, 43(3), 795–807. Advance online publication. DOI: 10.1007/s11245-024-10018-x

Haque, M. D. R., & Rubya, S. (2023). An Overview of Chatbot-Based Mobile Mental Health Apps: Insights From App Description and User Reviews. *JMIR mHealth and uHealth*, 11, e44838. DOI: 10.2196/44838 PMID: 37213181

Hasal, M. (2020). Chatbots: Security, privacy, data protection, and social aspects. *Concurrency and Computation*. Advance online publication. DOI: 10.1002/cpe.6426

Healio. (2019, September 26). 2019 health care data breaches setting records. Retrieved from https://www.healio.com/news/primary-care/20190926/2019-health-care-data-breaches-setting-records

HealthITSecurity. (2023). This year's largest healthcare data breaches. Retrieved from https://healthitsecurity.com/features/this-years-largest-healthcare-data-breaches

HealthITSecurity. (n.d.). What is the HIPAA Security Rule? Retrieved from https://healthitsecurity.com/features/what-is-the-hipaa-security-rule

Hungerbuehler, I., Daley, K., Cavanagh, K., Garcia Claro, H., & Kapps, M. (2021). Chatbot-Based Assessment of Employees' Mental Health: Design Process and Pilot Implementation. *JMIR Formative Research*, 5(4), e21678. DOI: 10.2196/21678 PMID: 33881403

Information Commissioner's Office (ICO). (n.d.-a). Personal data breaches: a guide. Retrieved from https://ico.org.uk/for-organisations/report-a-breach/personal-data-breach/personal-data-breaches-a-guide/

Information Commissioner's Office (ICO). (n.d.-b). Data protection by design and by default. Retrieved from https://ico.org.uk/for-organisations/law-enforcement/guide-to-le-processing/accountability-and-governance/data-protection-by-design-and-by-default/

Inkster, B., Knibbs, C., & Bada, M. (2023). Cybersecurity: A critical priority for digital mental health. Frontiers in Digital Health. https://www.frontiersin.org/journals/digital-health/articles/10.3389/fdgth.2023.1242264/full

Iwaya, L. H., Rashid, A., & Klein, J. (2022). On the privacy of mental health apps. Empirical Software Engineering. https://link.springer.com/article/10.1007/s10664-022-10236-0

Journal, H. I. P. A. A. (2019). Healthcare data breach report. Retrieved from https://www.hipaajournal.com/healthcare-data-breach-2019-report/

Journal, H. I. P. A. A. (2024a). What are the HIPAA Breach Notification Requirements? Retrieved from https://www.hipaajournal.com/hipaa-breach-notification-requirements/

Journal, H. I. P. A. A. (2024b). HIPAA Privacy Rule. Retrieved from https://www.hipaajournal.com/hipaa-privacy-rule/

Khalid, N., Qayyum, A., Bilal, M., Al-Fuqaha, A., & Qadir, J. (2023). Privacy-preserving artificial intelligence in healthcare: Techniques and applications. *Computers in Biology and Medicine*, 158, 106848. DOI: 10.1016/j.compbiomed.2023.106848 PMID: 37044052

Knapp, A. A., Cohen, K., Nicholas, J., Mohr, D. C., Carlo, A. D., Skerl, J. J., & Lattie, E. G. (2021). Integration of Digital Tools Into Community Mental Health Care Settings That Serve Young People: Focus Group Study. *JMIR Mental Health*, 8(8), e27379. DOI: 10.2196/27379 PMID: 34420928

Kshetri, N., Hughes, L., Slade, E. L., Jeyaraj, A., Kar, A. K., Baabdullah, A. M., & Miller, R. C. (2024). A systematic analysis of failures in protecting personal health data. *International Journal of Information Management*, 74, 102719. DOI: 10.1016/j.ijinfomgt.2023.102719

Labadze, L., Grigolia, M., & Machaidze, L. (2023). Role of AI chatbots in education: Systematic literature review. *International Journal of Educational Technology in Higher Education*, 20(56), 56. Advance online publication. DOI: 10.1186/s41239-023-00426-1

Lee, Y.-C., Cui, Y., Jamieson, J., Fu, W., & Yamashita, N. (2023). Exploring effects of chatbot-based social contact on reducing mental illness stigma. In *Proceedings of the 2023 CHI Conference on Human Factors in Computing Systems (CHI '23)*, April 23–28, 2023, Hamburg, Germany. ACM. DOI: 10.1145/3544548.3581384

Li, J. (2023). Security Implications of AI Chatbots in Health Care. *Journal of Medical Internet Research*, 25, e47551. DOI: 10.2196/47551 PMID: 38015597

Liu, H., Peng, H., Song, X., Xu, C., & Zhang, M. (2022). Using AI chatbots to provide self-help depression interventions for university students: A randomized trial of effectiveness. *Internet Interventions : the Application of Information Technology in Mental and Behavioural Health*, 27, 100495. DOI: 10.1016/j.invent.2022.100495 PMID: 35059305

Lustgarten, S. D., Garrison, Y. L., Sinnard, M. T., & Flynn, A. W. (2020). Digital privacy in mental healthcare: Current issues and recommendations for technology use. *Current Opinion in Psychology*, 36, 25–31. DOI: 10.1016/j.copsyc.2020.03.012 PMID: 32361651

Malwarebytes. (2020). Vastaamo psychotherapy data breach sees the most vulnerable victims extorted. https://www.malwarebytes.com/blog/news/2020/10/vastaamo-psychotherapy-data-breach-sees-the-most-vulnerable-victims-extorted

Metcalf, M. (2024). The best mental health chatbots in 2024. Retrieved from https://getmarlee.com/blog/mental-health-chatbot

mHealthIntelligence. (n.d.). Understanding the role of chatbots in virtual care delivery. Retrieved from https://mhealthintelligence.com/features/understanding-the-role-of-chatbots-in-virtual-care-delivery

Milmo, D. (2020). Tens of thousands of psychotherapy records hacked in Finland. The Guardian. https://www.theguardian.com/world/2020/oct/26/tens-of-thousands-psychotherapy-records-hacked-in-finland

MobiHealthNews. (n.d.). AI triage chatbots trekking toward standard care despite criticism. Retrieved from https://www.mobihealthnews.com/content/ai-triage-chatbots-trekking-toward-standard-care-despite-criticism

Moldstud. (n.d.). The role of security audits in assessing and strengthening cyber defenses. Retrieved from https://moldstud.com/articles/p-the-role-of-security-audits-in-assessing-and-strengthening-cyber-defenses

National Center for Biotechnology Information. (n.d.). HIPAA, the Privacy Rule, and Its Application to Health Research. Retrieved from https://www.ncbi.nlm.nih.gov/books/NBK9573/

New York University. (n.d.). IT security info breach notification. Retrieved from https://www.nyu.edu/about/policies-guidelines-compliance/policies-and-guidelines/it-security-info-breach-notification.html

Northern Illinois University. (n.d.). HIPAA Breach Notification Rule: Explanation and Guidance. Retrieved from https://www.niu.edu/doit/about/policies/hipaa-breach-notification-rule.shtml

Omarov, B., Zhumanov, Z., Gumar, A., & Kuntunova, L. (2023). Artificial Intelligence Enabled Mobile Chatbot Psychologist using AIML and Cognitive Behavioral Therapy. *International Journal of Advanced Computer Science and Applications*, 14(6). Advance online publication. DOI: 10.14569/IJACSA.2023.0140616

OneTrust. (n.d.). The GDPR Data Subject Rights. Retrieved from https://www.onetrust.com/blog/the-gdpr-data-subject-rights/

ProProfs Chat. (n.d.). Healthcare chatbot use cases. Retrieved from https://www.proprofschat.com/blog/healthcare-chatbot-use-cases/

Regan, M. (2020, October 27). Therapy patients in Finland blackmailed after hackers stole their records. CNN. https://edition.cnn.com/2020/10/27/tech/finland-therapy-patients-blackmailed-data-breach-intl/index.html

REPHRAIN: National Research Centre on Privacy, Harm Reduction and Adversarial Influence Online. (2024). On the privacy of mental health apps: An empirical investigation and recommendations. PubMed. https://pubmed.ncbi.nlm.nih.gov/36407814/

Sabour, S., Zhang, W., Xiao, X., Zhang, Y., Zheng, Y., Wen, J., Zhao, J., & Huang, M. (2023). A chatbot for mental health support: Exploring the impact of Emohaa on reducing mental distress in China. *Frontiers in Digital Health*, 5, 1133987. Advance online publication. DOI: 10.3389/fdgth.2023.1133987 PMID: 37214342

Sanvello, Woebot, Happify, Youper, & Bloom. (2021). Quality evaluation of stress, anxiety and depression apps for COVID-19. ScienceDirect. https://www.sciencedirect.com/science/article/pii/S2666915321001815

Schueller, S. M., & Histon, T. (2023). Digital Tools for Youth Mental Health. *Frontiers for Young Minds*, 11, 1169684. DOI: 10.3389/frym.2023.1169684

Securiti.ai. (n.d.). What are GDPR Data Subject Rights? Retrieved from https://securiti.ai/gdpr-data-subject-rights/

Security Boulevard. (2020). Therapy Center Hacked, 40,000 Patients Sent Ransom Demands. https://securityboulevard.com/2020/10/therapy-center-hacked-40000-patients-sent-ransom-demands/

Selaskowski, B., Reiland, M., Schulze, M., Aslan, B., Kannen, K., Wiebe, A., Wallbaum, T., Boll, S., Lux, S., Philipsen, A., & Braun, N. (2023). Chatbot-supported psychoeducation in adult attention-deficit hyperactivity disorder: Randomised controlled trial. *BJPsych Open*, 9(6), e192. DOI: 10.1192/bjo.2023.573 PMID: 37827996

Software, B. G. O. (n.d.). The process behind mental health app development. Retrieved from https://www.bgosoftware.com/blog/mental-health-app-development/

Sprinto. (2024). HIPAA Breach Notification Rule [Quick Guide]. Retrieved from https://sprinto.com/blog/hipaa-breach-notification-rule/

Steve, M. (2023). Why mental health apps need to take privacy more seriously. (2023, November 30). Brookings Institution. Retrieved from https://www.brookings.edu/articles/why-mental-health-apps-need-to-take-privacy-more-seriously/

The Verge. (2023). Mental health apps are still failing their privacy checkups. Retrieved from https://www.theverge.com/2023/5/4/23710840/mental-health-therapy-apps-mozilla-report-privacy-data-security

Thoropass. (n.d.). Understanding the GDPR breach notification timeline. Retrieved from https://thoropass.com/blog/compliance/gdpr-breach-notification-timeline/

Van der Schyff, E. L., Ridout, B., Amon, K. L., Forsyth, R., & Campbell, A. J. (2023). Providing Self-Led Mental Health Support Through an Artificial Intelligence-Powered Chat Bot (Leora) to Meet the Demand of Mental Health Care. *Journal of Medical Internet Research*, 25, e46448. DOI: 10.2196/46448 PMID: 37335608

Williams, R. (2024, February 5). A chatbot helped more people access mental-health services. Technology Review. Retrieved from https://www.technologyreview.com/2024/02/05/1087690/a-chatbot-helped-more-people-access-mental-health-services/

Zscaler. (n.d.). What Is the HIPAA Security Rule? Retrieved from https://www.zscaler.com/zpedia/what-is-hipaa-security-rule

Compilation of References

Abadi, M., Agarwal, A., Barham, P., Brevdo, E., Chen, Z., Citro, C., Corrado, G. S., Davis, A., Dean, J., Devin, M., & Associates. (2016). Tensorflow: Large-scale machine learning on heterogeneous distributed systems. *arXiv Preprint arXiv:1603.04467.*

Abd-Alrazaq, A. A., Alajlani, M., Ali, N., Denecke, K., Bewick, B. M., & Househ, M. (2021). Perceptions and opinions of patients about mental health chatbots: Scoping review. *Journal of Medical Internet Research. Journal of Medical Internet Research, 23*(1), e17828. DOI: 10.2196/17828 PMID: 33439133

Abd-Alrazaq, A. A., Rababeh, A., Alajlani, M., Bewick, B. M., & Househ, M. (2020). Effectiveness and Safety of Using Chatbots to Improve Mental Health: Systematic Review and Meta-Analysis. *Journal of Medical Internet Research, 22*(7), e16021. DOI: 10.2196/16021 PMID: 32673216

Abisha, D., Mahalakshmi, M., Pritiga, T., & Thanusiya, M. (2024). Revolutionizing Rural Healthcare in India: AI-Powered Chatbots for Affordable Symptom Analysis and Medical Guidance. 2024 International Conference on Inventive Computation Technologies (ICICT).

Actionbot. (n.d.). Chatbots in healthcare. Retrieved from https://action.bot/blog/chatbots-in-healthcare/

Adetayo, A. J. (2023). Artificial intelligence chatbots in academic libraries: The rise of ChatGPT. *Library Hi Tech News, 40*(3), 18–21. DOI: 10.1108/LHTN-01-2023-0007

Adewumi, T. P., Liwicki, F., & Liwicki, M. (2019). Conversational systems in machine learning from the point of view of the philosophy of science—Using alime chat and related studies. *Philosophies, 4*(3), 41. DOI: 10.3390/philosophies4030041

Adiukwu, F., de Filippis, R., Orsolini, L., Gashi Bytyçi, D., Shoib, S., Ransing, R., Slaih, M., Jaguga, F., Handuleh, J. I. M., Ojeahere, M. I., Ullah, I., Karaliuniene, R., Nagendrappa, S., Vahdani, B., Ashrafi, A., Ori, D., Noël, C., Abbass, Z., Jatchavala, C., & Shalbafan, M. (2022). Scaling up global mental health services during the COVID-19 pandemic and beyond. *Psychiatric Services (Washington, D.C.)*, *73*(2), 231–234. DOI: 10.1176/appi.ps.202000774 PMID: 34235945

Adiwardana, D., Luong, M.-T., So, D. R., Hall, J., Fiedel, N., Thoppilan, R., Yang, Z., Kulshreshtha, A., Nemade, G., Lu, Y., & Le, Q. V. (2020). *Towards a Human-like Open-Domain Chatbot.*

Agathokleous, E., Saitanis, C. J., Fang, C., & Yu, Z. (2023). Use of ChatGPT: What does it mean for biology and environmental science? *The Science of the Total Environment*, *888*, 164154. DOI: 10.1016/j.scitotenv.2023.164154 PMID: 37201835

Aggarwal, A., Tam, C. C., Wu, D., Li, X., & Qiao, S. (2023). Artificial intelligence–based chatbots for promoting health behavioral changes: Systematic review. *Journal of Medical Internet Research*, *25*, e40789. DOI: 10.2196/40789 PMID: 36826990

AgileBlue. (n.d.). What is a cybersecurity audit & why is it important? Retrieved from https://agileblue.com/what-is-a-cybersecurity-audit-why-is-it-important/

Ahmed, N., Liu, X., Al-Hazwani, I., & Huang, E. M. (2024). Cultural dimensions and mental health technology: A systematic review of hofstede's dimensions in shaping mental health experiences. *Extended Abstracts of the CHI Conference on Human Factors in Computing Systems.*

Ahmed, A., Hassan, A., Aziz, S., Abd-Alrazaq, A. A., Ali, N., Alzubaidi, M., Al-Thani, D., Elhusein, B., Siddig, M. A., Ahmed, M., & Househ, M. (2023). Chatbot features for anxiety and depression: A scoping review. *Health Informatics Journal*, *29*(1). Advance online publication. DOI: 10.1177/14604582221146719 PMID: 36693014

Alabdulatif, A., Al Asqah, M., Moulahi, T., & Zidi, S. (2023). Leveraging artificial intelligence in blockchain-based E-health for safer decision making framework. *Applied Sciences (Basel, Switzerland)*, *13*(2), 1035. DOI: 10.3390/app13021035

Alanzi, T., Alsalem, A. A., Alzahrani, H., Almudaymigh, N., Alessa, A., Mulla, R., AlQahtani, L., Bajonaid, R., Alharthi, A., Alnahdi, O., & Alanzi, N. (2023). AI-powered mental health virtual assistants acceptance: An empirical study on influencing factors among generations X, Y, and Z. *Cureus*. Advance online publication. DOI: 10.7759/cureus.49486 PMID: 38156169

Alimour, S. A., Alnono, E., Aljasmi, S., Farran, H. E., Alqawasmi, A. A., Alrabeei, M. M., Shwedeh, F., & Aburayya, A. (2024). The quality traits of artificial intelligence operations in predicting mental healthcare professionals' perceptions: A case study in the psychotherapy division. *Journal of Autonomous Intelligence*, *7*(4). Advance online publication. DOI: 10.32629/jai.v7i4.1438

Allen, B. (2024). The Promise of Explainable AI in Digital Health for Precision Medicine: A Systematic Review. *Journal of Personalized Medicine*, *14*(3), 277. DOI: 10.3390/jpm14030277 PMID: 38541019

Alowais, S. A., Alghamdi, S. S., Alsuhebany, N., Alqahtani, T., Alshaya, A. I., Almohareb, S. N., Aldairem, A., Alrashed, M., Bin Saleh, K., Badreldin, H. A., Al Yami, M. S., Al Harbi, S., & Albekairy, A. M. (2023). Revolutionizing healthcare: The role of artificial intelligence in clinical practice. *BMC Medical Education*, *23*(1), 689. DOI: 10.1186/s12909-023-04698-z PMID: 37740191

AlQudah, A. A., Al-Emran, M., & Shaalan, K. (2021). Technology acceptance in healthcare: A systematic review. *Applied Sciences (Basel, Switzerland)*, *11*(22), 10537. DOI: 10.3390/app112210537

Alshammari, N., Sarker, M. N. I., Kamruzzaman, M., Alruwaili, M., Alanazi, S. A., Raihan, M. L., & AlQahtani, S. A. (2022). Technology-driven 5G enabled e-healthcare system during COVID-19 pandemic. *IET Communications*, *16*(5), 449–463. DOI: 10.1049/cmu2.12240

American Medical Association. (n.d.). HIPAA Privacy Rule. Retrieved from https://www.ama-assn.org/practice-management/hipaa/hipaa-privacy-rule

Anand, V., Verma, L., Aggarwal, A., Nanjundappa, P., & Rai, H. (2021). COVID-19 and psychological distress: Lessons for India. *PLoS One*, *16*(8), e0255683. DOI: 10.1371/journal.pone.0255683 PMID: 34347847

Anders, B. A. (2023). Is using ChatGPT cheating, plagiarism, both, neither, or forward thinking? *Patterns (New York, N.Y.)*, *4*(3), 100694. DOI: 10.1016/j.patter.2023.100694 PMID: 36960444

Anderson, C. M., Hogarty, G. E., & Reiss, D. J. (1980). Family treatment of adult schizophrenic patients: A psycho-educational approach. *Schizophrenia Bulletin*, *6*(3), 490–505. DOI: 10.1093/schbul/6.3.490 PMID: 7403810

Anderson, M., & Anderson, S. L. (2019). How should AI be developed, validated, and implemented in patient care? *AMA Journal of Ethics*, *21*(2), 125–130. DOI: 10.1001/amajethics.2019.125 PMID: 30794121

Andersson, S., Bathula, D. R., Iliadis, S. I., Walter, M., & Skalkidou, A. (2021). Predicting women with depressive symptoms postpartum with machine learning methods. *Scientific Reports*, *11*(1), 7877. DOI: 10.1038/s41598-021-86368-y PMID: 33846362

Andrade-Arenas, L., Yactayo-Arias, C., & Pucuhuayla-Revatta, F. (2024). therapy and emotional support through a chatbot. *International Journal of Online and Biomedical Engineering*, *20*(2), 114–130. DOI: 10.3991/ijoe.v20i02.45377

Andrade, L. H., Alonso, J., Mneimneh, Z., Wells, J. E., Al-Hamzawi, A., Borges, G., Bromet, E., Bruffaerts, R., de Girolamo, G., de Graaf, R., Florescu, S., Gureje, O., Hinkov, H. R., Hu, C., Huang, Y., Hwang, I., Jin, R., Karam, E. G., Kovess-Masfety, V., & Kessler, R. C. (2013). Barriers to mental health treatment: Results from the WHO World Mental Health (WMH) surveys. *Psychological Medicine*, *44*(6), 1303–1317. DOI: 10.1017/S0033291713001943 PMID: 23931656

Andrew, J., Rudra, M., Eunice, J., & Belfin, R. V. (2023). Artificial intelligence in adolescents mental health disorder diagnosis, prognosis, and treatment. *Frontiers in Public Health*, *11*, 1110088. DOI: 10.3389/fpubh.2023.1110088 PMID: 37064712

Antes, A. L., Burrous, S., Sisk, B. A., Schuelke, M. J., Keune, J. D., & DuBois, J. M. (2021). Exploring perceptions of healthcare technologies enabled by artificial intelligence: An online, scenario-based survey. *BMC Medical Informatics and Decision Making*, *21*(1), 221. Advance online publication. DOI: 10.1186/s12911-021-01586-8 PMID: 34284756

Anton, M. T., & Jones, D. J. (2017). Adoption of technology-enhanced treatments: Conceptual and practical considerations. *Clinical Psychology : a Publication of the Division of Clinical Psychology of the American Psychological Association*, *24*(3), 223–240. DOI: 10.1111/cpsp.12197 PMID: 28966479

Appaji, A., Nagendra, B., Chako, D. M., Padmanabha, A., Jacob, A., Hiremath, C. V., Varambally, S., Kesavan, M., Venkatasubramanian, G., Rao, S. V., Webers, C. A. B., Berendschot, T. T. J. M., & Rao, N. P. (2019). Examination of retinal vascular trajectory in schizophrenia and bipolar disorder. *Psychiatry and Clinical Neurosciences*, *73*(12), 738–744. DOI: 10.1111/pcn.12921 PMID: 31400288

Arrieta, A. B. (2019). Explainable artificial intelligence (XAI): Concepts. *Taxonomies, Opportunities and challenges toward responsible. AI*, 11.

Ayano, G., Demelash, S., Yohannes, Z., Haile, K., Tulu, M., Assefa, D., Tesfaye, A., Haile, K., Solomon, M., Chaka, A., & Tsegay, L. (2021). Misdiagnosis, detection rate, and associated factors of severe psychiatric disorders in specialized psychiatry centers in Ethiopia. *Annals of General Psychiatry*, *20*(1), 1–10. DOI: 10.1186/s12991-021-00333-7 PMID: 33531016

Ay, B., Yildirim, O., Talo, M., Baloglu, U. B., Aydin, G., Puthankattil, S. D., & Acharya, U. R. (2019). Automated depression detection using deep representation and sequence learning with EEG signals. *Journal of Medical Systems*, *43*(7), 1–12. DOI: 10.1007/s10916-019-1345-y PMID: 31139932

Bajwa, R. S. (2024). *Parenting in the Age of Artificial Intelligence: Digital Guardians. Exploring Youth Studies in the Age of AI*. IGI Global. DOI: 10.4018/979-8-3693-3350-1.ch003

Bakator, M., & Radosav, D. (2018). Deep learning and medical diagnosis: A review of literature. *Multimodal Technologies and Interaction*, *2*(3), 47. DOI: 10.3390/mti2030047

Bak, M., Madai, V. I., Fritzsche, M. C., Mayrhofer, M. T., & McLennan, S. (2022). You can't have ai both ways: Balancing health data privacy and access fairly. *Frontiers in Genetics*, *13*, 929453. DOI: 10.3389/fgene.2022.929453 PMID: 35769991

Balan, R., Dobrean, A., & Poetar, C. R. (2024). Use of automated conversational agents in improving young population mental health: A scoping review. *NPJ Digital Medicine*, *7*(1), 1–9. DOI: 10.1038/s41746-024-01072-1 PMID: 38503909

Balcombe, L. (2023, October). AI chatbots in digital mental health. [). MDPI.]. *Informatics (MDPI)*, *10*(4), 82. DOI: 10.3390/informatics10040082

Bamgboje-Ayodele, A., Avery, S., Pearson, J., Mak, M., Smith, K., Rincones, O., Vinod, S., Bray, V., Ducinoska, I., McCarthy, K., Williamson, K., Delaney, G. P., & Girgis, A. (2022). Adapting an integrated care pathway for implementing electronic patient reported outcomes assessment in routine oncology care: Lessons learned from a case study. *Journal of Evaluation in Clinical Practice*, *28*(6), 1072–1083. DOI: 10.1111/jep.13688 PMID: 35470525

Bangor, A., Kortum, P., & Miller, J. (2009). Determining what individual SUS scores mean: Adding an adjective rating scale. *Journal of Usability Studies*, *4*(3), 114–123.

Bansal, D., Chhikara, R., Khanna, K., & Gupta, P. (2018). Comparative analysis of various machine learning algorithms for detecting dementia. *Procedia Computer Science*, *132*, 1497–1502. DOI: 10.1016/j.procs.2018.05.102

Bao, R., Zhang, A., & Li, S. (2020). COVID-19 pandemic and intrahepatic cholestasis of pregnancy: A case report. *BMC Pregnancy and Childbirth*, *20*(1), 1–3. https://www.ncbi.nlm.nih.gov/pmc/articles/PMC7256567/

Barak-Corren, Y., Wolf, R., Rozenblum, R., Creedon, J. K., Lipsett, S. C., Lyons, T. W., Michelson, K. A., Miller, K. A., Shapiro, D. J., Reis, B. Y., & Fine, A. M. (2024). Harnessing the Power of Generative AI for Clinical Summaries: Perspectives From Emergency Physicians. *Annals of Emergency Medicine*, *84*(2), 128–138. DOI: 10.1016/j.annemergmed.2024.01.039 PMID: 38483426

Barnett, A., Savic, M., Pienaar, K., Carter, A., Warren, N., Sandral, E., Manning, V., & Lubman, D. I. (2021). Enacting 'more-than-human' care: Clients' and counsellors' views on the multiple affordances of chatbots in alcohol and other drug counselling. *The International Journal on Drug Policy*, *94*, 102910. DOI: 10.1016/j.drugpo.2020.102910 PMID: 33059955

Baron, P. (2024). Are AI detection and plagiarism similarity scores worthwhile in the age of ChatGPT and other Generative AI? *Scholarship of Teaching and Learning in the South*, *8*(2), 151–179. DOI: 10.36615/sotls.v8i2.411

Barron, D. S., Baker, J. T., Budde, K. S., Eickhoff, S. B., Friston, K. J., Fox, P. T., & Krystal, J. H. (2021). Decision models and technology can help psychiatry develop biomarkers. *Frontiers in Psychiatry*, *12*, 706655. DOI: 10.3389/fpsyt.2021.706655 PMID: 34566711

Baumgartner, J., Zannettou, S., Keegan, B., Squire, M., & Blackburn, J. (2020). *The Pushshift Reddit Dataset.*

Baumgartner, R. (2021). Precision medicine and digital phenotyping: Digital medicine's way from more data to better health. *Big Data & Society*, *8*(2). DOI: 10.1177/20539517211066452

Baveye, P. C. (2024). Authorship for chatbots on scholarly publications: The time has not yet come. *European Science Editing*, *50*, e139657. DOI: 10.3897/ese.2024.e139657

Baye, M. R., De los Santos, B., & Wildenbeest, M. R. (2016). Search engine optimization: What drives organic traffic to retail sites? *Journal of Economics & Management Strategy*, *25*(1), 6–31. DOI: 10.1111/jems.12141

Beauchamp, T. (2008). The principle of beneficence in applied ethics.

Beauchamp, T. L., & Childress, J. F. (1994). The capacity for autonomous choice. *Principles of Biomedical Ethics*, 120-142.

Becker's Hospital Review. (2019). 27 hospital, health system data breaches in 2019. Retrieved from https://www.beckershospitalreview.com/cybersecurity/27-hospital-health-system-data-breaches-in-2019.html

Beg, M. J., & Verma, M. K. (2023). *The Mind and Machine: An Introduction to Artificial Intelligence: Exploring the Intersection of Artificial Intelligence, Human Cognition, Psychology and Robotics.* Amazon International.

Belda-Medina, J., & Calvo-Ferrer, J. R. (2022). Using chatbots as AI conversational partners in language learning. *Applied Sciences (Basel, Switzerland)*, *12*(17), 8427. DOI: 10.3390/app12178427

Bendig, E., Erb, B., Schulze-Thuesing, L., & Baumeister, H. (2022). The next generation: Chatbots in clinical psychology and psychotherapy to foster mental health – a scoping review. *Verhaltenstherapie*, *32*(1, Suppl. 1), 64–76. DOI: 10.1159/000501812

Bennett, S., Cuijpers, P., Ebert, D., McKenzie, M., Coughtrey, A., Heyman, I., Manzotti, G., & Shafran, R. (2019). Practitioner review: Unguided and guided self-help interventions for common mental health disorders in children and adolescents: A systematic review and meta-analysis. *Journal of Child Psychology and Psychiatry, and Allied Disciplines*, *60*(8), 828–847. DOI: 10.1111/jcpp.13010 PMID: 30775782

Benotti, L., Martnez, M. C., & Schapachnik, F. (2017). A tool for introducing computer science with automatic formative assessment. *IEEE Transactions on Learning Technologies*, *11*(2), 179–192. DOI: 10.1109/TLT.2017.2682084

Bezerra, A. C. V., de Mendonça, R. D., Lamborda, T. C., & César, C. L. G. (2018). Trends in prevalence of overweight and obesity in adults in 26 Brazilian state capitals and the Federal District from 2006 to 2016. *BMC Public Health*, *18*(1), 1–10. DOI: 10.1186/s12889-018-5235-x

Bhagyashree, S. I. R., Nagaraj, K., Prince, M., Fall, C. H., & Krishna, M. (2018). Diagnosis of Dementia by Machine learning methods in Epidemiological studies: A pilot exploratory study from south India. *Social Psychiatry and Psychiatric Epidemiology*, *53*(1), 77–86. DOI: 10.1007/s00127-017-1410-0 PMID: 28698926

Bhargava, I., & Mor, N. (2024, February 15). *The future of mental health: Emerging trends and innovations.* Economics Times. https://health.economictimes.indiatimes.com/news/industry/the-future-of-mental-health-emerging-trends-and-innovations/107673809

Bhatnagr, P., Rajesh, A., & Misra, R. (2024). Continuous intention usage of artificial intelligence enabled digital banks: A review of expectation confirmation model. *Journal of Enterprise Information Management*, *37*(6), 1763–1787. DOI: 10.1108/JEIM-11-2023-0617

Bhise, A., Munshi, A., Rodrigues, A., & Sawant, V. (2022). Overview of AI in education. In *Artificial Intelligence in Higher Education* (pp. 31–62). CRC Press. DOI: 10.1201/9781003184157-2

Bickmore, T. W., & Giorgino, T. (2006). Health dialog systems for patients and consumers. *Journal of Biomedical Informatics*, *39*(5), 556–571. DOI: 10.1016/j.jbi.2005.12.004 PMID: 16464643

Bin-Nashwan, S. A., Sadallah, M., & Bouteraa, M. (2023). Use of ChatGPT in academia: Academic integrity hangs in the balance. *Technology in Society*, *75*, 102370. DOI: 10.1016/j.techsoc.2023.102370

Binns, R.'It's Reducing a Human Being to a Percentage' Perceptions of Justice in Algorithmic Decisions. *Proceedings of the 2018 Chi conference on human factors in computing systems*. DOI: 10.1145/3173574.3173951

Biringer, E., Davidson, L., Sundfør, B., Lier, H. Ø., & Borg, M. (2016). Coping with mental health issues: Subjective experiences of self-help and helpful contextual factors at the start of mental health treatment. *Journal of Mental Health (Abingdon, England)*, *25*(1), 23–27. DOI: 10.3109/09638237.2015.1078883 PMID: 26484831

Biro, J., Linder, C., & Neyens, D. (2023). The effects of a health care chatbot's complexity and persona on user trust, perceived usability, and effectiveness: Mixed methods study. *JMIR Human Factors*, *10*(1), e41017. DOI: 10.2196/41017 PMID: 36724004

Biswas, M. (2018). Wit.ai and Dialogflow. In *Beginning AI Bot Frameworks: Getting Started with Bot Development* (pp. 67–100). Apress. DOI: 10.1007/978-1-4842-3754-0_3

Biswas, S. (2023). Role of ChatGPT in Computer Programming. *Mesopotamian Journal of Computer Science*, *2023*, 9–15. DOI: 10.58496/MJCSC/2023/002

Blackwell, S. E., Heisig, S., & Kuckertz, J. M. (2021). Optimizing delivery of recovery-oriented online self-help for depression: A randomized controlled trial. *Psychotherapy and Psychosomatics*, *90*, 25–37.

Blackwell, S. E., Woud, M. L., & Margraf, J. (2020). A meta-analysis of cognitive-behavioural interventions for anxiety and depression in children and adolescents. *Child and Adolescent Mental Health*, *25*, 37–46.

Blaze Information Security. (n.d.). Cybersecurity risks of digital health applications. Retrieved from https://www.blazeinfosec.com/post/cybersecurity-risks-digital-health-apps/

Bolukbasi, T. (2016). Man is to computer programmer as woman is to homemaker? debiasing word embeddings. *Advances in Neural Information Processing Systems*, 29.

Bonner, R. L., & Rich, A. R. (1990). Psychosocial vulnerability, life stress, and suicide ideation in a jail population: A cross-validation study. *Suicide & Life-Threatening Behavior*, *20*(3), 213–224. DOI: 10.1111/j.1943-278X.1990.tb00106.x PMID: 2238014

Boonstra, T. W., Nicholas, J., Wong, Q. J. J., Shaw, F., Townsend, S., & Christensen, H. (2018). Using mobile phone sensor technology for mental health research: Integrated analysis to identify hidden challenges and potential solutions. *Journal of Medical Internet Research*, *20*(7), e10131. DOI: 10.2196/10131 PMID: 30061092

Botella, C., Díaz-García, A., Baños, R. M., & Quero, S. (2009). Cybertherapy: Advantages, limitations, and ethical issues.

Boucher, E. M., Harake, N. R., Ward, H. E., Stoeckl, S. E., Vargas, J., Minkel, J., Parks, A. C., & Zilca, R. (2021). Artificially intelligent chatbots in digital mental health interventions: a review. *Expert Review of Medical Devices, 18*(sup1), 37–49. DOI: 10.1080/17434440.2021.2013200

Braun, M., Hummel, P., Beck, S., & Dabrock, P. (2021). Primer on an ethics of AI-based decision support systems in the clinic. *Journal of Medical Ethics*, *47*(12), e3–e3. DOI: 10.1136/medethics-2019-105860 PMID: 32245804

Brin, S., & Page, L. (1998). The anatomy of a large-scale hypertextual Web search engine. *Computer Networks and ISDN Systems*, *30*(1), 107–117. DOI: 10.1016/S0169-7552(98)00110-X

Brookings Institution. (2023). Why mental health apps need to take privacy more seriously. Retrieved from https://www.brookings.edu/articles/why-mental-health-apps-need-to-take-privacy-more-seriously/

Brown, A., Kumar, A. T., Melamed, O., Ahmed, I., Wang, Y. H., Deza, A., Morcos, M., Zhu, L., Maslej, M., Minian, N., Sujaya, V., Wolff, J., Doggett, O., Iantorno, M., Ratto, M., Selby, P., & Rose, J. (2023). A motivational interviewing chatbot with generative reflections for increasing readiness to quit smoking: Iterative development study. *JMIR Mental Health*, *10*(1), e49132. DOI: 10.2196/49132 PMID: 37847539

Brown, E. L., Ruggiano, N., Allala, S. C., Clarke, P. J., Davis, D., Roberts, L., Framil, C. V., Muñoz, M. T. H., Hough, M. S., & Bourgeois, M. S. (2023). Developing a Memory and Communication App for Persons Living With Dementia: An 8-Step Process. *JMIR Aging*, *6*, e44007. DOI: 10.2196/44007 PMID: 36920462

Brown, T. B., Mann, B., Ryder, N., Subbiah, M., Kaplan, J., Dhariwal, P., Neelakantan, A., Shyam, P., Sastry, G., Askell, A., Agarwal, S., Herbert-Voss, A., Krueger, G., Henighan, T., Child, R., Ramesh, A., Ziegler, D. M., Wu, J., Winter, C., & Amodei, D. (2020). Language Models Are Few-Shot Learners. *Proceedings of the 34th International Conference on Neural Information Processing Systems.*

Bucaioni, A., Ekedahl, H., Helander, V., & Nguyen, P. T. (2024). Programming with ChatGPT: How far can we go? *Machine Learning with Applications*, *15*, 100526. DOI: 10.1016/j.mlwa.2024.100526

Buruk, B., Ekmekci, P. E., & Arda, B. (2020). A critical perspective on guidelines for responsible and trustworthy artificial intelligence. *Medicine, Health Care, and Philosophy*, *23*(3), 387–399. DOI: 10.1007/s11019-020-09948-1 PMID: 32236794

Butler, R. (2000). What learners want to know: The role of achievement goals in shaping information seeking, learning, and interest. In Sansone, C., & Harackiewicz, J. M. (Eds.), *Intrinsic and Extrinsic Motivation* (pp. 161–194). Academic Press. DOI: 10.1016/B978-012619070-0/50029-5

Bzdok, D., & Meyer-Lindenberg, A. (2018). Machine learning for precision psychiatry: Opportunities and challenges. *Biological Psychiatry: Cognitive Neuroscience and Neuroimaging*, *3*(3), 223–230. DOI: 10.1016/j.bpsc.2017.11.007 PMID: 29486863

Cahan, P., & Treutlein, B. (2023). A conversation with ChatGPT on the role of computational systems biology in stem cell research. *Stem Cell Reports*, *18*(1), 1–2. DOI: 10.1016/j.stemcr.2022.12.009 PMID: 36630899

Camacho, E., & Torous, J. (2022). Assessment of mental health services available through smartphone apps. JAMA Network Open. https://www.ncbi.nlm.nih.gov/pmc/articles/PMC9857226/

Cambria, E., & White, B. (2014). Jumping NLP Curves: A Review of Natural Language Processing Research [Review Article]. *IEEE Computational Intelligence Magazine*, *9*(2), 48–57. DOI: 10.1109/MCI.2014.2307227

Cao, B., Zheng, L., Zhang, C., Yu, P. S., Piscitello, A., Zulueta, J., & Leow, A. D. (2017, August). Deepmood: modeling mobile phone typing dynamics for mood detection. In *Proceedings of the 23rd ACM SIGKDD international conference on knowledge discovery and data mining* (pp. 747-755). DOI: 10.1145/3097983.3098086

Castelvecchi, D. (2022). Are ChatGPT and AlphaCode going to replace programmers? *Nature*. Advance online publication. DOI: 10.1038/d41586-022-04383-z PMID: 36481949

Cavoukian, A. (2011). *Privacy by design: Best practices for privacy and the smart grid. ISSE 2010 Securing Electronic Business Processes: Highlights of the Information Security Solutions Europe 2010 Conference*. Wiesbaden: Vieweg+ Teubner.

Chagas, B. A., Pagano, A. S., Prates, R. O., Praes, E. C., Ferreguetti, K., Vaz, H., Reis, Z. S. N., Ribeiro, L. B., Ribeiro, A. L. P., Pedroso, T. M., Beleigoli, A., Oliveira, C. R. A., & Marcolino, M. S. (2023). Evaluating user experience with a Chatbot designed as a public health response to the COVID-19 pandemic in Brazil: Mixed methods study. *JMIR Human Factors*, *10*(1), e43135. DOI: 10.2196/43135 PMID: 36634267

Chan, A. H. Y., & Honey, M. L. L. (2022). User perceptions of mobile digital apps for mental health: Acceptability and usability - An integrative review. *Journal of Psychiatric and Mental Health Nursing*, *29*(1), 147–168. DOI: 10.1111/jpm.12744 PMID: 33604946

Chang, S., Sambasivam, R., Seow, E., Tan, G. C.-Y., Lu, S. H., Assudani, H., Chong, S. A., Subramaniam, M., & Vaingankar, J. A. (2021). "We are all trying to find a way to help ourselves": A look at self-help strategies among psychotherapy clients. *Frontiers in Psychology*, *12*, 621085. Advance online publication. DOI: 10.3389/fpsyg.2021.621085 PMID: 34690850

Chauncey, S. A., & McKenna, H. P. (2023). A framework and exemplars for ethical and responsible use of AI Chatbot technology to support teaching and learning. *Computers and Education: Artificial Intelligence*, *5*, 100182. DOI: 10.1016/j.caeai.2023.100182

Chauvin, J., Perera, Y., & Clarke, M. (2016). Digital technologies for population health and health equity gains: The perspective of public health associations. *Journal of Public Health Policy*, *37*(S2), 232–248. DOI: 10.1057/s41271-016-0013-4 PMID: 27899798

Cheddak, A., Ait Baha, T., Es-Saady, Y., El Hajji, M., & Baslam, M. (2024). BERTopic for Enhanced Idea Management and Topic Generation in Brainstorming Sessions. *Information (Basel)*, *15*(6), 365. DOI: 10.3390/info15060365

Cheng, Y., & Jiang, H. (2020). AI-Powered mental health chatbots: Examining users' motivations, active communicative action and engagement after mass-shooting disasters. *Journal of Contingencies and Crisis Management*, *28*(3), 339–354. DOI: 10.1111/1468-5973.12319

Chen, T., Tachmazidis, I., Batsakis, S., Adamou, M., Papadakis, E., & Antoniou, G. (2023). Diagnosing attention-deficit hyperactivity disorder (ADHD) using artificial intelligence: A clinical study in the UK. *Frontiers in Psychiatry*, *14*, 1164433. DOI: 10.3389/fpsyt.2023.1164433 PMID: 37363182

Chen, Y., Lin, Q., Chen, X., Liu, T., Ke, Q., Yang, Q., Guan, B., & Ming, W. K. (2023). Need assessment for history-taking instruction program using chatbot for nursing students: A qualitative study using focus group interviews. *Digital Health*, *29*(9), 20552076231185435. DOI: 10.1177/20552076231185435 PMID: 37426591

Chen, Y., Lorenzi, N., Nyemba, S., Schildcrout, J. S., & Malin, B. (2014). We work with them? Healthcare workers interpretation of organizational relations mined from electronic health records. *International Journal of Medical Informatics*, *83*(7), 495–506. DOI: 10.1016/j.ijmedinf.2014.04.006 PMID: 24845147

Chew, H. S. J., & Achananuparp, P. (2022). Perceptions and needs of Artificial intelligence in health care to increase adoption: Scoping review. *Journal of Medical Internet Research*, *24*(1), e32939. DOI: 10.2196/32939 PMID: 35029538

Chicago Sun-Times. (2024, May 29). Email hack exposed University of Chicago Medical Center patient information. Retrieved from https://chicago.suntimes.com/health/2024/05/29/email-hack-exposed-university-chicago-medical-center-patient-information-data-breach-security-health

Chicago Tribune. (2019, March 4). Rush reports data breach involving 45,000 patients. Retrieved from https://www.chicagotribune.com/2019/03/04/rush-reports-data-breach-involving-45000-patients/

Chin, H., Song, H., Baek, G., Shin, M., Jung, C., Cha, M., Choi, J., & Cha, C. (2023). The potential of chatbots for emotional support and promoting mental well-being in different cultures: Mixed methods study. *Journal of Medical Internet Research*, *25*, e51712. Advance online publication. DOI: 10.2196/51712 PMID: 37862063

Cho, J., & Garcia-Molina, H. (2002). Parallel crawlers. *The Web Conference*.

Chowdhary, K., & Chowdhary, K. (2020). Natural language processing. *Fundamentals of artificial intelligence*, 603-649.

Chuang, C.-H., Lo, J.-H., & Wu, Y.-K. (2023). Integrating chatbot and augmented reality technology into biology learning during COVID-19. *Electronics (Basel)*, *12*(1), 222. DOI: 10.3390/electronics12010222

Chung, M., Ko, E., Joung, H., & Kim, S. J. (2020). Chatbot e-service and customer satisfaction regarding luxury brands. *Journal of Business Research*, *117*, 587–595. DOI: 10.1016/j.jbusres.2018.10.004

Chun-Hung, L., Guan-Hsiung, L., Wu-Chuan, Y., & Yu-Hsin, L. (2023). Chatbot-assisted therapy for patients with methamphetamine use disorder: A preliminary randomized controlled trial. *Frontiers in Psychiatry*, *14*, 1159399. Advance online publication. DOI: 10.3389/fpsyt.2023.1159399 PMID: 37484677

Cicek, G., & Akan, A. (2021, November). Deep Learning Approach Versus Traditional Machine Learning for ADHD Classification. In *2021 Medical Technologies Congress (TIPTEKNO)* (pp. 1-4). IEEE. DOI: 10.1109/TIPTEKNO53239.2021.9632940

Cimpanu, C. (2020). Finnish psychotherapy data breach sees the most vulnerable victims extorted. CyberScoop. https://cyberscoop.com/finnish-psychotherapy-data-breach-vastaamo/

Cinelli, M., Quattrociocchi, W., Galeazzi, A., Valensise, C. M., Brugnoli, E., Schmidt, A. L., Zola, P., Zollo, F., & Scala, A. (2020). The COVID-19 social media infodemic. *Scientific Reports*, *10*(1), 1–10. DOI: 10.1038/s41598-020-73510-5 PMID: 33024152

Clark, L., Pantidi, N., Cooney, O., Doyle, P., Garaialde, D., Edwards, J., Spillane, B., Gilmartin, E., Murad, C., Munteanu, C., Wade, V., & Cowan, B. R. (2019). What Makes a Good Conversation? Challenges in Designing Truly Conversational Agents. *Proceedings of the 2019 CHI Conference on Human Factors in Computing Systems*, 1–12. DOI: 10.1145/3290605.3300705

Codecademy. (n.d.). *What are chatbots?* https://www.codecademy.com/article/what-are-chatbots

Coghlan, S., Leins, K., Sheldrick, S., Cheong, M., Gooding, P., & D'Alfonso, S. (2023). To chat or bot to chat: Ethical issues with using chatbots in mental health. *Digital Health*, *9*, 20552076231183542. DOI: 10.1177/20552076231183542 PMID: 37377565

Colizzi, M., Lasalvia, A., & Ruggeri, M. (2020). Prevention and early intervention in youth mental health: Is it time for a multidisciplinary and trans-diagnostic model for care? *International Journal of Mental Health Systems*, *14*(1), 1–14. DOI: 10.1186/s13033-020-00356-9 PMID: 32226481

Co, M., Yuen, T. H. J., & Cheung, B. H. H. (2022). Using clinical history taking chatbot mobile app for clinical bedside teachings – A prospective case control study. *Heliyon*, *8*(6), e09751. DOI: 10.1016/j.heliyon.2022.e09751 PMID: 35770149

Compliancy Group. (n.d.). HIPAA Security Rule Requirements Explained. Retrieved from https://compliancy-group.com/hipaa-security-rule/

Consolo, L., Basile, I., Colombo, S., Rusconi, D., Pasquot, L., Campa, T., Caraceni, A., & Lusignani, M. (2024). Exploring patient perspectives on electronic patient-reported outcome measures in home-based cancer palliative care: A qualitative study. *Digital Health*, *10*. DOI: 10.1177/20552076241249962 PMID: 38665884

Coronado, M., Iglesias, C. A., Carrera, Á., & Mardomingo, A. (2018). A cognitive assistant for learning java featuring social dialogue. *International Journal of Human-Computer Studies*, *117*, 55–67. DOI: 10.1016/j.ijhcs.2018.02.004

Costello, E. J. (2016). Early detection and prevention of mental health problems: Developmental epidemiology and systems of support. *Journal of Clinical Child and Adolescent Psychology*, *45*(6), 710–717. DOI: 10.1080/15374416.2016.1236728 PMID: 27858462

Cropley, D. (2023). Is artificial intelligence more creative than humans?: ChatGPT and the divergent association task. *Learning Letters*, *2*, 13–13. DOI: 10.59453/ll.v2.13

Cunningham-Nelson, S., Boles, W., Trouton, L., & Margerison, E. (2019). *A Review of Chatbots in Education: Practical Steps Forward*. Engineers Australia. https://search.informit.org/doi/10.3316/informit.068364390172788

Cyber Security Cooperative Research Centre. (n.d.). Mental health apps: Privacy risks. Retrieved from https://cybersecuritycrc.org.au/mental-health-apps-privacy-risks

Cynet. (n.d.). GDPR Data Breach Notifications: Everything You Need to Know. Retrieved from https://www.cynet.com/cynet-for-compliance/gdpr-data-breach-notifications-everything-you-need-to-know/

D'Alfonso, S. (2020). AI in mental health. *Current Opinion in Psychology*, *36*, 112–117. DOI: 10.1016/j.copsyc.2020.04.005 PMID: 32604065

da Fona Costa, L., & Cesar Jr, R. M. (2018). *Shape classification and analysis: theory and practice*. Crc Press. DOI: 10.1201/9781315222325

Dana, R., & Gavril, R. (2023). Exploring the psychological implications of chatGPT: A qualitative study. *Journal Plus Education*, *32*(1), 43–55.

Danieli, M., Ciulli, T., Mousavi, S. M., Silvestri, G., Barbato, S., Di Natale, L., & Riccardi, G. (2022). Assessing the impact of conversational artificial intelligence in the treatment of stress and anxiety in aging adults: Randomized controlled trial. *JMIR Mental Health*, *9*(9), e38067. DOI: 10.2196/38067 PMID: 36149730

Dao, X., & Le, N. (2023). Investigating the effectiveness of ChatGPT in mathematical reasoning and problem solving: Evidence from the Vietnamese national high school graduation examination. /arxiv.2306.06331DOI: 10.48550

Data Privacy Manager. (n.d.). What are 8 Data Subject rights according to the GDPR. Retrieved from https://dataprivacymanager.net/what-are-data-subject-rights-according-to-the-gdpr/

Data Protection Commission. (n.d.). Quick Guide to GDPR Breach Notifications. Retrieved from https://www.dataprotection.ie/en/organisations/know-your-obligations/quick-guide-gdpr-breach-notifications

Daud, S. H. M., Teo, N. H. I., & Zain, N. H. M. (2020). Ejava chatbot for learning programming language: Apost-pandemic alternative virtual tutor. *International Journal (Toronto, Ont.)*, *8*(7), 3290–3298.

Davis, F. D. (1989). Perceived usefulness, perceived ease of use, and user acceptance of information technology. *Management Information Systems Quarterly*, *13*(3), 319. DOI: 10.2307/249008

De Bruyn, M., Lotfi, E., Buhmann, J., & Daelemans, W. (2020, August). *BART for Knowledge Grounded Conversations.*

De Freitas, J., Uğuralp, A. K., Oğuz-Uğuralp, Z., & Puntoni, S. (2022). Chatbots and mental health: Insights into the safety of generative AI. *Journal of Consumer Psychology.*

De Gruttola, V. G., Clax, P., DeMets, D. L., Downing, G. J., Ellenberg, S. S., Friedman, L., Gail, M. H., Prentice, R., Wittes, J., & Zeger, S. L. (2001). Considerations in the evaluation of surrogate endpoints in clinical trials: Summary of a National Institutes of Health workshop. *Controlled Clinical Trials*, *22*(5), 485–502. DOI: 10.1016/S0197-2456(01)00153-2 PMID: 11578783

de Vasconcellos, V. G. (2023). *Artificial Intelligence and Co-Authorship of Scientific Manuscripts: Discussions about Using ChatGPT in Scientific Research and Writing* (Vol. 9). HeinOnline.

Deady, M., Glozier, N., Calvo, R., Johnston, D., Mackinnon, A., Milne, D., Choi, I., Gayed, A., Peters, D., Bryant, R., Christensen, H., & Harvey, S. B. (2022). Preventing depression using a smartphone app: A randomized controlled trial. *Psychological Medicine*, *52*(3), 457–466. DOI: 10.1017/S0033291720002081 PMID: 32624013

Deiana, G., Dettori, M., Arghittu, A., Azara, A., Gabutti, G., & Castiglia, P. (2023). Artificial intelligence and public health: Evaluating ChatGPT responses to vaccination myths and misconceptions. *Vaccines*, *11*(7), 1217. DOI: 10.3390/vaccines11071217 PMID: 37515033

Devlin, J., Chang, M.-W., Lee, K., & Toutanova, K. (2019). *BERT: Pre-training of Deep Bidirectional Transformers for Language Understanding.*

Dev, P., Winzelberg, A. J., Celio, A., & Taylor, C. B. (1999). Student bodies: Psycho-education communities on the web. *Proc AMIA Symp*, 510–514. PMID: 10566411

Di Pelino, S., Lamarche, L., Carr, T., Datta, J., Gaber, J., Oliver, D., Gallagher, J., Dragos, S., Price, D., & Mangin, D. (2022). Lessons learned through two phases of developing and implementing a technology supporting integrated care: Case study. *JMIR Formative Research*, *6*(4), e34899. DOI: 10.2196/34899 PMID: 35404253

Dig8ital. (n.d.). Boost your security: The importance of network security audits. Retrieved from https://dig8ital.com/post/network-security-audits/

Dinan, E., Roller, S., Shuster, K., Fan, A., Auli, M., & Weston, J. (2019). *Wizard of Wikipedia: Knowledge-Powered Conversational agents*.

Ding, M., Huo, Y., Hu, J., & Lu, Z. (2018). DeepInsight: Multi-Task Multi-Scale Deep Learning for Mental Disorder Diagnosis. In *BMVC* (p. 115).

DOWN, LAYING, and INTELLIGENCE ACT. "Proposal for a Regulation of the European Parliament and of the Council laying down harmonised rules on Artificial Intelligence (Artificial Intelligence Act) and amending certain Union legislative acts." (2021).

Dsouza, R., Sahu, S., Patil, R., & Kalbande, D. R. (2019). Chat with bots intelligently: A critical review & analysis. *2019 International Conference on Advances in Computing, Communication and Control (ICAC3)*, 1–6. DOI: 10.1109/ICAC347590.2019.9036844

Durall, E., & Kapros, E. (2020). Co-design for a competency self-assessment chatbot and survey in science education. *Learning and Collaboration Technologies. Human and Technology Ecosystems: 7th International Conference, LCT 2020, Held as Part of the 22nd HCI International Conference, HCII 2020, Copenhagen, Denmark, July 19–24, 2020. Proceedings*, *22*(Part II), 13–24.

Egger, R., Neuburger, L., & Mattuzzi, M. (2022). Data science and ethical issues: between knowledge gain and ethical responsibility. In *Applied Data Science in Tourism: Interdisciplinary Approaches, Methodologies, and Applications* (pp. 51–66). Springer International Publishing. DOI: 10.1007/978-3-030-88389-8_4

Ehrenpreis, M., & DeLooper, J. (2022). Implementing a chatbot on a library website. *Journal of Web Librarianship*, *16*(2), 120–142. DOI: 10.1080/19322909.2022.2060893

Eisner, E., Berry, N., & Bucci, S. (2023). Digital tools to support mental health: A survey study in psychosis. *BMC Psychiatry*, *23*(1), 726. DOI: 10.1186/s12888-023-05114-y PMID: 37803367

Elmasri, D., & Maeder, A. (2016). A conversational agent for an online mental health intervention. In *Brain Informatics and Health:International Conference, BIH 2016,Omaha, NE, USA,October 13-16, 2016Proceedings* (pp. 243-251). Springer International Publishing. DOI: 10.1007/978-3-319-47103-7_24

Else, H. (2023). Abstracts written by ChatGPT fool scientists. *Nature, 613*(7944), 423. DOI: 10.1038/d41586-023-00056-7 PMID: 36635510

Elyoseph, Z., Hadar-Shoval, D., Asraf, K., & Lvovsky, M. (2023). ChatGPT outperforms humans in emotional awareness evaluations. *Frontiers in Psychology, 14*, 1199058. DOI: 10.3389/fpsyg.2023.1199058 PMID: 37303897

Eom, S., Wen, J., & Ashill, N. (2006). The Determinants of Students' Perceived Learning Outcomes and Satisfaction in University Online Education: An Empirical Investigation. *Decision Sciences Journal of Innovative Education, 4*(2), 215–235. DOI: 10.1111/j.1540-4609.2006.00114.x

Ettman, C. K., & Galea, S. (2023). The potential influence of AI on population mental health. *JMIR Mental Health, 10*, e49936. DOI: 10.2196/49936 PMID: 37971803

Eubanks, V. (2018). *Automating inequality: How high-tech tools profile, police, and punish the poor*. St. Martin's Press.

European Commission. (2019). Directorate General for Communications Networks, Content and Technology. *Ethics guidelines for trustworthy AI.*

European Commission. (n.d.). What does data protection 'by design' and 'by default' mean? Retrieved from https://commission.europa.eu/law/law-topic/data-protection/reform/rules-business-and-organisations/obligations/what-does-data-protection-design-and-default-mean_en

European Journal of Privacy Law & Technologies. (n.d.). Announcements. https://universitypress.unisob.na.it/ojs/index.php/ejplt/announcement/view/125

Fadhil, A., Wang, Y., & Reiterer, H. (2019). Assistive conversational agent for health coaching: A validation study. *Methods of Information in Medicine, 58*(1), 9–23. DOI: 10.1055/s-0039-1688757

Farid, A. A., Selim, G. I., & Khater, H. A. A. (2020). Applying artificial intelligence techniques to improve clinical diagnosis of Alzheimer's disease. *European Journal of Engineering Science and Technology, 3*(2), 58–79. DOI: 10.33422/ejest.v3i2.487

Farooq, A., Anwar, S., Awais, M., & Alnowami, M. (2017, September). Artificial intelligence based smart diagnosis of Alzheimer's disease and mild cognitive impairment. In *2017 International Smart cities conference (ISC2)* (pp. 1-4). IEEE. DOI: 10.1109/ISC2.2017.8090871

Farvolden, P. (2024, February). AI chatbots break down barriers to much-needed mental health treatments. Retrieved from https://www.rgare.com/knowledge-center/article/ai-chatbots-break-down-barriers-to-much-needed-mental-health-treatments

Federal Trade Commission. (2016). Mobile health app developers: FTC best practices. Retrieved from https://www.ncbi.nlm.nih.gov/pmc/articles/PMC6371412/

Feldman, M. J., Hoffer, E. P., Barnett, G. O., Kim, R. J., Famiglietti, K. T., & Chueh, H. C. (2012). Impact of a computer-based diagnostic decision support tool on the differential diagnoses of medicine residents. *Journal of Graduate Medical Education*, *4*(2), 227–231. DOI: 10.4300/JGME-D-11-00180.1 PMID: 23730446

Fernández-Arteaga, V., Tovilla-Zárate, C. A., Fresán, A., González-Castro, T. B., Juárez-Rojop, I. E., López-Narváez, L., & Hernández-Díaz, Y. (2016). Association between completed suicide and environmental temperature in a Mexican population, using the Knowledge Discovery in Database approach. *Computer Methods and Programs in Biomedicine*, *135*, 219–224. DOI: 10.1016/j.cmpb.2016.08.002 PMID: 27586493

Ferreri, F., Bourla, A., Mouchabac, S., & Karila, L. (2018). e-Addictology: An overview of new technologies for assessing and intervening in addictive behaviors. *Frontiers in Psychiatry*, *9*, 348832. DOI: 10.3389/fpsyt.2018.00051 PMID: 29545756

Financial Express. (2023). How mental health apps are yet to fulfil the promise of user data privacy. Retrieved from https://www.financialexpress.com/business/digital-transformation-how-mental-health-apps-are-yet-to-fulfil-the-promise-of-user-data-privacy-3378043/

Fiske, A., Henningsen, P., & Buyx, A. (2019). Your robot therapist will see you now: Ethical implications of embodied artificial intelligence in psychiatry, psychology, and psychotherapy. *Journal of Medical Internet Research*, *21*(5), e13216. DOI: 10.2196/13216 PMID: 31094356

Fitzpatrick, K. K., Darcy, A., & Vierhile, M. (2017). Delivering cognitive behavior therapy to young adults with symptoms of depression and anxiety using a fully automated conversational agent (Woebot): A randomized controlled trial. *JMIR Mental Health*, *4*(2), e7785. DOI: 10.2196/mental.7785 PMID: 28588005

Fleming, T. M., de Beurs, D., Khazaal, Y., Gaggioli, A., Riva, G., Botella, C., Baños, R. M., Aschieri, F., Bavin, L. M., Kleiboer, A., Merry, S., Lau, H. M., & Riper, H. (2016). Maximizing the impact of e-therapy and serious gaming: Time for a paradigm shift. *Frontiers in Psychiatry, 7,* 65. DOI: 10.3389/fpsyt.2016.00065 PMID: 27148094

Flora, K., Raftopoulos, A., & Pontikes, T. (2010). A look at the evolution of the self-help movement. *Journal of Groups in Addiction & Recovery, 5*(3-4), 214–225. DOI: 10.1080/1556035X.2010.523349

Floridi & Cowls. (2022). A unified framework of five principles for AI in society. *Machine learning and the city: Applications in architecture and urban design*, 535-545.

Floridi, L., Cowls, J., Beltrametti, M., Chatila, R., Chazerand, P., Dignum, V., Luetge, C., Madelin, R., Pagallo, U., Rossi, F., Schafer, B., Valcke, P., & Vayena, E. (2018). AI4People—an ethical framework for a good AI society: Opportunities, risks, principles, and recommendations. *Minds and Machines, 28*(4), 689–707. DOI: 10.1007/s11023-018-9482-5 PMID: 30930541

Følstad, A., & Taylor, C. (2021). Investigating the user experience of customer service chatbot interaction: A framework for qualitative analysis of chatbot dialogues. *Quality and User Experience, 6*(1), 6. DOI: 10.1007/s41233-021-00046-5

France, B. (2016, November 23). *The importance of choosing the right therapist.* Medium. https://medium.com/@BenFrance/the-importance-of-choosing-the-right-therapist-5622d4f22a13

Frey, B. (2024, March 27). *Earkick: AI-powered mental health support.* Earkick. https://blog.earkick.com/earkick-ai-powered-mental-health-support/

Frieder, S., Pinchetti, L., Griffiths, R. R., Salvatori, T., Lukasiewicz, T., Petersen, P. C., . . . Berner, J. (2023). Mathematical capabilities of ChatGPT. *arXiv preprint arXiv:2301.13867.*

Fulmer, R., Joerin, A., Gentile, B., Lakerink, L., & Rauws, M. (2018). Using psychological artificial intelligence (Tess) to relieve symptoms of depression and anxiety: Randomized controlled trial. *JMIR Mental Health, 5*(4), e9782. DOI: 10.2196/mental.9782 PMID: 30545815

Fusar-Poli, P., De Pablo, G. S., De Micheli, A., Nieman, D. H., Correll, C. U., Kessing, L. V., Pfennig, A., Bechdolf, A., Borgwardt, S., Arango, C., & van Amelsvoort, T. (2020). What is good mental health? A scoping review. *European Neuropsychopharmacology, 31,* 33–46. DOI: 10.1016/j.euroneuro.2019.12.105 PMID: 31901337

Gamble, A. (2020). Artificial intelligence and mobile apps for mental healthcare: A social informatics perspective. *Proceedings of the International Conferences on Internet Technologies & Society (ITS 2020) and Sustainability, Technology and Education (STE 2020).*

Gammoh, L. A. (2024). ChatGPT in academia: Exploring university students' risks, misuses, and challenges in Jordan. *Journal of Further and Higher Education*, *48*(6), 608–624. DOI: 10.1080/0309877X.2024.2378298

Gao, J., Galley, M., & Li, L. (2019). *Neural approaches to conversational AI: Question answering, task-oriented dialogues and social chatbots*. Now Foundations and Trends. DOI: 10.1561/9781680835533

Garattini, L., Badinella Martini, M., & Zanetti, M. (2021). More room for telemedicine after COVID-19: Lessons for primary care? *The European Journal of Health Economics*, *22*(2), 183–186. DOI: 10.1007/s10198-020-01248-y PMID: 33231825

Garg, K., Kumar, C. N., & Chandra, P. S. (2019). Number of psychiatrists in India: Baby steps forward, but a long way to go. *Indian Journal of Psychiatry*, *61*(1), 104–105. PMID: 30745666

Gavin, B., Lyne, J., & McNicholas, F. (2020). Mental health and the COVID-19 pandemic: Looking back and moving forward. *Irish Journal of Psychological Medicine*, *37*(4), 247–249. DOI: 10.1017/ipm.2020.128 PMID: 33323135

Gcore. (2023). What is an AI chatbot? Retrieved from https://gcore.com/learning/what-is-an-ai-chatbot/

GDPR-Info.eu. (n.d.). Chapter 3 – Rights of the data subject. Retrieved from https://gdpr-info.eu/chapter-3/

GDPR-Info.eu. (n.d.). Notification of a personal data breach to the supervisory authority. Retrieved from https://gdpr-info.eu/art-33-gdpr/

GDPR-Info.eu. (n.d.). Privacy by Design. Retrieved from https://gdpr-info.eu/issues/privacy-by-design/

GDPR-Text.com. (n.d.). Article 25 GDPR. Data protection by design and by default. Retrieved from https://gdpr-text.com/read/article-25/

Gellatly, J., Bower, P., Hennessy, S., Richards, D., Gilbody, S., & Lovell, K. (2007). What makes self-help interventions effective in the management of depressive symptoms? Meta-analysis and meta-regression. *Psychological Medicine*, *37*(9), 1217–1228. DOI: 10.1017/S0033291707000062 PMID: 17306044

George, A. S., Muralikrishnan, G., Ninan, L. R., Varrier, P. S., & Dhanya, L. (2021). Survey on the design and development of Indian language chatbots. 2021 International Conference on Communication, Control and Information Sciences (ICCISc).

Gerlich, M. (2023). Perceptions and acceptance of artificial intelligence: A multidimensional study. *Social Sciences (Basel, Switzerland)*, *12*(9), 502. DOI: 10.3390/socsci12090502

Gillan, C. M., & Whelan, R. (2017). What big data can do for treatment in psychiatry. *Current Opinion in Behavioral Sciences*, *18*, 34–42. DOI: 10.1016/j.cobeha.2017.07.003

Glauner, P. (2022). An assessment of the ai regulation proposed by the european commission. In *The future circle of healthcare: AI, 3D printing, longevity, ethics, and uncertainty mitigation* (pp. 119–127). Springer International Publishing. DOI: 10.1007/978-3-030-99838-7_7

Golbin, I., Rao, A. S., Hadjarian, A., & Krittman, D. (2020, December). Responsible AI: a primer for the legal community. In *2020 IEEE international conference on big data (big data)* (pp. 2121-2126). IEEE. DOI: 10.1109/BigData50022.2020.9377738

Goodwin, G., Haddad, P., Ferrier, I., Aronson, J. K., Barnes, T. R. H., Cipriani, A., Coghill, D. R., Fazel, S., Geddes, J. R., Grunze, H., Holmes, E. A., Howes, O., Hudson, S., Hunt, N., Jones, I., Macmillan, I. C., McAllister-Williams, H., Miklowitz, D. R., Morriss, R., & Young, A. H. (2016). *Evidence-based guidelines for treating bipolar disorder*: Revised third edition recommendations from the British Association for Psychopharmacology. *Journal of Psychopharmacology*, *30*(6), 495-553. DOI: 10.1177/0269881116636545

Gordon, J. S. (2021). AI and law: ethical, legal, and socio-political implications. *ai & Society*, *36*, 403-404.

Goto, A., & Katanoda, K. (2023). Should we acknowledge ChatGPT as an author? *Journal of Epidemiology*, *33*(7), 333–334. DOI: 10.2188/jea.JE20230078 PMID: 37032108

Gould, R., & Clum, G. (1993). A meta-analysis of self-help treatment approaches. *Clinical Psychology Review*, *13*(2), 169–186. DOI: 10.1016/0272-7358(93)90039-O

Graham, F. (2022). Daily briefing: Will ChatGPT kill the essay assignment? *Nature*. Advance online publication. DOI: 10.1038/d41586-022-04437-2 PMID: 36517680

Graham, S., Depp, C., Lee, E. E., Nebeker, C., Tu, X., Kim, H. C., & Jeste, D. V. (2019). Artificial intelligence for mental health and mental illnesses: An overview. *Current Psychiatry Reports, 21*(11), 1–18. DOI: 10.1007/s11920-019-1094-0 PMID: 31701320

Greenberg, A. (2020). A Hacker is Trying to Extort Patients in a Massive Psychotherapy Data Breach. Wired. https://www.wired.com/story/vastaamo-psychotherapy-patients-hack-data-breach/

Greer, S., Ramo, D., Chang, Y.-J., Fu, M., Moskowitz, J., & Haritatos, J. (2019). Use of the chatbot "vivibot" to deliver positive psychology skills and promote well-being among young people after cancer treatment: Randomized controlled feasibility trial. *JMIR mHealth and uHealth, 7*(10), e15018. DOI: 10.2196/15018 PMID: 31674920

Grist, R., Croker, A., Denne, M., & Stallard, P. (2018). Technology delivered interventions for depression and anxiety in children and adolescents: A systematic review and meta-analysis. *Clinical Child and Family Psychology Review, 22*(2), 147–171. DOI: 10.1007/s10567-018-0271-8 PMID: 30229343

Grodniewicz, J. P., & Hohol, M. (2024). Therapeutic Chatbots as Cognitive-Affective Artifacts. *Topoi, 43*(3), 795–807. Advance online publication. DOI: 10.1007/s11245-024-10018-x

Grudin, J., & Jacques, R. (2019). Chatbots, Humbots, and the Quest for Artificial General Intelligence. *Proceedings of the 2019 CHI Conference on Human Factors in Computing Systems*, 1–11. DOI: 10.1145/3290605.3300439

Guidance, W. H. O. (2021). *Ethics and governance of artificial intelligence for health.* World Health Organization.

Gu, J., Wang, Y., Cho, K., & Li, V. (2017). Search Engine Guided Non-Parametric Neural Machine Translation. *Proceedings of the AAAI Conference on Artificial Intelligence,* 32. DOI: 10.1609/aaai.v32i1.12013

Gupta, T. (2023, October 26). *The role of generative AI in natural language processing.* eLearning Industry. https://elearningindustry.com/role-of-generative-ai-in-natural-language-processing#:~:text=In%20the%20context%20of%20Natural,Pre%2Dtrained%20Transformer)%20series.

Gupta, M. D., Jha, M. K., Bansal, A., Yadav, R., Ramakrishanan, S., Girish, M. P., Sarkar, P. G., Qamar, A., Kumar, S., Kumar, S., Jain, A., Saijpaul, R., Gupta, V., Kansal, D., Garg, S., Arora, S., Biswas, P. S., Yusuf, J., Malhotra, R. K., & Gupta, A. (2021). COVID 19-related burnout among healthcare workers in India and ECG based predictive machine learning model: Insights from the BRUCEE-Li study. *Indian Heart Journal*, *73*(6), 674–681. DOI: 10.1016/j.ihj.2021.10.002 PMID: 34673026

Hahn, T., Nierenberg, A. A., & Whitfield-Gabrieli, S. (2017). Predictive analytics in mental health: Applications, guidelines, challenges and perspectives. *Molecular Psychiatry*, *22*(1), 37–43. DOI: 10.1038/mp.2016.201 PMID: 27843153

Halms, T., Strasser, M., Kunz, M., & Hasan, A. (2022). How to reduce mental health burden in health care workers during COVID-19?–a scoping review of guideline recommendations. *Frontiers in Psychiatry*, *12*, 770193. DOI: 10.3389/fpsyt.2021.770193 PMID: 35126194

Haman, M., & Školník, M. (2024). Using ChatGPT to conduct a literature review. *Accountability in Research*, *31*(8), 1244–1246. DOI: 10.1080/08989621.2023.2185514 PMID: 36879536

Hamburg, M. A., & Collins, F. S. (2010). The path to personalized medicine. *The New England Journal of Medicine*, *363*(4), 301–304. DOI: 10.1056/NEJMp1006304 PMID: 20551152

Hanna, R. (2023). *Philosophy That Can't Be Done By Chatbots: Rational Anthropology*. Unpublished MS. https://www. academia. edu/74562370/Philosophy_That_Can_t_Be_Done_By_Chatbots_ Rational_Anthropology_April_2023_version_

Haque, M. R., & Rubya, S. (2023). An overview of chatbot-based mobile mental health apps: Insights from app description and user reviews. *JMIR mHealth and uHealth*, *11*(1), e44838. DOI: 10.2196/44838 PMID: 37213181

Haristiani, N. (2019). Artificial Intelligence (AI) Chatbot as Language Learning Medium: An inquiry. *Journal of Physics: Conference Series*, *1387*(1), 012020. https://api.semanticscholar.org/CorpusID:213284963. DOI: 10.1088/1742-6596/1387/1/012020

Hasal, M. (2020). Chatbots: Security, privacy, data protection, and social aspects. *Concurrency and Computation*. Advance online publication. DOI: 10.1002/cpe.6426

Hassanipour, S., Nayak, S., Bozorgi, A., Keivanlou, M.-H., Dave, T., Alotaibi, A., & Kuriyakose, D. (2024). The ability of ChatGPT in paraphrasing texts and reducing plagiarism: A descriptive analysis. *JMIR Medical Education*, *10*(1), e53308. DOI: 10.2196/53308 PMID: 38989841

Healio. (2019, September 26). 2019 health care data breaches setting records. Retrieved from https://www.healio.com/news/primary-care/20190926/2019-health-care-data-breaches-setting-records

HealthITSecurity. (2023). This year's largest healthcare data breaches. Retrieved from https://healthitsecurity.com/features/this-years-largest-healthcare-data-breaches

HealthITSecurity. (n.d.). What is the HIPAA Security Rule? Retrieved from https://healthitsecurity.com/features/what-is-the-hipaa-security-rule

Herrera, S. N., Sarac, C., Phili, A., Gorman, J., Martin, L., Lyallpuri, R., Dobbs, M. F., DeLuca, J. S., Mueser, K. T., Wyka, K. E., Yang, L. H., Landa, Y., & Corcoran, C. M. (2023). Psychoeducation for individuals at clinical high risk for psychosis: A scoping review. *Schizophrenia Research*, *252*, 148–158. DOI: 10.1016/j.schres.2023.01.008 PMID: 36652831

He, Z. (2023). From ELIZA to ChatGPT: The Evolution of Chatbots in Public Health. *XRDS: Crossroads. The ACM Magazine for Students*, *29*(3), 59–59.

Hilal, A. M., Issaoui, I., Obayya, M., Al-Wesabi, F. N., Nemri, N., Hamza, M. A., & Zamani, A. S. (2022). Modeling of Explainable Artificial Intelligence for Biomedical Mental Disorder Diagnosis. *Computers, Materials & Continua*, *71*(2).

Hirschtritt, M. E., & Insel, T. R. (2018). Digital technologies in psychiatry: Present and future. *Focus (San Francisco, Calif.)*, *16*(3), 251–258. DOI: 10.1176/appi.focus.20180001 PMID: 31975919

Hirunyawipada, T., & Paswan, A. K. (2006). Consumer innovativeness and perceived risk: Implications for high technology product adoption. *Journal of Consumer Marketing*, *23*(4), 182–198. DOI: 10.1108/07363760610674310

Ho, A., Hancock, J., & Miner, A. S. (2018). Psychological, Relational, and Emotional Effects of Self-Disclosure After Conversations With a Chatbot. *Journal of Communication*, *68*(4), 712–733. DOI: 10.1093/joc/jqy026 PMID: 30100620

Hollis, C., Falconer, C. J., Martin, J., Whittington, C., Stockton, S., Glazebrook, C., & Davies, E. B. (2017). Annual research review: Digital health interventions for children and young people with mental health problems – a systematic and meta-review. *Journal of Child Psychology and Psychiatry, and Allied Disciplines*, *58*(4), 474–503. DOI: 10.1111/jcpp.12663 PMID: 27943285

Holmes, S., Moorhead, A., Bond, R., Zheng, H., Coates, V., & Mctear, M. (2019). Usability testing of a healthcare chatbot: Can we use conventional methods to assess conversational user interfaces? *Proceedings of the 31st European Conference on Cognitive Ergonomics - ECCE 2019*. DOI: 10.1145/3335082.3335094

Holohan, M., & Fiske, A. (2021). "Like I'm talking to a real person": Exploring the meaning of transference for the use and design of AI-based applications in psychotherapy. *Frontiers in Psychology*, *12*, 720476. DOI: 10.3389/fpsyg.2021.720476 PMID: 34646209

Ho, M.-T., Mantello, P., & Ho, M.-T. (2023). An analytical framework for studying attitude towards emotional AI: The three-pronged approach. *MethodsX*, *10*(102149), 102149. DOI: 10.1016/j.mex.2023.102149 PMID: 37091958

Hone, K., & El Said, G. (2016). Exploring the factors affecting MOOC retention: A survey study. *Computers & Education*, *98*, 157–168. Advance online publication. DOI: 10.1016/j.compedu.2016.03.016

Hopfield, J. J. (1982). Neural networks and physical systems with emergent collective computational abilities. *Proceedings of the National Academy of Sciences of the United States of America*, *79*(8), 2554–2558. DOI: 10.1073/pnas.79.8.2554 PMID: 6953413

Hörnemalm, A. (2023). Chatgpt as a software development tool: The future of development.

Horvitz, E., & Mulligan, D. (2015). Data, privacy, and the greater good. *Science*, *349*(6245), 253–255. DOI: 10.1126/science.aac4520 PMID: 26185242

How Long Will It Take Google to Index My Site? | Safari Digital. (n.d.). Retrieved November 17, 2022, from https://www.safaridigital.com.au/blog/how-long-will-it-take-google-to-index-my-site/

Hswen, Y., Gopaluni, A., Brownstein, J. S., & Hawkins, J. B. (2019). Using Twitter to detect psychological characteristics of self-identified persons with autism spectrum disorder: A feasibility study. *JMIR mHealth and uHealth*, *7*(2), e12264. DOI: 10.2196/12264 PMID: 30747718

Huang, W., Hew, K. F., & Fryer, L. K. (2022). Chatbots for language learning—Are they really useful? A systematic review of chatbot-supported language learning. *Journal of Computer Assisted Learning*, *38*(1), 237–257. DOI: 10.1111/jcal.12610

Huckvale, K., Venkatesh, S., & Christensen, H. (2019). Toward clinical digital phenotyping: A timely opportunity to consider purpose, quality, and safety. *NPJ Digital Medicine*, *2*(1), 1–11. DOI: 10.1038/s41746-019-0166-1 PMID: 31508498

Huda, F. A., Mathewos, K., Mahmood, H. R., Faruk, O., Hirschhorn, L. R., & Binagwaho, A. (2024). Examining the implementation of facility-based integrated management of childhood illness and insecticide treated nets in Bangladesh: Lessons learned through implementation research. *BMC Pediatrics*, *23*(S1, Suppl 1), 653. DOI: 10.1186/s12887-023-04389-0 PMID: 38413880

Huh, S. (2023). Are ChatGPT's knowledge and interpretation ability comparable to those of medical students in Korea for taking a parasitology examination?: A descriptive study. *Journal of Educational Evaluation for Health Professions*, *20*, 1. DOI: 10.3352/jeehp.2023.20.01 PMID: 36627845

Hungerbuehler, I., Daley, K., Cavanagh, K., Garcia Claro, H., & Kapps, M. (2021). Chatbot-Based Assessment of Employees' Mental Health: Design Process and Pilot Implementation. *JMIR Formative Research*, *5*(4), e21678. DOI: 10.2196/21678 PMID: 33881403

Hussain, A., & Ahmad, S. (2024). Mapping the literature on artificial intelligence in academic libraries: A bibliometrics approach. *Science & Technology Libraries*, *43*(2), 131–146. DOI: 10.1080/0194262X.2023.2238198

Hutchens, J. L. (1997). *How to Pass the Turing Test by Cheating*.

IBM. (n.d.). *What is a chatbot?*https://www.ibm.com/topics/chatbots

Ibrahim, F. A., Pahuja, E., Dinakaran, D., Manjunatha, N., Kumar, C. N., & Math, S. B. (2020). The future of telepsychiatry in India. *Indian Journal of Psychological Medicine*, *42*(5, suppl), 112S–117S. DOI: 10.1177/0253717620959255 PMID: 33354056

Ide, K., Hawke, P., & Nakayama, T. (2023). Can ChatGPT be considered an author of a medical article? *Journal of Epidemiology*, *33*(7), 381–382. DOI: 10.2188/jea.JE20230030 PMID: 37032109

Information Commissioner's Office (ICO). (n.d.-a). Personal data breaches: a guide. Retrieved from https://ico.org.uk/for-organisations/report-a-breach/personal-data-breach/personal-data-breaches-a-guide/

Information Commissioner's Office (ICO). (n.d.-b). Data protection by design and by default. Retrieved from https://ico.org.uk/for-organisations/law-enforcement/guide-to-le-processing/accountability-and-governance/data-protection-by-design-and-by-default/

Iniesta, R., Stahl, D., & McGuffin, P. (2016). Machine learning, statistical learning and the future of biological research in psychiatry. *Psychological Medicine*, *46*(12), 2455–2465. DOI: 10.1017/S0033291716001367 PMID: 27406289

Inkster, B., Knibbs, C., & Bada, M. (2023). Cybersecurity: A critical priority for digital mental health. Frontiers in Digital Health. https://www.frontiersin.org/journals/digital-health/articles/10.3389/fdgth.2023.1242264/full

Intelliverse.ai. (2023, September 12). *How AI is making mental healthcare more accessible.* LinkedIn. https://www.linkedin.com/pulse/how-ai-making-mental-healthcare-more-accessible/

Ip, P., Chim, D., Chan, K. L., Li, T. M., Ho, F. K. W., Van Voorhees, B. W., Tiwari, A., Tsang, A., Chan, C. W. L., Ho, M., Tso, W., & Wong, W. H. S. (2016). Effectiveness of a culturally attuned Internet-based depression prevention program for Chinese adolescents: A randomized controlled trial. *Depression and Anxiety, 33*(12), 1123–1131. DOI: 10.1002/da.22554 PMID: 27618799

Ismail, M., & Ade-Ibijola, A. (2019). Lecturer's apprentice: A chatbot for assisting novice programmers. *2019 International Multidisciplinary Information Technology and Engineering Conference (IMITEC)*, 1–8. DOI: 10.1109/IMITEC45504.2019.9015857

Iwaya, L. H., Rashid, A., & Klein, J. (2022). On the privacy of mental health apps. Empirical Software Engineering. https://link.springer.com/article/10.1007/s10664-022-10236-0

Jackson-Triche, M., Vetal, D., Turner, E.-M., Dahiya, P., & Mangurian, C. (2023). Meeting the behavioral health needs of health care workers during COVID-19 by leveraging chatbot technology: Development and usability study. *Journal of Medical Internet Research, 25*, e40635. DOI: 10.2196/40635 PMID: 37146178

Jacobson, N. C., Weingarden, H., & Wilhelm, S. (2019). Using digital phenotyping to accurately detect depression severity. *The Journal of Nervous and Mental Disease, 207*(10), 893–896. DOI: 10.1097/NMD.0000000000001042 PMID: 31596769

Jameson, J. L., & Longo, D. L. (2015). Precision medicine—Personalized, problematic, and promising. *Obstetrical & Gynecological Survey, 70*(10), 612–614. DOI: 10.1097/01.ogx.0000472121.21647.38 PMID: 26014593

Jang, S., Kim, J. J., Kim, S. J., Hong, J., Kim, S., & Kim, E. (2021). Mobile app-based chatbot to deliver cognitive behavioral therapy and psychoeducation for adults with attention deficit: A development and feasibility/usability study. *International Journal of Medical Informatics, 150*, 104440. DOI: 10.1016/j.ijmedinf.2021.104440 PMID: 33799055

Jan, J., Alshare, K. A., & Lane, P. L. (2024). Hofstede's cultural dimensions in technology acceptance models: A meta-analysis. *Universal Access in the Information Society, 23*(2), 717–741. DOI: 10.1007/s10209-022-00930-7

Janssen, R. J., Mourão-Miranda, J., & Schnack, H. G. (2018). Making individual prognoses in psychiatry using neuroimaging and machine learning. *Biological Psychiatry: Cognitive Neuroscience and Neuroimaging*, *3*(9), 798–808. DOI: 10.1016/j.bpsc.2018.04.004 PMID: 29789268

Jarrah, A. M., Wardat, Y., & Fidalgo, P. (2023). Using ChatGPT in academic writing is (not) a form of plagiarism: What does the literature say. *Online Journal of Communication and Media Technologies*, *13*(4), e202346. DOI: 10.30935/ojcmt/13572

Järvelä, K., Takala, P., Michard, F., & Vikatmaa, L. (2022). Clinical evaluation of a wearable sensor for mobile monitoring of respiratory rate on hospital wards. *Journal of Clinical Monitoring and Computing*, *36*(1), 81–86. DOI: 10.1007/s10877-021-00753-6 PMID: 34476669

Jauhiainen, J. S., & Guerra, A. G. (2023). Generative AI and ChatGPT in school children's education: Evidence from a school lesson. *Sustainability (Basel)*, *15*(18), 14025. DOI: 10.3390/su151814025

Javaid, M., Haleem, A., & Singh, R. P. (2023). ChatGPT for healthcare services: An emerging stage for an innovative perspective. *BenchCouncil Transactions on Benchmarks. Standards and Evaluations*, *3*(1), 100105.

Jeon, J., Lee, S., & Choe, H. (2023). Beyond ChatGPT: A conceptual framework and systematic review of speech-recognition chatbots for language learning. *Computers & Education*, *206*, 104898. DOI: 10.1016/j.compedu.2023.104898

Jiang, F., Jiang, Y., Zhi, H., Dong, Y., Li, H., Ma, S., Wang, Y., Dong, Q., Shen, H., & Wang, Y. (2017). Artificial intelligence in healthcare: Past, present and future. *Stroke and Vascular Neurology*, *2*(4), 230–243. DOI: 10.1136/svn-2017-000101 PMID: 29507784

Jiang, X., Li, Y., Jokinen, J. P., Hirvola, V. B., Oulasvirta, A., & Ren, X. (2020, April). How we type: Eye and finger movement strategies in mobile typing. In *Proceedings of the 2020 CHI conference on human factors in computing systems* (pp. 1-14). DOI: 10.1145/3313831.3376711

Jin, K. W., Li, Q., Xie, Y., & Xiao, G. (2023). Artificial intelligence in mental healthcare: An overview and future perspectives. *The British Journal of Radiology*, *96*(1150), 20230213. DOI: 10.1259/bjr.20230213 PMID: 37698582

Jin, S. V., & Youn, S. (2022). Social Presence and Imagery Processing as Predictors of Chatbot Continuance Intention in Human-AI-Interaction. *International Journal of Human-Computer Interaction*, 1–13. DOI: 10.1080/10447318.2022.2129277

Johnson, N. (2024, January 3). *Mental Illness Could Now be Detected Through an App*. YR Media. https://yr.media/health/mental-health/brain-mental-illness-biaffect-depression-bipolar-alex-leow/

Jorm, A. F., & Griffiths, K. M. (2006). Population promotion of informal self-help strategies for early intervention against depression and anxiety. *Psychological Medicine*, *36*(1), 3–6. DOI: 10.1017/S0033291705005659 PMID: 16356291

Joshi, M. A., & Patel, P. (2018). Google page rank algorithm and it's updates. *International Conference on Emerging Trends in Science, Engineering and Management, ICETSEM-2018*.

Journal, H. I. P. A. A. (2019). Healthcare data breach report. Retrieved from https://www.hipaajournal.com/healthcare-data-breach-2019-report/

Journal, H. I. P. A. A. (2024a). What are the HIPAA Breach Notification Requirements? Retrieved from https://www.hipaajournal.com/hipaa-breach-notification-requirements/

Journal, H. I. P. A. A. (2024b). HIPAA Privacy Rule. Retrieved from https://www.hipaajournal.com/hipaa-privacy-rule/

Jurdak, M. (2016). *Learning and teaching real world problem solving in school mathematics: A multiple-perspective framework for crossing the boundary*. Springer International Publishing. DOI: 10.1007/978-3-319-08204-2

Jurdak, M. E. (2006). Contrasting perspectives and performance of high school students on problem solving in real world situated, and school contexts. *Educational Studies in Mathematics*, *63*(3), 283–301. DOI: 10.1007/s10649-005-9008-y

Jurdak, M., & Shahin, I. (1999). An ethnographic study of the computational strategies of a group of young street vendors in beirut. *Educational Studies in Mathematics*, *40*(2), 155–172. DOI: 10.1023/A:1003894908704

Jurdak, M., & Shahin, I. (2001). Problem solving activity in the workplace and the school: The case of constructing solids. *Educational Studies in Mathematics*, *47*(3), 297–315. DOI: 10.1023/A:1015106804646

Kamita, T., Ito, T., Matsumoto, A., Munakata, T., & Inoue, T. (2018). A chatbot system for mental healthcare based on SAT counseling method. *Mobile Information Systems*, 9517321:1-9517321:11. DOI: 10.1155/2019/9517321

Kamita, T., Matsumoto, A., Sun, B., & Inoue, T. (2020). Promotion of continuous use of a self-guided mental healthcare system by a chatbot. *Companion Publication of the 2020 Conference on Computer Supported Cooperative Work and Social Computing,* 293–298. DOI: 10.1145/3406865.3418343

Karimian, G., Petelos, E., & Evers, S. M. (2022). The ethical issues of the application of artificial intelligence in healthcare: A systematic scoping review. *AI and Ethics, 2*(4), 539–551. DOI: 10.1007/s43681-021-00131-7

Karthik, S., & Sudha, M. (2021). Predicting bipolar disorder and schizophrenia based on non-overlapping genetic phenotypes using deep neural network. *Evolutionary Intelligence, 14*(2), 619–634. DOI: 10.1007/s12065-019-00346-y

Kashefi, A., & Mukerji, T. (2023). ChatGPT for programming numerical methods. *Journal of Machine Learning for Modeling and Computing, 4*(2), 1–74. DOI: 10.1615/JMachLearnModelComput.2023048492

Kaur, S., Singh, S., Arun, P., Kaur, D., & Bajaj, M. (2020). Phase space reconstruction of EEG signals for classification of ADHD and control adults. *Clinical EEG and Neuroscience, 51*(2), 102–113. DOI: 10.1177/1550059419876525 PMID: 31533446

Kaushal, V., & Yadav, R. (2022). The role of chatbots in academic libraries: An experience-based perspective. *Journal of the Australian Library and Information Association, 71*(3), 215–232. DOI: 10.1080/24750158.2022.2106403

Kazi, H., Chowdhry, B. S., & Memon, Z. (2012). *MedChatBot: An UMLS based chatbot for medical students.*

Kelly, S., Kaye, S.-A., & Oviedo-Trespalacios, O. (2023). What factors contribute to the acceptance of artificial intelligence? A systematic review. *Telematics and Informatics, 77*(101925), 101925. DOI: 10.1016/j.tele.2022.101925

KEMP. S. (n.d.-a). *The Latest Facebook Messenger Statistics: Everything You Need to Know—DataReportal – Global Digital Insights.* Retrieved March 23, 2023, from https://datareportal.com/essential-facebook-messenger-stats

KEMP. S. (n.d.-b). *The Latest Facebook Statistics: Everything You Need to Know.* DataReportal – Global Digital Insights. Retrieved February 9, 2023, from https://datareportal.com/essential-facebook-stats

Kerasidou, A. (2020). Artificial intelligence and the ongoing need for empathy, compassion and trust in healthcare. *Bulletin of the World Health Organization, 98*(4), 245–250. DOI: 10.2471/BLT.19.237198 PMID: 32284647

Khalid, N., Qayyum, A., Bilal, M., Al-Fuqaha, A., & Qadir, J. (2023). Privacy-preserving artificial intelligence in healthcare: Techniques and applications. *Computers in Biology and Medicine, 158*, 106848. DOI: 10.1016/j.compbiomed.2023.106848 PMID: 37044052

Khawaja, Z., & Bélisle-Pipon, J. C. (2023). Your robot therapist is not your therapist: Understanding the role of AI-powered mental health chatbots. *Frontiers in Digital Health, 5*, 1278186. DOI: 10.3389/fdgth.2023.1278186 PMID: 38026836

Khosravi, M., Zare, Z., Mojtabaeian, S. M., & Izadi, R. (2024). Ethical challenges of using artificial intelligence in healthcare delivery: A thematic analysis of a systematic review of reviews. *Journal of Public Health (Berlin)*, •••, 1–11. DOI: 10.1007/s10389-024-02219-w

Kim, B., Ahn, J., & Kim, G. (2020). *Sequential Latent Knowledge Selection for Knowledge-Grounded Dialogue.*

Kim, S.-K. A., & Wong, U.-H. (2023). *ChatGPT impacts on academia.* Paper presented at the 2023 International Conference on System Science and Engineering (ICSSE). DOI: 10.1109/ICSSE58758.2023.10227188

Kim, H. M., Xu, Y., & Wang, Y. (2022). Overcoming the mental health stigma through m-health apps: Results from the healthy minds study. *Telemedicine Journal and e-Health, 28*(10), 1534–1540. DOI: 10.1089/tmj.2021.0418 PMID: 35254886

Kim, J. W., Jones, K. L., & D'Angelo, E. (2019). How to prepare prospective psychiatrists in the era of artificial intelligence. *Academic Psychiatry, 43*(3), 337–339. DOI: 10.1007/s40596-019-01025-x PMID: 30659443

Kim, T. W., Hooker, J., & Donaldson, T. (2021). Taking principles seriously: A hybrid approach to value alignment in artificial intelligence. *Journal of Artificial Intelligence Research, 70*, 871–890. DOI: 10.1613/jair.1.12481

King, M. R. (2022). The Future of AI in Medicine: A Perspective from a Chatbot. *Annals of Biomedical Engineering*. Advance online publication. DOI: 10.1007/s10439-022-03121-w PMID: 36572824

King, M. R., & Chat, G. P. T. (2023). A conversation on artificial intelligence, chatbots, and plagiarism in higher education. *Cellular and Molecular Bioengineering, 16*(1), 1–2. DOI: 10.1007/s12195-022-00754-8 PMID: 36660590

Klainin-Yobas, P., Ng, S. H., Stephen, P. D. M., & Lau, Y. (2016). Efficacy of psychosocial interventions on psychological outcomes among people with cardiovascular diseases: A systematic review and meta-analysis. *Patient Education and Counseling, 99*(4), 512–521. DOI: 10.1016/j.pec.2015.10.020 PMID: 27045976

Kleine, A.-K., Kokje, E., Lermer, E., & Gaube, S. (2023). Attitudes toward the adoption of 2 artificial intelligence–enabled mental health tools among prospective psychotherapists: Cross-sectional study. *JMIR Human Factors*, *10*, e46859. DOI: 10.2196/46859 PMID: 37436801

Knapp, A. A., Cohen, K., Nicholas, J., Mohr, D. C., Carlo, A. D., Skerl, J. J., & Lattie, E. G. (2021). Integration of Digital Tools Into Community Mental Health Care Settings That Serve Young People: Focus Group Study. *JMIR Mental Health*, *8*(8), e27379. DOI: 10.2196/27379 PMID: 34420928

Ko, D. W., & Yang, J. J. (2022). EEG-Based schizophrenia diagnosis through time series image conversion and deep learning. *Electronics (Basel)*, *11*(14), 2265. DOI: 10.3390/electronics11142265

Korinek, A. (2023). Generative AI for economic research: Use cases and implications for economists. *Journal of Economic Literature*, *61*(4), 1281–1317. DOI: 10.1257/jel.20231736

Koulouri, T., Macredie, R. D., & Olakitan, D. (2022). Chatbots to support young adults' mental health: An exploratory study of acceptability. *ACM Transactions on Interactive Intelligent Systems*, *12*(2), 1–39. DOI: 10.1145/3485874

Kretzschmar, K., Tyroll, H., Pavarini, G., Manzini, A., & Singh, I. (2019). Can your phone be your therapist? Young people's ethical perspectives on the use of fully automated conversational agents (chatbots) in mental health support. *Biomedical Informatics Insights*, *11*, 1178222619829083. DOI: 10.1177/1178222619829083 PMID: 30858710

Kshetri, N., Hughes, L., Slade, E. L., Jeyaraj, A., Kar, A. K., Baabdullah, A. M., & Miller, R. C. (2024). A systematic analysis of failures in protecting personal health data. *International Journal of Information Management*, *74*, 102719. DOI: 10.1016/j.ijinfomgt.2023.102719

Kuang, D., & He, L. (2014, November). Classification on ADHD with deep learning. In *2014 International Conference on Cloud Computing and Big Data* (pp. 27-32). IEEE. DOI: 10.1109/CCBD.2014.42

Kuhn, E., & Owen, J. E. (2020). Advances in PTSD treatment delivery: The role of digital technology in PTSD treatment. *Current Treatment Options in Psychiatry*, *7*(2), 88–102. DOI: 10.1007/s40501-020-00207-x

Kulkarni, R., & Jaiswal, R. C. (2023). A survey on AI chatbots. *International Journal for Research in Applied Science and Engineering Technology*, *11*(9), 1738–1744. DOI: 10.22214/ijraset.2023.55911

Kunnumpurath, B., Menon, V. A., & Paul, A. (2024). ChatGPT and virtual experience: Student engagement in online script writing - an experimental investigation among media students. In *Advances in Computational Intelligence and Robotics* (pp. 32–50). IGI Global.

Kunnumpurath, B., Prasad, A., Menon, V. A., & Thomas, J. (2024). Cultivating self-esteem: Exploring the intersection of culture, neurocognition, and behavior among female media professionals. In *Cognitive Behavioral Neuroscience in Organizational Settings* (pp. 65–82). IGI Global. DOI: 10.4018/979-8-3693-1858-4.ch004

Kuo, Y.-F., Wu, C.-M., & Deng, W.-J. (2009). The relationships among service quality, perceived value, customer satisfaction, and post-purchase intention in mobile value-added services. *Computers in Human Behavior*, *25*(4), 887–896. DOI: 10.1016/j.chb.2009.03.003

Labadze, L., Grigolia, M., & Machaidze, L. (2023). Role of AI chatbots in education: Systematic literature review. *International Journal of Educational Technology in Higher Education*, *20*(56), 56. Advance online publication. DOI: 10.1186/s41239-023-00426-1

Lahmiri, S., & Shmuel, A. (2019). Performance of machine learning methods applied to structural MRI and ADAS cognitive scores in diagnosing Alzheimer's disease. *Biomedical Signal Processing and Control*, *52*, 414–419. DOI: 10.1016/j.bspc.2018.08.009

Landau, A. Y., Ferrarello, S., Blanchard, A., Cato, K., Atkins, N., Salazar, S., Patton, D. U., & Topaz, M. (2022). Developing machine learning-based models to help identify child abuse and neglect: Key ethical challenges and recommended solutions. *Journal of the American Medical Informatics Association : JAMIA*, *29*(3), 576–580. DOI: 10.1093/jamia/ocab286 PMID: 35024859

Landim, A., Pereira, A., & Vieira, T., de B. Costa, E., Moura, J., Wanick, V., & Bazaki, E. (. (2022). Chatbot design approaches for fashion E-commerce: An interdisciplinary review. *International Journal of Fashion Design, Technology and Education*, *15*(2), 200–210. DOI: 10.1080/17543266.2021.1990417

Lane, E., D'Arcey, J., Kidd, S., Onyeaka, H., Alon, N., Joshi, D., & Torous, J. (2023). Digital Phenotyping in Adults with Schizophrenia: A Narrative Review. *Current Psychiatry Reports*, *25*(11), 699–706. DOI: 10.1007/s11920-023-01467-z PMID: 37861979

Laven, S. (1996). Claude-by brian mclaughlin. *Retrieved from The Simon Laven Page:*Https://Www. Simonlaven. Com/Claude. *Htm*.

Lavrič, F., & Škraba, A. (2023). *Group Brainstorming Support by ChatGPT & Ayoa at the Design of Regional Development Plan.* Paper presented at the 42th International Conference on Organizational Science Development, Portorož, Slovenia. DOI: 10.18690/um.fov.3.2023.43

Laymouna, M., Ma, Y., Lessard, D., Schuster, T., Engler, K., & Lebouché, B. (2024). Roles, Users, Benefits, and Limitations of Chatbots in Health Care: Rapid Review. *Journal of Medical Internet Research, 26*, e56930. DOI: 10.2196/56930 PMID: 39042446

Le Glaz, A., Haralambous, Y., Kim-Dufor, D. H., Lenca, P., Billot, R., Ryan, T. C., Marsh, J., DeVylder, J., Walter, M., Berrouiguet, S., & Lemey, C. (2021). Machine learning and natural language processing in mental health: Systematic review. *Journal of Medical Internet Research, 23*(5), e15708. DOI: 10.2196/15708 PMID: 33944788

Lee, D., & Yeo, S. (2022). Developing an AI-based chatbot for practicing responsive teaching in mathematics. *Computers & Education, 191*, 104646. DOI: 10.1016/j.compedu.2022.104646

Lee, D., & Yoon, S. N. (2021). Application of artificial intelligence-based technologies in the healthcare industry: Opportunities and challenges. *International Journal of Environmental Research and Public Health, 18*(1), 271. DOI: 10.3390/ijerph18010271 PMID: 33401373

Lee, E. E., Torous, J., De Choudhury, M., Depp, C. A., Graham, S. A., Kim, H.-C., Paulus, M. P., Krystal, J. H., & Jeste, D. V. (2021). Artificial intelligence for mental health care: Clinical applications, barriers, facilitators, and artificial wisdom. *Biological Psychiatry: Cognitive Neuroscience and Neuroimaging, 6*(9), 856–864. DOI: 10.1016/j.bpsc.2021.02.001 PMID: 33571718

Lee, H. (2024). The rise of ChatGPT: Exploring its potential in medical education. *Anatomical Sciences Education, 17*(5), 926–931. DOI: 10.1002/ase.2270 PMID: 36916887

Lee, J. Y. (2023). Can an artificial intelligence chatbot be the author of a scholarly article? *Journal of Educational Evaluation for Health Professions*, 20. PMID: 36842449

Lee, Y.-C., Cui, Y., Jamieson, J., Fu, W., & Yamashita, N. (2023). Exploring effects of chatbot-based social contact on reducing mental illness stigma. In *Proceedings of the 2023 CHI Conference on Human Factors in Computing Systems (CHI '23)*, April 23–28, 2023, Hamburg, Germany. ACM. DOI: 10.1145/3544548.3581384

Leo, A. J., Schuelke, M. J., Hunt, D. M., Metzler, J. P., Miller, J. P., Areán, P. A., Armbrecht, M. A., & Cheng, A. L. (2022). A digital mental health intervention in an orthopedic setting for patients with symptoms of depression and/or anxiety: Feasibility prospective cohort study. *JMIR Formative Research*, *6*(2), e34889. DOI: 10.2196/34889 PMID: 35039278

Leondes, C. T. (Ed.). (2001). *Expert systems: the technology of knowledge management and decision making for the 21st century*. Elsevier.

Leshkevich, T., & Motozhanets, A. (2022). Social perception of artificial intelligence and digitization of cultural heritage: Russian context. *Applied Sciences (Basel, Switzerland)*, *12*(5), 2712. DOI: 10.3390/app12052712

Li, Y., Qu, S., Shen, J., Min, S., & Yu, Z. (2023). Curriculum-Driven Edubot: A Framework for Developing Language Learning Chatbots Through Synthesizing Conversational Data. *arXiv preprint arXiv:2309.16804*.

Liao, Q. V., Geyer, W., Muller, M., & Khazaen, Y. (2020). Conversational Interfaces for Information Search. In Fu, W. T., & van Oostendorp, H. (Eds.), *Understanding and Improving Information Search: A Cognitive Approach* (pp. 267–287). Springer International Publishing. DOI: 10.1007/978-3-030-38825-6_13

Li, H., Zhang, R., Lee, Y.-C., Kraut, R. E., & Mohr, D. C. (2023). Systematic review and meta-analysis of AI-based conversational agents for promoting mental health and well-being. *NPJ Digital Medicine*, *6*(1), 1. Advance online publication. DOI: 10.1038/s41746-023-00979-5 PMID: 38114588

Li, J. (2023). Digital technologies for mental health improvements in the COVID-19 pandemic: A scoping review. *BMC Public Health*, *23*(1), 413. DOI: 10.1186/s12889-023-15302-w PMID: 36859184

Li, J. (2023). Security Implications of AI Chatbots in Health Care. *Journal of Medical Internet Research*, *25*, e47551. DOI: 10.2196/47551 PMID: 38015597

Limberg, L., & Alexandersson, M. (2010). Learning and Information Seeking. In *Encyclopedia of Library and Information Science* (pp. 3252–3262). Taylor and Francis Group. DOI: 10.1081/E-ELIS3-120044669

Lin, C.-C., Huang, A. Y., & Yang, S. J. (2023). A review of ai-driven conversational chatbots implementation methodologies and challenges (1999–2022). *Sustainability (Basel)*, *15*(5), 4012. DOI: 10.3390/su15054012

Lin, M. P.-C., & Chang, D. (2020). Enhancing post-secondary writers' writing skills with a chatbot. *Journal of Educational Technology & Society*, *23*(1), 78–92.

Liu, Y., Ott, M., Goyal, N., Du, J., Joshi, M., Chen, D., Levy, O., Lewis, M., Zettlemoyer, L., & Stoyanov, V. (2019). *RoBERTa: A Robustly Optimized BERT Pretraining Approach.*

Liu, H., Peng, H., Song, X., Xu, C., & Zhang, M. (2022). Using AI chatbots to provide self-help depression interventions for university students: A randomized trial of effectiveness. *Internet Interventions : the Application of Information Technology in Mental and Behavioural Health, 27*, 100495. DOI: 10.1016/j.invent.2022.100495 PMID: 35059305

Liu, J. (2024). ChatGPT: Perspectives from human–computer interaction and psychology. *Frontiers in Artificial Intelligence, 7*, 1418869. DOI: 10.3389/frai.2024.1418869 PMID: 38957452

Li, W., Chen, J., Chen, F., Liang, J., & Yu, H. (2024). Exploring the potential of ChatGPT-4 in responding to common questions about abdominoplasty: An AI-based case study of a plastic surgery consultation. *Aesthetic Plastic Surgery, 48*(8), 1571–1583. DOI: 10.1007/s00266-023-03660-0 PMID: 37770637

Liyanage, H., Liaw, S. T., Jonnagaddala, J., Schreiber, R., Kuziemsky, C., Terry, A. L., & de Lusignan, S. (2019). Artificial intelligence in primary health care: perceptions, issues, and challenges. *Yearbook of medical informatics, 28*(01), 041-046.

Loh, H. W., Ooi, C. P., Barua, P. D., Palmer, E. E., Molinari, F., & Acharya, U. R. (2022). Automated detection of ADHD: Current trends and future perspective. *Computers in Biology and Medicine, 146*, 105525. DOI: 10.1016/j.compbiomed.2022.105525 PMID: 35468405

Lopes, E., Jain, G., Carlbring, P., & Pareek, S. (2023). Talking Mental Health: A Battle of Wits Between Humans and AI. *Journal of Technology in Behavioral Science, 9*(4), 1–11. DOI: 10.1007/s41347-023-00359-6

Lueken, U., & Hahn, T. (2020). Personalized mental health: Artificial intelligence technologies for treatment response prediction in anxiety disorders. In *Personalized Psychiatry* (pp. 201–213). Academic Press. DOI: 10.1016/B978-0-12-813176-3.00017-1

Luger, E., & Sellen, A. (2016). "Like Having a Really Bad PA" The Gulf between User Expectation and Experience of Conversational Agents. *Proceedings of the 2016 CHI conference on human factors in computing systems*. DOI: 10.1145/2858036.2858288

Lukens, E. P., & McFarlane, W. R. (2006). Psychoeducation as evidence-based practice: Considerations for practice, research, and policy. In Roberts, A. R., & Yeager, K. R. (Eds.), *Foundations of evidence-based social work practice* (pp. 291–313). Oxford University Press. DOI: 10.1093/oso/9780195305944.003.0022

Lustgarten, S. D., Garrison, Y. L., Sinnard, M. T., & Flynn, A. W. (2020). Digital privacy in mental healthcare: Current issues and recommendations for technology use. *Current Opinion in Psychology*, *36*, 25–31. DOI: 10.1016/j.copsyc.2020.03.012 PMID: 32361651

Luxton, D. D. (2014). Artificial intelligence in psychological practice: Current and future applications and implications. *Professional Psychology, Research and Practice*, *45*(5), 332–339. DOI: 10.1037/a0034559

Luxton, D. D. (2020). Ethical implications of conversational agents in global public health. *Bulletin of the World Health Organization*, *98*(4), 285–287. DOI: 10.2471/BLT.19.237636 PMID: 32284654

Ly, K. H., Ly, A. M., & Andersson, G. (2017). A fully automated conversational agent for promoting mental well-being: A pilot RCT using mixed methods. *Internet Interventions : the Application of Information Technology in Mental and Behavioural Health*, *10*, 39–46. DOI: 10.1016/j.invent.2017.10.002 PMID: 30135751

Mabunda, K. (2020). *An intelligent chatbot for guiding visitors and locating venues*. University of Johannesburg.

Mahato, S., Goyal, N., Ram, D., & Paul, S. (2020). Detection of depression and scaling of severity using six channel EEG data. *Journal of Medical Systems*, *44*(7), 1–12. DOI: 10.1007/s10916-020-01573-y PMID: 32435986

Mahendran, N., Vincent, P. D. R., Srinivasan, K., Sharma, V., & Jayakody, D. K. (2020). Realizing a stacking generalization model to improve the prediction accuracy of major depressive disorder in adults. *IEEE Access : Practical Innovations, Open Solutions*, *8*, 49509–49522. DOI: 10.1109/ACCESS.2020.2977887

Maher, C. A., Davis, C. R., Curtis, R. G., Short, C. E., & Murphy, K. J. (2020). A physical activity and diet program delivered by artificially intelligent virtual health coach: Proof-of-concept study. *JMIR mHealth and uHealth*, *8*(7), e17558. DOI: 10.2196/17558 PMID: 32673246

Mains, J. A., & Scogin, F. R. (2003). The effectiveness of self-administered treatments: A practice-friendly review of the research. *Journal of Clinical Psychology*, *59*(2), 237–246. DOI: 10.1002/jclp.10145 PMID: 12552632

Malwarebytes. (2020). Vastaamo psychotherapy data breach sees the most vulnerable victims extorted. https://www.malwarebytes.com/blog/news/2020/10/vastaamo-psychotherapy-data-breach-sees-the-most-vulnerable-victims-extorted

Maniruzzaman, M., Shin, J., & Hasan, M. A. M. (2022). Predicting children with ADHD using behavioral activity: A machine learning analysis. *Applied Sciences (Basel, Switzerland)*, *12*(5), 2737. DOI: 10.3390/app12052737

Manríquez Roa, T., Biller-Andorno, N., & Trachsel, M. (2019). The ethics of artificial intelligence in psychotherapy.

Marks, I. M., Cavanagh, K., & Gega, L. (2007). Computer-aided psychotherapy: Revolution or bubble? *The British Journal of Psychiatry*, *191*(6), 471–473. DOI: 10.1192/bjp.bp.107.041152 PMID: 18055948

Maroengsit, W., Piyakulpinyo, T., Phonyiam, K., Pongnumkul, S., Chaovalit, P., & Theeramunkong, T. (2019). A Survey on Evaluation Methods for Chatbots. *Proceedings of the 2019 7th International Conference on Information and Education Technology*, 111–119. DOI: 10.1145/3323771.3323824

Math, S. B., Gowda, G. S., Basavaraju, V., Manjunatha, N., Kumar, C. N., Enara, A., Gowda, M., & Thirthalli, J. (2019). Cost estimation for the implementation of the Mental Healthcare Act 2017. *Indian Journal of Psychiatry*, *61*(10, Suppl 4), S650–S659. DOI: 10.4103/psychiatry.IndianJPsychiatry_188_19 PMID: 31040453

Matthias, A. (2004). The responsibility gap: Ascribing responsibility for the actions of learning automata. *Ethics and Information Technology*, *6*(3), 175–183. DOI: 10.1007/s10676-004-3422-1

Mbunge, E., Batani, J., Gaobotse, G., & Muchemwa, B. (2022). Virtual healthcare services and digital health technologies deployed during coronavirus disease 2019 (COVID-19) pandemic in South Africa: A systematic review. *Global Health Journal (Amsterdam, Netherlands)*, *6*(2), 102–113. DOI: 10.1016/j.glohj.2022.03.001 PMID: 35282399

McCarthy, J. (1989). *Artificial Intelligence*. Logic and Formalizing Common Sense.

McCorduck, P., & Cfe, C. (2004). *Machines who think: A personal inquiry into the history and prospects of artificial intelligence*. AK Peters/CRC Press. DOI: 10.1201/9780429258985

McGorry, P. D., Nelson, B., Goldstone, S., & Yung, A. R. (2010). Clinical staging: A heuristic and practical strategy for new research and better health and social outcomes for psychotic and related mood disorders. *Canadian Journal of Psychiatry*, *55*(8), 486–497. DOI: 10.1177/070674371005500803 PMID: 20723276

Mckie, I. A. S., & Narayan, B. (2019). Enhancing the academic library experience with chatbots: An exploration of research and implications for practice. *Journal of the Australian Library and Information Association, 68*(3), 268–277. DOI: 10.1080/24750158.2019.1611694

Meehan, A. J., Lewis, S. J., Fazel, S., Fusar-Poli, P., Steyerberg, E. W., Stahl, D., & Danese, A. (2022). Clinical prediction models in psychiatry: A systematic review of two decades of progress and challenges. *Molecular Psychiatry, 27*(6), 2700–2708. DOI: 10.1038/s41380-022-01528-4 PMID: 35365801

Meghrajani, V. R., Marathe, M., Sharma, R., Potdukhe, A., Wanjari, M. B., & Taksande, A. B. (2023). A comprehensive analysis of mental health problems in India and the role of mental asylums. *Cureus, 15*(7), e42559. DOI: 10.7759/cureus.42559 PMID: 37637646

Mehrabi, N., Morstatter, F., Saxena, N., Lerman, K., & Galstyan, A. (2021). A survey on bias and fairness in machine learning. *ACM Computing Surveys, 54*(6), 1–35. DOI: 10.1145/3457607

Mehta, A., Kumar, H., Yazji, K., Wireko, A. A., Nagarajan, J. S., Ghosh, B., Nahas, A., Ojeda, L. M., Anand, A., & Sharath, M. (2023). Effectiveness of artificial intelligence-assisted colonoscopy in early diagnosis of colorectal cancer: A systematic review. *International Journal of Surgery, 109*(4), 946–952. DOI: 10.1097/JS9.0000000000000285 PMID: 36917126

Melián-González, S., Gutiérrez-Taño, D., & Bulchand-Gidumal, J. (2021). Predicting the intentions to use chatbots for travel and tourism. *Current Issues in Tourism, 24*(2), 192–210. DOI: 10.1080/13683500.2019.1706457

Memmert, L. (2024). Brainstorming with a Generative Language Model: Understanding Performance Through Brainstorming Group Effects.

Mendoza, S., Sánchez-Adame, L., Urquiza-Yllescas, J., González-Beltrán, B., & Decouchant, D. (2022). A Model to Develop Chatbots for Assisting the Teaching and Learning Process. *Sensors (Basel), 22*(15), 5532. DOI: 10.3390/s22155532 PMID: 35898035

Menon, V. A., Prasad, A., Puthur, L. A., K K, S., & Joseph, L. (2023). Social media dependency and Facebook usage among the older adults of Kerala. *Studies in Media and Communication, 11*(4), 202. DOI: 10.11114/smc.v11i4.6060

Meskó, B. (2023, August 10). *Top 10 health chatbots.* LinkedIn. https://www.linkedin.com/pulse/top-10-health-chatbots-bertalan-mesk%C3%B3-md-phd/

Metcalf, M. (2024). The best mental health chatbots in 2024. Retrieved from https://getmarlee.com/blog/mental-health-chatbot

mHealthIntelligence. (n.d.). Understanding the role of chatbots in virtual care delivery. Retrieved from https://mhealthintelligence.com/features/understanding-the-role-of-chatbots-in-virtual-care-delivery

Mhlanga, D. (2023). ChatGPT in education: Exploring opportunities for emerging economies to improve education with ChatGPT. *Available atSSRN* 4355758. DOI: 10.2139/ssrn.4355758

Mijwil, M. M., Hiran, K. K., Doshi, R., Dadhich, M., Al-Mistarehi, A.-H., & Bala, I. (2023). ChatGPT and the future of academic integrity in the artificial intelligence era: A new frontier. *Al-Salam Journal for Engineering and Technology*, *2*(2), 116–127. DOI: 10.55145/ajest.2023.02.02.015

Mijwil, M. M., & Shukur, B. S. (2022). A scoping review of machine learning techniques and their utilisation in predicting heart diseases. *Ibn AL-Haitham Journal For Pure and Applied Sciences*, *35*(3), 175–189. DOI: 10.30526/35.3.2813

Miklosik, A. (2018). *Search Engine Marketing Strategies: Google Answer Box-Related Search Visibility Factors* (pp. 463–485).

Miklosik, A., Hlavatý, I., Daňo, F., & Červenka, P. (2016). *Google answer box keyword-related analysis a case study.*

Miller, D. D., & Brown, E. W. (2018). Artificial intelligence in medical practice: The question to the answer? *The American Journal of Medicine*, *131*(2), 129–133. DOI: 10.1016/j.amjmed.2017.10.035 PMID: 29126825

Milmo, D. (2020). Tens of thousands of psychotherapy records hacked in Finland. The Guardian. https://www.theguardian.com/world/2020/oct/26/tens-of-thousands-psychotherapy-records-hacked-in-finland

Milne-Ives, M., Selby, E., Inkster, B., Lam, C., & Meinert, E. (2022). Artificial intelligence and machine learning in mobile apps for mental health: A scoping review. *PLOS Digital Health*, *1*(8), e0000079. DOI: 10.1371/journal.pdig.0000079 PMID: 36812623

Miner, A. S., Milstein, A., Schueller, S., Hegde, R., Mangurian, C., & Linos, E. (2016). Smartphone-based conversational agents and responses to questions about mental health, interpersonal violence, and physical health. *JAMA Internal Medicine*, *176*(5), 619–625. DOI: 10.1001/jamainternmed.2016.0400 PMID: 26974260

Mittal, A., Dumka, L., & Mohan, L. (2023). A comprehensive review on the use of artificial intelligence in mental health care. *2023 14th International Conference on Computing Communication and Networking Technologies (ICCCNT).*

MobiHealthNews. (n.d.). AI triage chatbots trekking toward standard care despite criticism. Retrieved from https://www.mobihealthnews.com/content/ai-triage-chatbots-trekking-toward-standard-care-despite-criticism

Mogaji, E., Balakrishnan, J., Nwoba, A. C., & Nguyen, N. P. (2021). Emerging-market consumers' interactions with banking chatbots. *Telematics and Informatics, 65*, 101711. DOI: 10.1016/j.tele.2021.101711

Moghadasi, M. N., Zhuang, Y., & Gellban, H. (2020, July). Robo: A counselor chatbot for opioid addicted patients. In *Proceedings of the 2020 2nd Symposium on Signal Processing Systems* (pp. 91-95). DOI: 10.1145/3421515.3421525

Moghimi, E., Stephenson, C., Gutierrez, G., Jagayat, J., Layzell, G., Patel, C., McCart, A., Gibney, C., Langstaff, C., Ayonrinde, O., Khalid-Khan, S., Milev, R., Snelgrove-Clarke, E., Soares, C., Omrani, M., & Alavi, N. (2023). Mental health challenges, treatment experiences, and care needs of post-secondary students: A cross-sectional mixed-methods study. *BMC Public Health, 23*(1), 655. DOI: 10.1186/s12889-023-15452-x PMID: 37020282

Mohr, D. C., Zhang, M., & Schueller, S. M. (2017). Personal sensing: Understanding mental health using ubiquitous sensors and machine learning. *Annual Review of Clinical Psychology, 13*(1), 23–47. DOI: 10.1146/annurev-clinpsy-032816-044949 PMID: 28375728

Moldstud. (n.d.). The role of security audits in assessing and strengthening cyber defenses. Retrieved from https://moldstud.com/articles/p-the-role-of-security-audits-in-assessing-and-strengthening-cyber-defenses

Monash University. (2021, March 19). *All you need is Ash: Chatbot designed to boost teen mental health at school.* https://www.monash.edu/news/articles/all-you-need-is-ash-chatbot-designed-to-boost-teen-mental-health-at-school

Mooghali, M., Stroud, A. M., Yoo, D. W., Barry, B. A., Grimshaw, A. A., Ross, J. S., Zhu, X., & Miller, J. E. (2023). Barriers and Facilitators to Trustworthy and Ethical AI-enabled Medical Care From Patient and Healthcare Provider Perspectives: A Literature Review. medRxiv, 2023.2010. 2002.23296447.

Moral-Sánchez, S. N., Rey, F. J. R., & Cebrián-de-la-Serna, M. (2023). Analysis of artificial intelligence chatbots and satisfaction for learning in mathematics education. *IJERI: International Journal of Educational Research and Innovation*, (20), 1–14. DOI: 10.46661/ijeri.8196

Mörch, C. M., Gupta, A., & Mishara, B. L. (2020). Canada protocol: An ethical checklist for the use of artificial Intelligence in suicide prevention and mental health. *Artificial Intelligence in Medicine*, *108*, 101934. DOI: 10.1016/j.artmed.2020.101934 PMID: 32972663

Morley, J., Floridi, L., Kinsey, L., & Elhalal, A. (2020). From what to how: An initial review of publicly available AI ethics tools, methods and research to translate principles into practices. *Science and Engineering Ethics*, *26*(4), 2141–2168. DOI: 10.1007/s11948-019-00165-5 PMID: 31828533

Morley, J., Machado, C. C., Burr, C., Cowls, J., Joshi, I., Taddeo, M., & Floridi, L. (2020). The ethics of AI in health care: A mapping review. *Social Science & Medicine*, *260*, 113172. DOI: 10.1016/j.socscimed.2020.113172 PMID: 32702587

Motlova, L. B., Balon, R., Beresin, E. V., Brenner, A. M., Coverdale, J. H., Guerrero, A. P. S., Louie, A. K., & Roberts, L. W. (2017). Psychoeducation as an opportunity for patients, psychiatrists, and psychiatric educators: Why do we ignore it? *Academic Psychiatry*, *41*(4), 447–451. DOI: 10.1007/s40596-017-0728-y PMID: 28536990

Mulder, R., Newton-Howes, G., & Coid, J. W. (2016). The futility of risk prediction in psychiatry. *The British Journal of Psychiatry*, *209*(4), 271–272. DOI: 10.1192/bjp.bp.116.184960 PMID: 27698212

Murthy, R. S. (2017). National Mental Health Survey of India 2015-2016. *Indian Journal of Psychiatry*, *59*(1), 21–26. DOI: 10.4103/psychiatry.IndianJPsychiatry_102_17 PMID: 28529357

Mzwri, K., & Turcsányi-Szabó, M. (2023). Chatbot Development using APIs and Integration into the MOOC. *Central-European Journal of New Technologies in Research. Education and Practice*, *5*(1), 18–30. DOI: 10.36427/CEJNTREP.5.1.5041

National Center for Biotechnology Information. (n.d.). HIPAA, the Privacy Rule, and Its Application to Health Research. Retrieved from https://www.ncbi.nlm.nih.gov/books/NBK9573/

National Research Council, Division on Earth, Life Studies, Board on Life Sciences, & Committee on A Framework for Developing a New Taxonomy of Disease. (2011). Toward precision medicine: building a knowledge network for biomedical research and a new taxonomy of disease.

Naveed, M., Majeed, M., Jabeen, K., Hanif, N., Naveed, R., Saleem, S., & Khan, N. (2024). Plant Disease Diagnosis with Artificial Intelligence (AI). In *Microbial Data Intelligence and Computational Techniques for Sustainable Computing* (pp. 217-234). Springer.

Nebeker, C., Torous, J., & Bartlett Ellis, R. J. (2019). Building the case for actionable ethics in digital health research supported by artificial intelligence. *BMC Medicine*, *17*(1), 1–7. DOI: 10.1186/s12916-019-1377-7 PMID: 31311535

Nehme, M., Schneider, F., Perrin, A., Sum Yu, W., Schmitt, S., Violot, G., Ducrot, A., Tissandier, F., Posfay-Barbe, K., & Guessous, I. (2023). The Development of a Chatbot Technology to Disseminate Post–COVID-19 Information: Descriptive Implementation Study. *Journal of Medical Internet Research*, *25*, e43113. DOI: 10.2196/43113 PMID: 37195688

New York University. (n.d.). IT security info breach notification. Retrieved from https://www.nyu.edu/about/policies-guidelines-compliance/policies-and-guidelines/it-security-info-breach-notification.html

Newell, S., & Jordan, Z. (2015). The patient experience of patient-centered communication with nurses in the hospital setting: A qualitative systematic review protocol. *JBI Evidence Synthesis*, *13*(1), 76–87. PMID: 26447009

Ngai, E. W. T., Lee, M. C. M., Luo, M., Chan, P. S. L., & Liang, T. (2021). An intelligent knowledge-based chatbot for customer service. *Electronic Commerce Research and Applications*, *50*, 101098. DOI: 10.1016/j.elerap.2021.101098

Ng, J., Haller, E., & Murray, A. (2022). The ethical chatbot: A viable solution to socio-legal issues. *Alternative Law Journal*, *47*(4), 308–313. DOI: 10.1177/1037969X221113598

Nicol, G., Wang, R., Graham, S., Dodd, S., & Garbutt, J. (2022). Chatbot-delivered cognitive behavioral therapy in adolescents with depression and anxiety during the COVID-19 pandemic: Feasibility and acceptability study. *JMIR Formative Research*, *6*(11), e40242. DOI: 10.2196/40242 PMID: 36413390

Niederkrotenthaler, T., Eisenwort, B., Till, B., Sonneck, G., Tran, U. S., & Sonneck, G. (2021). Applying language models for suicide prevention: Evaluating news article adherence to WHO reporting guidelines. *Crisis*. Advance online publication. DOI: 10.1027/0227-5910/a000811

Niloy, A. C., Akter, S., Sultana, N., Sultana, J., & Rahman, S. I. U. (2024). Is Chatgpt a menace for creative writing ability? An experiment. *Journal of Computer Assisted Learning*, *40*(2), 919–930. DOI: 10.1111/jcal.12929

Niss, M., Blum, W., & Galbraith, P. (2007). Part 1 Introduction. In Blum, W., Galbraith, P., Henn, H., & Niss, M. (Eds.), *Modeling and applications in mathematics education: The 14th ICMI study* (pp. 3–33). Springer. DOI: 10.1007/978-0-387-29822-1_1

Norcross, J. C. (2000). Here comes the self-help revolution in mental heath. *Psychotherapy (Chicago, Ill.), 37*(4), 370–377. DOI: 10.1037/0033-3204.37.4.370

Northern Illinois University. (n.d.). HIPAA Breach Notification Rule: Explanation and Guidance. Retrieved from https://www.niu.edu/doit/about/policies/hipaa-breach-notification-rule.shtml

Noy, N., Gao, Y., Jain, A., Narayanan, A., Patterson, A., & Taylor, J. (2019). Industry-Scale Knowledge Graphs: Lessons and Challenges: Five Diverse Technology Companies Show How It's Done. *ACM Queue; Tomorrow's Computing Today, 17*(2), 48–75. DOI: 10.1145/3329781.3332266

Nussey, C., Pistrang, N., & Murphy, T. (2013). How does psychoeducation help? A review of the effects of providing information about Tourette syndrome and attention-deficit/hyperactivity disorder. *Child: Care, Health and Development, 39*(5), 617–627. DOI: 10.1111/cch.12039 PMID: 23461278

O'Connor, S. (2023). Open artificial intelligence platforms in nursing education: Tools for academic progress or abuse? *Nurse Education in Practice, 66*, 103537. DOI: 10.1016/j.nepr.2022.103537 PMID: 36549229

O'neil, C. (2017). *Weapons of math destruction: How big data increases inequality and threatens democracy*. Crown.

Obasa, A. E. (2023). The Ethics of Artificial Intelligence in Healthcare Settings.

Ojha, A. K. (2023). Technological innovations in mental health: Enhancing access and affordability for improved well-being. *Journal of Mental Health Issues and Behavior, 33*(33), 5–11. DOI: 10.55529/jmhib.33.5.11

Okonkwo, C. W., & Ade-Ibijola, A. (2020). *Python-Bot: A Chatbot for Teaching Python Programming*.

Okonkwo, C. W., & Ade-Ibijola, A. (2021). Chatbots applications in education: A systematic review. *Computers and Education: Artificial Intelligence, 2*, 100033. DOI: 10.1016/j.caeai.2021.100033

Olawade, D. B., Wada, O. Z., Odetayo, A., David-Olawade, A. C., Asaolu, F., & Eberhardt, J. (2024). Enhancing mental health with Artificial Intelligence: Current trends and future prospects. *Journal of Medicine, Surgery, and Public Health, 3*(100099), 100099. DOI: 10.1016/j.glmedi.2024.100099

Oliver, D., Spada, G., Colling, C., Broadbent, M., Baldwin, H., Patel, R., Stewart, R., Stahl, D., Dobson, R., McGuire, P., & Fusar-Poli, P. (2021). Real-world implementation of precision psychiatry: Transdiagnostic risk calculator for the automatic detection of individuals at-risk of psychosis. *Schizophrenia Research, 227*, 52–60. DOI: 10.1016/j.schres.2020.05.007 PMID: 32571619

Omarov, B., Zhumanov, Z., Gumar, A., & Kuntunova, L. (2023). Artificial Intelligence Enabled Mobile Chatbot Psychologist using AIML and Cognitive Behavioral Therapy. *International Journal of Advanced Computer Science and Applications, 14*(6). Advance online publication. DOI: 10.14569/IJACSA.2023.0140616

Omrani, N., Rivieccio, G., Fiore, U., Schiavone, F., & Agreda, S. G. (2022). To trust or not to trust? An assessment of trust in AI-based systems: Concerns, ethics and contexts. *Technological Forecasting and Social Change, 181*, 121763. DOI: 10.1016/j.techfore.2022.121763

Ondáš, S., Pleva, M., & Hládek, D. (2019). How chatbots can be involved in the education process. *2019 17th International Conference on Emerging Elearning Technologies and Applications (ICETA)*, 575–580.

OneTrust. (n.d.). The GDPR Data Subject Rights. Retrieved from https://www.onetrust.com/blog/the-gdpr-data-subject-rights/

Oracle Cloud Infrastructure (OCI). (n.d.). *What is a chatbot?*https://www.oracle.com/in/chatbots/what-is-a-chatbot/

Pandey, A., & Misra, M. (2023). Artificial Intelligence in Mental Health Care. In Yadav, D. K., & Gulati, A. (Eds.), *Artificial Intelligence and Machine Learning in Healthcare*. Springer. DOI: 10.1007/978-981-99-6472-7_8

Panesar, A., & Panesar, H. (2021). Artificial intelligence and machine learning in global healthcare. In *Handbook of Global Health* (pp. 1775–1813). Springer International Publishing. DOI: 10.1007/978-3-030-45009-0_75

Pang, Z., Yuan, H., Zhang, Y. T., & Packirisamy, M. (2018). Guest editorial health engineering driven by the industry 4.0 for aging society. *IEEE Journal of Biomedical and Health Informatics, 22*(6), 1709–1710. DOI: 10.1109/JBHI.2018.2874081

Papadopoulos, I., & Koulouglioti, C. (2018). The influence of culture on attitudes towards humanoid and animal-like robots: An integrative review. *Journal of Nursing Scholarship*, *50*(6), 653–665. DOI: 10.1111/jnu.12422 PMID: 30242796

Parviainen, J., & Rantala, J. (2022). Chatbot breakthrough in the 2020s? An ethical reflection on the trend of automated consultations in health care. *Medicine, Health Care, and Philosophy*, *25*(1), 61–71. DOI: 10.1007/s11019-021-10049-w PMID: 34480711

Passos, I. C., Mwangi, B., Cao, B., Hamilton, J. E., Wu, M. J., Zhang, X. Y., Zunta-Soares, G. B., Quevedo, J., Kauer-Sant'Anna, M., Kapczinski, F., & Soares, J. C. (2016). Identifying a clinical signature of suicidality among patients with mood disorders: A pilot study using a machine learning approach. *Journal of Affective Disorders*, *193*, 109–116. DOI: 10.1016/j.jad.2015.12.066 PMID: 26773901

Peacock, S. M., Goodwin, I. H., Wood, R. K., McBride, C. J., Brock, A. C., Erekson, D. M., & Boyd, Z. M. (2021). *MATCH: Client-therapist matching with machine learning*. Brigham Young University.

Peng, D., Wang, Z., & Xu, Y. (2020). Challenges and opportunities in mental health services during the COVID-19 pandemic. *General Psychiatry*, *33*(5), e100275. DOI: 10.1136/gpsych-2020-100275 PMID: 32914056

Pennycook, G., Bear, A., Collins, E. T., & Rand, D. G. (2020). The implied truth effect: Attaching warnings to a subset of fake news headlines increases perceived accuracy of headlines without warnings. *Management Science*, *66*(11), 4944–4957. DOI: 10.1287/mnsc.2019.3478

Pérez, J. Q., Daradoumis, T., & Puig, J. M. M. (2020). Rediscovering the use of chatbots in education: A systematic literature review. *Computer Applications in Engineering Education*, *28*(6), 1549–1565. DOI: 10.1002/cae.22326

Perna, G., Grassi, M., Caldirola, D., & Nemeroff, C. B. (2018). The revolution of personalized psychiatry: Will technology make it happen sooner? *Psychological Medicine*, *48*(5), 705–713. DOI: 10.1017/S0033291717002859 PMID: 28967349

Perrone, M. (2024, March 23). *Ready or not, AI chatbots are here to help with Gen Z's mental health struggles.* AP News. https://apnews.com/article/chatbots-mental-health-therapy-counseling-ai-73feb819ff52a51d53fee117c3207219

Peters, M. A., Jackson, L., Papastephanou, M., Jandrić, P., Lazaroiu, G., Evers, C. W., & Tesar, M. (2024). AI and the future of humanity: ChatGPT-4, philosophy and education–Critical responses. *Educational Philosophy and Theory*, *56*(9), 828–862. DOI: 10.1080/00131857.2023.2213437

Pham, K. T., Nabizadeh, A., & Selek, S. (2022). Artificial intelligence and chatbots in psychiatry. *The Psychiatric Quarterly*, *93*(1), 249–253. DOI: 10.1007/s11126-022-09973-8 PMID: 35212940

Pham, M. T., & Avnet, T. (2004). Ideals and oughts and the reliance on affect versus substance in persuasion. *The Journal of Consumer Research*, *30*(4), 503–518. DOI: 10.1086/380285

Piao, M., Ryu, H., Lee, H., & Kim, J. (2020). Use of the healthy lifestyle coaching chatbot app to promote stair-climbing habits among office workers: Exploratory randomized controlled trial. *JMIR mHealth and uHealth*, *8*(5), e15085. DOI: 10.2196/15085 PMID: 32427114

Pillai, R., & Sivathanu, B. (2020). Adoption of AI-based chatbots for hospitality and tourism. *International Journal of Contemporary Hospitality Management*, *32*(10), 3199–3226. DOI: 10.1108/IJCHM-04-2020-0259

Pitychoutis, K. (2024). Harnessing AI Chatbots for EFL Essay Writing: A Paradigm Shift in Language Pedagogy. *Arab World English Journal.*

Prabhakar, S. K., Rajaguru, H., & Sun-Hee, K. (2020). Schizophrenia EEG signal classification based on swarm intelligence computing. *Computational Intelligence and Neuroscience: CIN, 2020.*

Prakash, A. V. (2020). Intelligent Conversational Agents in Mental Healthcare Services: A Thematic Analysis of User Perceptions Authors. *Pacific Asia Journal of the Association for Information Systems, 12.*

Prescott, M. R., Sagui-Henson, S. J., Welcome Chamberlain, C. E., Castro Sweet, C., & Altman, M. (2022). Real world effectiveness of digital mental health services during the COVID-19 pandemic. *PLoS One*, *17*(8), e0272162. DOI: 10.1371/journal.pone.0272162 PMID: 35980879

Prochaska, J. J., Vogel, E. A., Chieng, A., Baiocchi, M., Maglalang, D. D., Pajarito, S., Weingardt, K. R., Darcy, A., & Robinson, A. (2021). A randomized controlled trial of a therapeutic relational agent for reducing substance misuse during the COVID-19 pandemic. *Drug and Alcohol Dependence*, *227*, 108986. DOI: 10.1016/j.drugalcdep.2021.108986 PMID: 34507061

Prochaska, J. J., Vogel, E. A., Chieng, A., Kendra, M., Baiocchi, M., Pajarito, S., & Robinson, A. (2021). A therapeutic relational agent for reducing problematic substance use (Woebot): Development and usability study. *Journal of Medical Internet Research*, *23*(3), e24850. DOI: 10.2196/24850 PMID: 33755028

ProProfs Chat. (n.d.). Healthcare chatbot use cases. Retrieved from https://www.proprofschat.com/blog/healthcare-chatbot-use-cases/

Qiu, M., Li, F.-L., Wang, S., Gao, X., Chen, Y., Zhao, W., Chen, H., Huang, J., & Chu, W. (2017). Alime chat: A sequence to sequence and rerank based chatbot engine. *Proceedings of the 55th Annual Meeting of the Association for Computational Linguistics(*Volume 2*: Short Papers)*, 498–503. DOI: 10.18653/v1/P17-2079

Rai, M., & Pandey, J. K. (Eds.). (2024). *Using Machine Learning to Detect Emotions and Predict Human Psychology*. IGI Global. DOI: 10.4018/979-8-3693-1910-9

Rajagopalan, S. S., Bhardwaj, S., Panda, R., Reddam, V. R., Ganne, C., Kenchaiah, R., & Bharath, R. D. (2018). Machine learning detects EEG microstate alterations in patients living with temporal lobe epilepsy. *Seizure*, *61*, 8–13. DOI: 10.1016/j.seizure.2018.07.007 PMID: 30044996

Rajaram, A. K. P., Saproo, S., & Bansal, S. (2023). A Novel 4A Framework for Measuring Outcomes of Technological Implementation in The Healthcare Industry. *Int. J. Life Sci. Pharma Res,13*(2), P135-P143.

Rajpurkar, P., Zhang, J., Lopyrev, K., & Liang, P. (2016). Squad: 100,000+ questions for machine comprehension of text. *arXiv Preprint arXiv:1606.05250*. DOI: 10.18653/v1/D16-1264

Rane, N. (2023). ChatGPT and similar Generative Artificial Intelligence (AI) for building and construction industry: Contribution, Opportunities and Challenges of large language Models for Industry 4.0, Industry 5.0, and Society 5.0. *Opportunities and Challenges of Large Language Models for Industry, 4*.

Rane, M. S., Robertson, M. M., Westmoreland, D. A., Teasdale, C. A., Grov, C., & Nash, D. (2022). Intention to vaccinate children against COVID-19 among vaccinated and unvaccinated US parents. *JAMA Pediatrics*, *176*(2), 201–203. DOI: 10.1001/jamapediatrics.2021.5153 PMID: 34870702

Ranoliya, B. R., Raghuwanshi, N., & Singh, S. (2017). Chatbot for university related FAQs. *2017 International Conference on Advances in Computing, Communications and Informatics (ICACCI)*, 1525–1530. DOI: 10.1109/ICACCI.2017.8126057

Rashkin, H., Smith, E. M., Li, M., & Boureau, Y.-L. (2019). Towards Empathetic Open-domain Conversation Models: A New Benchmark and Dataset. *Proceedings of the 57th Annual Meeting of the Association for Computational Linguistics*, 5370–5381. DOI: 10.18653/v1/P19-1534

Ray, A., Bhardwaj, A., Malik, Y. K., Singh, S., & Gupta, R. (2022). Artificial intelligence and Psychiatry: An overview. *Asian Journal of Psychiatry, 70*, 103021. DOI: 10.1016/j.ajp.2022.103021 PMID: 35219978

Razzaki, S., Baker, A., Perov, Y., Middleton, K., Baxter, J., Mullarkey, D., Sangar, D., Taliercio, M., Butt, M., Majeed, A., & Associates. (2018). A comparative study of artificial intelligence and human doctors for the purpose of triage and diagnosis. *arXiv Preprint arXiv:1806.10698.*

Reddy, S., Allan, S., Coghlan, S., & Cooper, P. (2020). A governance model for the application of AI in health care. *Journal of the American Medical Informatics Association : JAMIA, 27*(3), 491–497. DOI: 10.1093/jamia/ocz192 PMID: 31682262

Regan, M. (2020, October 27). Therapy patients in Finland blackmailed after hackers stole their records. CNN. https://edition.cnn.com/2020/10/27/tech/finland-therapy-patients-blackmailed-data-breach-intl/index.html

Reitzle, L., Schmidt, C., Färber, F., Huebl, L., Wieler, L. H., Ziese, T., & Heidemann, C. (2021). Perceived access to health care services and relevance of telemedicine during the COVID-19 pandemic in Germany. *International Journal of Environmental Research and Public Health, 18*(14), 7661. DOI: 10.3390/ijerph18147661 PMID: 34300110

REPHRAIN: National Research Centre on Privacy, Harm Reduction and Adversarial Influence Online. (2024). On the privacy of mental health apps: An empirical investigation and recommendations. PubMed. https://pubmed.ncbi.nlm.nih.gov/36407814/

Rivas, P., & Zhao, L. (2023). Marketing with chatgpt: Navigating the ethical terrain of gpt-based chatbot technology. *AI, 4*(2), 375–384. DOI: 10.3390/ai4020019

Robards, F., Kang, M., Luscombe, G., Hawke, C., Sanci, L., Steinbeck, K., Zwi, K., Towns, S., & Usherwood, T. (2020). Intersectionality: Social marginalisation and self-reported health status in young people. *International Journal of Environmental Research and Public Health, 17*(21), 8104. DOI: 10.3390/ijerph17218104 PMID: 33153094

Rodrigues Vasconcelos, M. A., & dos Santos, R. P. (2023). Enhancing STEM learning with ChatGPT and Bing chat as objects to think with: A case study. Cornell University Library. DOI: 10.29333/ejmste/13313

Rogan, J., Bucci, S., & Firth, J. (2024). Health care professionals' views on the use of passive sensing, AI, and machine learning in mental health care: Systematic review with meta-synthesis. *JMIR Mental Health, 11*, e49577. DOI: 10.2196/49577 PMID: 38261403

Roller, S., Dinan, E., Goyal, N., Ju, D., Williamson, M., Liu, Y., Xu, J., Ott, M., Shuster, K., Smith, E. M., Boureau, Y.-L., & Weston, J. (2020). *Recipes for building an open-domain chatbot.*

Rosen, G. (1993). Self-help or hype? comments on psychology's failure to advance self-care. *Professional Psychology, Research and Practice*, *24*(3), 340–345. DOI: 10.1037/0735-7028.24.3.340

Rotman, D. (2023). ChatGPT is about to revolutionize the economy. We need to decide what that looks like. *MIT Technology Review*.

Ruane, E., Birhane, A., & Ventresque, A. (2019). Conversational AI: Social and Ethical Considerations. *AICS*, *2563*, 104–115.

Russell, S. J., & Norvig, P. (2016). *Artificial intelligence: a modern approach.* Pearson.

Rutledge, R. B., Chekroud, A. M., & Huys, Q. J. (2019). Machine learning and big data in psychiatry: Toward clinical applications. *Current Opinion in Neurobiology*, *55*, 152–159. DOI: 10.1016/j.conb.2019.02.006 PMID: 30999271

Ryan, C., Nielssen, O., Paton, M., & Large, M. (2010). Clinical decisions in psychiatry should not be based on risk assessment. *Australasian Psychiatry*, *18*(5), 398–403. DOI: 10.3109/10398562.2010.507816 PMID: 20863176

Ryu, J., Heisig, S., & McLaughlin, C. (2022). A natural language processing approach reveals interpretable linguistic features of therapeutic alliance in psychotherapy. *iScience*, *24*, 102751.

Sabour, S., Zhang, W., Xiao, X., Zhang, Y., Zheng, Y., Wen, J., Zhao, J., & Huang, M. (2023). A chatbot for mental health support: Exploring the impact of Emohaa on reducing mental distress in China. *Frontiers in Digital Health*, *5*, 1133987. Advance online publication. DOI: 10.3389/fdgth.2023.1133987 PMID: 37214342

Sachdeva, N. (2023, July 12). *Chatbots as virtual therapists: The future of mental health care.* Daffodil Software Engineering Insights. https://insights.daffodilsw.com/blog/chatbots-the-future-of-mental-health-care

Sackett, D. L. (1997, February). Evidence-based medicine. *Seminars in Perinatology*, *21*(1), 3–5. DOI: 10.1016/S0146-0005(97)80013-4 PMID: 9190027

Salamanca-Buentello, F., Seeman, M. V., Daar, A. S., & Upshur, R. E. (2020). The ethical, social, and cultural dimensions of screening for mental health in children and adolescents of the developing world. *PLoS One*, *15*(8), e0237853. DOI: 10.1371/journal.pone.0237853 PMID: 32834012

Sallstrom, L., Morris, O., & Mehta, H. (2019). Artificial intelligence in Africa's healthcare: Ethical considerations. *ORF Issue Brief*, *312*, 1–11.

Salton, G., & Buckley, C. (1988). Term-weighting approaches in automatic text retrieval. *Information Processing & Management*, *24*(5), 513–523. DOI: 10.1016/0306-4573(88)90021-0

SAMHSA. (2022). *Adaptations and Innovations for Delivering Mental Health and Substance Use Disorder Treatment Services During the COVID-19 Pandemic*. https://www.samhsa.gov/sites/default/files/dtac-adaptations-innovations-covid-19-pandemic.pdf

Sands, D., & Wald, J. (2014). Transforming health care delivery through consumer engagement, health data transparency, and patient-generated health information. *Yearbook of Medical Informatics*, *23*(01), 170–176. DOI: 10.15265/IY-2014-0017 PMID: 25123739

Sandu, N., & Gide, E. (2019). Adoption of AI-Chatbots to Enhance Student Learning Experience in Higher Education in India. *2019 18th International Conference on Information Technology Based Higher Education and Training (ITHET)*, 1–5. DOI: 10.1109/ITHET46829.2019.8937382

Sanvello, Woebot, Happify, Youper, & Bloom. (2021). Quality evaluation of stress, anxiety and depression apps for COVID-19. ScienceDirect. https://www.sciencedirect.com/science/article/pii/S2666915321001815

Sarkhel, S., Singh, O. P., & Arora, M. (2020). Clinical practice guidelines for psychoeducation in psychiatric disorders general principles of psychoeducation. *Indian Journal of Psychiatry*, *62*(8, Suppl 2), S319–S323. DOI: 10.4103/psychiatry.IndianJPsychiatry_780_19 PMID: 32055073

Sau, A., & Bhakta, I. (2017). Predicting anxiety and depression in elderly patients using machine learning technology. *Healthcare Technology Letters*, *4*(6), 238–243. DOI: 10.1049/htl.2016.0096

Sawada, Y., Tanabe, A., & Nakada, Y. (2022). *A chatbot to search for similar fashion photos and reference fashion coordinators via body part and fashion item segmentations*. Paper presented at the 2022 IEEE Symposium Series on Computational Intelligence (SSCI). DOI: 10.1109/SSCI51031.2022.10022245

Scerbo, M. W. (2023). *Can Artificial Intelligence Be My Coauthor?* (Vol. 18). LWW.

Schmidhuber, J. (2015). Deep learning in neural networks: An overview. *Neural Networks*, *61*, 85–117. DOI: 10.1016/j.neunet.2014.09.003 PMID: 25462637

Schueller, S. M., & Histon, T. (2023). Digital Tools for Youth Mental Health. *Frontiers for Young Minds*, *11*, 1169684. DOI: 10.3389/frym.2023.1169684

Schulte-Nölke, H. (2023). The EU Digital Services Act and EU Consumer Law. *Harmonizing Digital Contract Law*. Nomos Verlagsgesellschaft mbH & Co. KG.

Schütze, H., Manning, C. D., & Raghavan, P. (2008). *Introduction to information retrieval* (Vol. 39). Cambridge University Press Cambridge.

Schwab, K. (2017). *The Fourth Industrial Revolution; Currency*. Google Scholar Google Scholar Digital Library Digital Library.

Sebastian, G., & Sebastian, S. R. (2024). Exploring ethical implications of ChatGPT and other AI chatbots and regulation of disinformation propagation. *Annals of Engineering Mathematics and Computational Intelligence*, *1*(1), 1–12.

Securiti.ai. (n.d.). What are GDPR Data Subject Rights? Retrieved from https://securiti.ai/gdpr-data-subject-rights/

Security Boulevard. (2020). Therapy Center Hacked, 40,000 Patients Sent Ransom Demands. https://securityboulevard.com/2020/10/therapy-center-hacked-40000-patients-sent-ransom-demands/

Segura, C., Palau, À., Luque, J., Costa-Jussà, M. R., & Banchs, R. E. (2019). Chatbol, a chatbot for the Spanish "La Liga." *9th International Workshop on Spoken Dialogue System Technology*, 319–330. DOI: 10.1007/978-981-13-9443-0_28

Selaskowski, B., Reiland, M., Schulze, M., Aslan, B., Kannen, K., Wiebe, A., Wallbaum, T., Boll, S., Lux, S., Philipsen, A., & Braun, N. (2023). Chatbot-supported psychoeducation in adult attention-deficit hyperactivity disorder: Randomised controlled trial. *BJPsych Open*, *9*(6), e192. DOI: 10.1192/bjo.2023.573 PMID: 37827996

Seo, M. J. (2022). Consumers' Negative Responses to the Communication Failure of Chatbots in Online Fashion Shopping Malls. *Fashion & Textile Research Journal*, *24*(2), 183–194. DOI: 10.5805/SFTI.2022.24.2.183

Series, T. L. H. S., Williams, A., Lee, J., Kadakia, K., Cupito, A., Cocchiola, M., Chukwurah, C. S., Chua, P. S., Bailey, A., & Ahmed, M. (2023). Digital health COVID-19 impact assessment: Lessons learned and compelling needs. In *Emerging Stronger from COVID-19: Priorities for Health System Transformation*. National Academies Press.

Shafi, I., Fatima, A., Afzal, H., Díez, I. T., Lipari, V., Breñosa, J., & Ashraf, I. (2023). A Comprehensive Review of Recent Advances in Artificial Intelligence for Dentistry E-Health. *Diagnostics (Basel), 13*(13), 2196. DOI: 10.3390/diagnostics13132196 PMID: 37443594

Shakarian, P., Koyyalamudi, A., Ngu, N., & Mareedu, L. (2023). An independent evaluation of ChatGPT on mathematical word problems (mwp). *arXiv preprint arXiv:2302.13814.*

Shao, C., Ciampaglia, G. L., Varol, O., Yang, K.-C., Flammini, A., & Menczer, F. (2018). The spread of low-credibility content by social bots. *Nature Communications, 9*(1), 1–9. DOI: 10.1038/s41467-018-06930-7 PMID: 30459415

Sharma, A., & Kumar, R. (2022). A constrained framework for context-aware remote E-healthcare (CARE) services. *Transactions on Emerging Telecommunications Technologies, 33*(8), e3649. DOI: 10.1002/ett.3649

Shatte, A. B., Hutchinson, D. M., & Teague, S. J. (2019). Machine learning in mental health: A scoping review of methods and applications. *Psychological Medicine, 49*(9), 1426–1448. DOI: 10.1017/S0033291719000151 PMID: 30744717

Shawar, B. A., & Atwell, E. (2015). ALICE Chatbot: Trials and Outputs. *Computación y Sistemas*, 19.

Shibata, T., & Wada, K. (2011). Robot therapy: A new approach for mental healthcare of the elderly–a mini-review. *Gerontology, 57*(4), 378–386. DOI: 10.1159/000319015 PMID: 20639620

Shin, J., & Bae, S. M. (2023). A systematic review of location data for depression prediction. *International Journal of Environmental Research and Public Health, 20*(11), 5984. DOI: 10.3390/ijerph20115984 PMID: 37297588

Shukla, D. (2022, April 20). *Why mental healthcare is less accessible to marginalized communities.* MedicalNewsToday. https://www.medicalnewstoday.com/articles/why-mental-healthcare-is-less-accessible-to-marginalized-communities

Sieck, C. J., Nicks, S. E., Salem, J., DeVos, T., Thatcher, E., & Hefner, J. L. (2022). Addressing Equity and Social Needs: The New Frontier of Patient Engagement Research. In *Responding to the Grand Challenges in Health Care via Organizational Innovation* (Vol. 21, pp. 151-165). Emerald Publishing Limited.

Singh, B., Olds, T., Brinsley, J., Dumuid, D., Virgara, R., Matricciani, L., Watson, A., Szeto, K., Eglitis, E., Miatke, A., Simpson, C. E. M., Vandelanotte, C., & Maher, C. (2023). Systematic review and meta-analysis of the effectiveness of chatbots on lifestyle behaviours. *NPJ Digital Medicine*, *6*(1), 1–10. DOI: 10.1038/s41746-023-00856-1 PMID: 37353578

Singh, J., Bansal, A., Mittal, S., & Kumari, A. C. (2023). Revitalizing Traditional Health Practices with HealingHands: An AI powered Chatbot. 2023 International Conference on Computational Intelligence and Sustainable Engineering Solutions (CISES).

Singh, O. P. (2019). Chatbots in psychiatry: Can treatment gap be lessened for psychiatric disorders in India. *Indian Journal of Psychiatry*, *61*(3), 225. DOI: 10.4103/0019-5545.258323 PMID: 31142896

Singh, V., Sarkar, S., Gaur, V., Grover, S., & Singh, O. P. (2024). Clinical Practice Guidelines on using artificial intelligence and gadgets for mental health and well-being. *Indian Journal of Psychiatry*, *66*(Suppl 2), S414–S419. DOI: 10.4103/indianjpsychiatry.indianjpsychiatry_926_23 PMID: 38445270

Sinha, S., Basak, S., Dey, Y., & Mondal, A. K. (2019). *An Educational Chatbot for Answering Queries*. Advances in Intelligent Systems and Computing.

Skinner, A. L., Attwood, A., Baddeley, R., Evans-Reeves, K., Bauld, L., & Munafo, M. (2017). Digital phenotyping and the development and delivery of health guidelines and behaviour change interventions. *Addiction (Abingdon, England)*, *112*(7), 1281–1285. DOI: 10.1111/add.13746 PMID: 28472848

Skjuve, M. B., & Brandtzæg, P. B. (2017). Chatbots as a new user interface for providing health information to young people. In Andersson, Y., Dahlquist, U., & Ohlsson, J. (Eds.), *Youth and news in a digital media environment – Nordic-Baltic perspectives*. Nordicom.

Smith, D. H.Ethics of Trust/worthiness in Autonomous Systems: a scoping review. *Proceedings of the First International Symposium on Trustworthy Autonomous Systems*. DOI: 10.1145/3597512.3600207

Smutny, P., & Schreiberova, P. (2020). Chatbots for learning: A review of educational chatbots for the Facebook Messenger. *Computers & Education*, *151*, 103862. DOI: 10.1016/j.compedu.2020.103862

Software, B. G. O. (n.d.). The process behind mental health app development. Retrieved from https://www.bgosoftware.com/blog/mental-health-app-development/

Sonderegger, S., & Seufert, S. (2022). *Chatbot-mediated Learning: Conceptual Framework for the Design of Chatbot Use Cases in Education* (pp. 207–215). DOI: 10.5220/0010999200003182

Søvold, L. E., Naslund, J. A., Kousoulis, A. A., Saxena, S., Qoronfleh, M. W., Grobler, C., & Münter, L. (2021). Prioritizing the mental health and well-being of healthcare workers: An urgent global public health priority. *Frontiers in Public Health*, *9*, 679397. DOI: 10.3389/fpubh.2021.679397 PMID: 34026720

Sprinto. (2024). HIPAA Breach Notification Rule [Quick Guide]. Retrieved from https://sprinto.com/blog/hipaa-breach-notification-rule/

Squires, M., Tao, X., Elangovan, S., Gururajan, R., Zhou, X., Acharya, U. R., & Li, Y. (2023). Deep learning and machine learning in psychiatry: A survey of current progress in depression detection, diagnosis and treatment. *Brain Informatics*, *10*(1), 10. DOI: 10.1186/s40708-023-00188-6 PMID: 37093301

Srite & Karahanna. (2006). The role of espoused national cultural values in technology acceptance. *MIS Quarterly: Management Information Systems, 30*(3), 679. DOI: 10.2307/25148745

Stephens, T. N., Joerin, A., Rauws, M., & Werk, L. N. (2019). Feasibility of pediatric obesity and prediabetes treatment support through Tess, the AI behavioral coaching chatbot. *Translational Behavioral Medicine*, *9*(3), 440–447. DOI: 10.1093/tbm/ibz043 PMID: 31094445

Steve, M. (2023). Why mental health apps need to take privacy more seriously. (2023, November 30). Brookings Institution. Retrieved from https://www.brookings.edu/articles/why-mental-health-apps-need-to-take-privacy-more-seriously/

Stokel-Walker, C. (2022). AI bot ChatGPT writes smart essays - should professors worry? *Nature*. Advance online publication. DOI: 10.1038/d41586-022-04397-7 PMID: 36494443

Strzelecki, A. (2019). Website removal from search engines due to copyright violation. *Aslib Journal of Information Management*, *71*(1), 54–71. DOI: 10.1108/AJIM-05-2018-0108

Sukums, F., Mzurikwao, D., Sabas, D., Chaula, R., Mbuke, J., Kabika, T., Kaswija, J., Ngowi, B., Noll, J., Winkler, A. S., & Andersson, S. W. (2023). The use of artificial intelligence-based innovations in the health sector in Tanzania: A scoping review. *Health Policy and Technology*, *12*(1), 100728. DOI: 10.1016/j.hlpt.2023.100728

Suppadungsuk, S., Thongprayoon, C., Miao, J., Krisanapan, P., Qureshi, F., Kashani, K., & Cheungpasitporn, W. (2023). Exploring the Potential of Chatbots in Critical Care Nephrology. *Medicines (Basel, Switzerland), 10*(10), 58. DOI: 10.3390/medicines10100058 PMID: 37887265

Suppadungsuk, S., Thongprayoon, C., Nikravangolsefid, N., Singh, W., Cheungpasitporn, W., Dong, Y., & Kashani, K. B. (2024). Magnesium Derangement among Critically Ill Patients with Acute Kidney Injury: An Association with Acute Kidney Disease. *Nephron, 148*(8), 553–562. DOI: 10.1159/000539674 PMID: 38861941

Swanberg, S. E. (2019). Psychological armor: The science news-letter warns against propaganda (1926–1965). *Journalism Studies, 20*(13), 1883–1902. DOI: 10.1080/1461670X.2018.1541754

Tachmazidis, I., Chen, T., Adamou, M., & Antoniou, G. (2020). A hybrid AI approach for supporting clinical diagnosis of attention deficit hyperactivity disorder (ADHD) in adults. *Health Information Science and Systems, 9*(1), 1. DOI: 10.1007/s13755-020-00123-7 PMID: 33235709

Tai-Seale, M., Downing, N. L., Jones, V. G., Milani, R. V., Zhao, B., Clay, B., Sharp, C. D., Chan, A. S., & Longhurst, C. A. (2019). Technology-enabled consumer engagement: Promising practices at four health care delivery organizations. *Health Affairs, 38*(3), 383–390. DOI: 10.1377/hlthaff.2018.05027 PMID: 30830826

Tajbakhsh, N., Shin, J. Y., Gurudu, S. R., Hurst, R. T., Kendall, C. B., Gotway, M. B., & Liang, J. (2016). Convolutional neural networks for medical image analysis: Full training or fine tuning? *IEEE Transactions on Medical Imaging, 35*(5), 1299–1312. DOI: 10.1109/TMI.2016.2535302 PMID: 26978662

Talaviya, A. (2023, November 6). *Machine learning algorithms used in creating AI chatbots.* Medium. https://medium.com/@avikumart_/machine-learning-algorithms-used-in-creating-ai-chatbots-3bac9fe27cb9

Talyshinskii, A., Naik, N., Hameed, B. Z., Juliebø-Jones, P., & Somani, B. K. (2024). Potential of AI-driven chatbots in urology: Revolutionizing patient care through artificial intelligence. *Current Urology Reports, 25*(1), 9–18. DOI: 10.1007/s11934-023-01184-3 PMID: 37723300

Tam-Seto, L., Wood, V. M., Linden, B., & Stuart, H. (2021). Perceptions of an AI-supported mobile app for military health in the Canadian armed forces. *Military Behavioral Health, 9*(3), 247–254. DOI: 10.1080/21635781.2020.1838364

Tanir, D., & Karakas, A. B. (2023). The Use of AI and Structural Magnetic Resonance Imaging in the Diagnosis of Major Depressive Disorder. In *Machine Learning and AI Techniques in Interactive Medical Image Analysis* (pp. 167–187). IGI Global.

Tanwar, S., Parekh, K., & Evans, R. (2020). Blockchain-based electronic healthcare record system for healthcare 4.0 applications. *Journal of Information Security and Applications*, *50*, 102407. DOI: 10.1016/j.jisa.2019.102407

Tao, D., Wang, T., Wang, T., Zhang, T., Zhang, X., & Qu, X. (2020). A systematic review and meta-analysis of user acceptance of consumer-oriented health information technologies. *Computers in Human Behavior*, *104*(106147), 106147. DOI: 10.1016/j.chb.2019.09.023

Thapa, R., van Teijlingen, E., Regmi, P. R., & Heaslip, V. (2021). Caste exclusion and health discrimination in South Asia: A systematic review. *Asia-Pacific Journal of Public Health*, *33*(8), 828–838. DOI: 10.1177/10105395211014648 PMID: 34024157

The Economic Times. (2022, October 10). *World Mental Health Day: 60-70 mn people in India suffer from common mental disorders; stigmatisation, financial barriers prevent timely treatment.* https://economictimes.indiatimes.com/magazines/panache/world-mental-health-day-60-70-mn-people-in-india-suffer-from-common-mental-disorders-stigmatisation-financial-barriers-prevent-timely-treatment/articleshow/104289268.cms?from=mdr

The Verge. (2023). Mental health apps are still failing their privacy checkups. Retrieved from https://www.theverge.com/2023/5/4/23710840/mental-health-therapy-apps-mozilla-report-privacy-data-security

Thieme, A., Belgrave, D., & Doherty, G. (2020). Machine learning in mental health: A systematic review of the HCI literature to support the development of effective and implementable ML systems. *ACM Transactions on Computer-Human Interaction*, *27*(5), 1–53. DOI: 10.1145/3398069

Thomas, L. P., Menon, V. A., Thomas, J., Ali, K. A. A., Soman, K. K., & Kumar, T. K. S. (2024). Towards a model: Exploring fatigue factors in ZOOM online classes. *2024 International Conference on Current Trends in Advanced Computing (ICCTAC)*. DOI: 10.1109/ICCTAC61556.2024.10581300

Thordardottir, B., Malmgren Fänge, A., Lethin, C., Rodriguez Gatta, D., & Chiatti, C. (2019). Acceptance and use of innovative Assistive Technologies among people with cognitive impairment and their caregivers: A systematic review. *BioMed Research International*, *2019*, 1–18. DOI: 10.1155/2019/9196729 PMID: 30956989

Thoropass. (n.d.). Understanding the GDPR breach notification timeline. Retrieved from https://thoropass.com/blog/compliance/gdpr-breach-notification-timeline/

Thorp, H. H. (2023). *ChatGPT is fun, but not an author* (Vol. 379). American Association for the Advancement of Science.

Tian, H., Lu, W., Li, T. O., Tang, X., Cheung, S.-C., Klein, J., & Bissyandé, T. F. (2023). Is ChatGPT the ultimate programming assistant—how far is it? *arXiv preprint arXiv:2304.11938*.

Tikka, S. K., Singh, B. K., Nizamie, S. H., Garg, S., Mandal, S., Thakur, K., & Singh, L. K. (2020). Artificial intelligence-based classification of schizophrenia: A high density electroencephalographic and support vector machine study. *Indian Journal of Psychiatry*, *62*(3), 273–282. DOI: 10.4103/psychiatry.IndianJPsychiatry_91_20 PMID: 32773870

Tolentino, J. C., & Schmidt, S. L. (2018). DSM-5 criteria and depression severity: Implications for clinical practice. *Frontiers in Psychiatry*, *9*, 412752. DOI: 10.3389/fpsyt.2018.00450 PMID: 30333763

Topol, E. (2019). *Deep medicine: how artificial intelligence can make healthcare human again.*

Torous, J., Bucci, S., Bell, I. H., Kessing, L. V., Faurholt-Jepsen, M., Whelan, P., Carvalho, A. F., Keshavan, M., Linardon, J., & Firth, J. (2021). The growing field of digital psychiatry: Current evidence and the future of apps, social media, chatbots, and virtual reality. *World Psychiatry; Official Journal of the World Psychiatric Association (WPA)*, *20*(3), 318–335. DOI: 10.1002/wps.20883 PMID: 34505369

Town, R., Hayes, D., March, A., Fonagy, P., & Stapley, E. (2023). Self-management, self-care, and self-help in adolescents with emotional problems: A scoping review. *European Child & Adolescent Psychiatry*, •••, 1–28. DOI: 10.1007/s00787-022-02134-z PMID: 36641785

Turing, A. M. (1950). Computing machinery and intelligence. *Mind*, *59*(October), 433–460. DOI: 10.1093/mind/LIX.236.433

Ukpabi, D. C., Aslam, B., & Karjaluoto, H. (2019). Chatbot adoption in tourism services: A conceptual exploration. In *Robots, artificial intelligence, and service automation in travel, tourism and hospitality* (pp. 105–121). Emerald Publishing Limited. DOI: 10.1108/978-1-78756-687-320191006

Uludag, K. (2023e). Revealing the hidden aspects of ChatGPT: An inquiry into concerns surrounding plagiarism rates.

Uludag, K. (2023). The use of AI-supported Chatbot in Psychology. *Available atSSRN* 4331367. DOI: 10.2139/ssrn.4331367

Uludag, K. (2023a). Brain Imaging Analysis with ChatGPT and Python's Powerful NumPy Package. *Available atSSRN* 4449615. DOI: 10.2139/ssrn.4449615

Uludag, K. (2023b). Chatbots Can Be Trained to Represent Humans after Death: Interview with ChatGPT. *Available atSSRN* 4399732. DOI: 10.2139/ssrn.4399732

Uludag, K. (2023b). How to Use ChatGPT in Brain Imaging Analysis. *Available atSSRN* 4440457. DOI: 10.2139/ssrn.4440457

Uludag, K. (2023c). ChatGPT Can Distinguish Paranoid Thoughts in Patients with Schizophrenia. *Available atSSRN* 4391941. DOI: 10.2139/ssrn.4391941

Uludag, K. (2023c). Learn Basic Statistical Analysis with Panda using Chatbots: ChatGPT in Programming Education. *Available atSSRN* 4428650. DOI: 10.2139/ssrn.4428650

Uludag, K. (2023d). ChatGPT Can Help to Distinguish Delusional Jealousy. *Available atSSRN* 4406212. DOI: 10.2139/ssrn.4406212

Uludag, K. (2023d). Testing creativity of ChatGPT in psychology: Interview with ChatGPT. *Available atSSRN* 4390872. DOI: 10.2139/ssrn.4390872

Uludag, K. (2023f). Understanding Sexting Addiction: Exploring the Role of Chatbots in Its Development and Definition. *Available atSSRN* 4398059. DOI: 10.2139/ssrn.4398059

Uludag, K. (2024). Exploring the Association Between Textual Parameters and Psychological and Cognitive Factors. *Psychology Research and Behavior Management*, *17*, 1139–1150. DOI: 10.2147/PRBM.S460503 PMID: 38505355

Uludag, K. (2024). Exploring the Scikit-Learn Package With ChatGPT. In *The Pioneering Applications of Generative AI* (pp. 251–273). IGI Global. DOI: 10.4018/979-8-3693-3278-8.ch012

US Food and Drug Administration. (2020). *Qualification Process for Drug Development Tools Guidance for Industry and FDA Staff.* https://www.fda.gov/media/133511/download

Vaidyam, A. N., Wisniewski, H., Halamka, J. D., Kashavan, M. S., & Torous, J. B. (2019). Chatbots and conversational agents in mental health: A review of the psychiatric landscape. *Canadian Journal of Psychiatry*, *64*(7), 456–464. DOI: 10.1177/0706743719828977 PMID: 30897957

Valera, S. (2023, March 8). *Best mood tracker apps.* Verwell Mind. https://www.verywellmind.com/best-mood-tracker-apps-5212922

Van der Schyff, E. L., Ridout, B., Amon, K. L., Forsyth, R., & Campbell, A. J. (2023). Providing Self-Led Mental Health Support Through an Artificial Intelligence-Powered Chat Bot (Leora) to Meet the Demand of Mental Health Care. *Journal of Medical Internet Research, 25*, e46448. DOI: 10.2196/46448 PMID: 37335608

Van Le, D., Montgomery, J., Kirkby, K. C., & Scanlan, J. (2018). Risk prediction using natural language processing of electronic mental health records in an inpatient forensic psychiatry setting. *Journal of Biomedical Informatics, 86*, 49–58. DOI: 10.1016/j.jbi.2018.08.007 PMID: 30118855

Vares, E. A., Salum, G. A., Spanemberg, L., Caldieraro, M. A., & Fleck, M. P. (2015). Depression dimensions: Integrating clinical signs and symptoms from the perspectives of clinicians and patients. *PLoS One, 10*(8), e0136037. DOI: 10.1371/journal.pone.0136037 PMID: 26313556

Venkatraman, M. P., & Price, L. L. (1990). Differentiating between cognitive and sensory innovativeness. *Journal of Business Research, 20*(4), 293–315. DOI: 10.1016/0148-2963(90)90008-2

Viduani, A., Cosenza, V., Araújo, R. M., & Kieling, C. (2023). Chatbots in the field of mental health: Challenges and opportunities. In Passos, I. C., Rabelo-da-Ponte, F. D., & Kapczinski, F. (Eds.), *Digital mental health.* Springer. DOI: 10.1007/978-3-031-10698-9_8

Vilaza, G. N., & McCashin, D. (2021). Is the automation of digital mental health ethical? Applying an ethical framework to chatbots for cognitive behaviour therapy. *Frontiers in Digital Health, 3*, 689736. DOI: 10.3389/fdgth.2021.689736 PMID: 34713163

Vinutha, N., Pattar, S., Sharma, S., Shenoy, P. D., & Venugopal, K. R. (2020). A machine learning framework for assessment of cognitive and functional impairments in Alzheimer's disease: Data preprocessing and analysis. *The Journal of Prevention of Alzheimer's Disease, 7*(2), 87–94. DOI: 10.14283/jpad.2020.7 PMID: 32236397

Wainberg, M. L., Scorza, P., Shultz, J. M., Helpman, L., Mootz, J. J., Johnson, K. A., Neria, Y., Bradford, J. E., Oquendo, M. A., & Arbuckle, M. R. (2017). Challenges and opportunities in global mental health: A research-to-practice perspective. *Current Psychiatry Reports, 19*(5), 28. DOI: 10.1007/s11920-017-0780-z PMID: 28425023

Walsh, D. (2023, June 21). *A Blueprint for Using AI in Psychotherapy.* Stanford HAI. https://hai.stanford.edu/news/blueprint-using-ai-psychotherapy

Wang, S., Claudy, M., & Yan, Q. (2024). Collaborating with AI in Brainstorming: How Gender Cues of Virtual Agents Affect User Idea Generation and Selection.

Wang, C., Liu, S., Yang, H., Guo, J., Wu, Y., & Liu, J. (2023). Ethical considerations of using ChatGPT in health care. *Journal of Medical Internet Research*, *25*, e48009. DOI: 10.2196/48009 PMID: 37566454

Wang, J., Cheng, Z., Yao, Q., Liu, L., Xu, D., & Hu, G. (2024). Bioinformatics and biomedical informatics with ChatGPT: Year one review. *Quantitative Biology*, *12*(4), 345–359. DOI: 10.1002/qub2.67 PMID: 39364207

Wardat, Y., Tashtoush, M. A., AlAli, R., & Jarrah, A. M. (2023). ChatGPT: A revolutionary tool for teaching and learning mathematics. *Eurasia Journal of Mathematics, Science and Technology Education*, *19*(7), em2286. DOI: 10.29333/ejmste/13272

Waring, O. M., & Majumder, M. S. (2020). Introduction to digital phenotyping for global health. *Leveraging data science for global health*, 251-261.

Warrier, U., Warrier, A., & Khandelwal, K. (2023). Ethical considerations in the use of artificial intelligence in mental health. *The Egyptian Journal of Neurology, Psychiatry and Neurosurgery*, *59*(1), 139. Advance online publication. DOI: 10.1186/s41983-023-00735-2

Wei, X., Cao, Y., Peng, X., & Prybutok, V. (2024). A meta-analysis of technology acceptance in healthcare from the consumer's perspective. *Health Marketing Quarterly*, *41*(2), 1–22. DOI: 10.1080/07359683.2024.2316425 PMID: 38421028

Weizenbaum, J. (1966). ELIZA—A computer program for the study of natural language communication between man and machine. *Communications of the ACM*, *9*(1), 36–45. DOI: 10.1145/365153.365168

Whittaker, M. (2018). *AI now report 2018*. AI Now Institute at New York University.

Wieland, B., de Wit, J., & de Rooij, A. (2022). Electronic brainstorming with a chatbot partner: A good idea due to increased productivity and idea diversity. *Frontiers in Artificial Intelligence*, *5*, 880673. DOI: 10.3389/frai.2022.880673 PMID: 36213166

Wies, B., Landers, C., & Ienca, M. (2021). Digital mental health for young people: A scoping review of ethical promises and challenges. *Frontiers in Digital Health*, *3*, 697072. DOI: 10.3389/fdgth.2021.697072 PMID: 34713173

Wijaya, T. T., Su, M., Cao, Y., Weinhandl, R., & Houghton, T. (2024). Examining Chinese preservice mathematics teachers' adoption of AI chatbots for learning: Unpacking perspectives through the UTAUT2 model. *Education and Information Technologies*, 1–29.

Wijekoon, A., Wiratunga, N., Corsar, D., Martin, K., Nkisi-Orji, I., Palihawadana, C., Caro-Martínez, M., Díaz-Agudo, B., Bridge, D., & Liret, A. (2024). iSee: Advancing Multi-Shot Explainable AI Using Case-based Recommendations. *arXiv preprint arXiv:2408.12941*. DOI: 10.3233/FAIA241057

Williams, R. (2024, February 5). A chatbot helped more people access mental-health services. Technology Review. Retrieved from https://www.technologyreview.com/2024/02/05/1087690/a-chatbot-helped-more-people-access-mental-health-services/

Williams, R. T. (2024). *The ethical implications of using generative chatbots in higher education.* Paper presented at the Frontiers in Education. DOI: 10.3389/feduc.2023.1331607

Woolley, S. C., & Howard, P. N. (Eds.). (2018). *Computational propaganda: Political parties, politicians, and political manipulation on social media.* Oxford University Press. DOI: 10.1093/oso/9780190931407.001.0001

World Health Organization. (2022). *Mental health and COVID-19: early evidence of the pandemic's impact: scientific brief, 2 March 2022* (No. WHO/2019 -nCoV/Sci_Brief/Mental_health/2022.1). World Health Organization.

World Mental Health Report: transforming mental health for all. (2022). World Health Organization.

Wu, D., Liang, S., & Yu, W. (2018). Collaborative Information Searching as Learning in Academic Group Work. *Aslib Journal of Information Management, 70*, 00–00. DOI: 10.1108/AJIM-03-2017-0063

Wube, H. D., Esubalew, S. Z., Weldesellasie, F. F., & Debelee, T. G. (2022). Text-Based Chatbot in Financial Sector: A Systematic Literature Review. *Data Science in Finance and Economics*, *2*(3), 232–259. DOI: 10.3934/DSFE.2022011

Wu, Y., Wang, G., Li, W., & Li, Z. (2008). Automatic chatbot knowledge acquisition from online forum via rough set and ensemble learning. *2008 IFIP International Conference on Network and Parallel Computing*, 242–246. DOI: 10.1109/NPC.2008.24

Xia, J., Merinder, L. B., & Belgamwar, M. R. (2011). Psychoeducation for schizophrenia. *Cochrane Database of Systematic Reviews*, *15*(6), CD002831. Advance online publication. DOI: 10.1002/14651858.CD002831.pub2 PMID: 21678337

XinhuaNet. (2021, July 16). *China launches new space station core module.*http://www.xinhuanet.com/english/2021-07/16/c_1310064630.htm

Xu, B., & Zhuang, Z. (2022). Survey on psychotherapy chatbots. *Concurrency and Computation*, *34*(7), e6170. DOI: 10.1002/cpe.6170

Xu, L., Sanders, L., Li, K., & Chow, J. C. (2021). Chatbot for health care and oncology applications using artificial intelligence and machine learning: Systematic review. *JMIR Cancer*, *7*(4), e27850. DOI: 10.2196/27850 PMID: 34847056

Yadav, K., & Hasija, Y. (2022). Artificial intelligence and technological development in behavioral and mental healthcare. *2022 International Conference for Advancement in Technology (ICONAT)*. DOI: 10.1109/ICONAT53423.2022.9726100

Yang, S. C. (1997). Information seeking as problem-solving using a qualitative approach to uncover the novice learners' information-seeking processes in a perseus hypertext system. *Library & Information Science Research*, *19*(1), 71–94. DOI: 10.1016/S0740-8188(97)90006-2

Yan, W. J., Ruan, Q. N., & Jiang, K. (2022). Challenges for artificial intelligence in recognizing mental disorders. *Diagnostics (Basel)*, *13*(1), 2. DOI: 10.3390/diagnostics13010002 PMID: 36611294

Yilmaz, R., & Yilmaz, F. G. K. (2023). Augmented intelligence in programming learning: Examining student views on the use of ChatGPT for programming learning. *Computers in Human Behavior: Artificial Humans*, *1*(2), 100005. DOI: 10.1016/j.chbah.2023.100005

Youper. (n.d.). *Effectiveness*. Youper. https://www.youper.ai/effectiveness

Yu, H. (2023). Reflection on whether Chat GPT should be banned by academia from the perspective of education and teaching. *Frontiers in Psychology*, *14*, 1181712. DOI: 10.3389/fpsyg.2023.1181712 PMID: 37325766

Yunus, A. P., Masago, Y., Hijioka, Y., & Saito, Y. (2020). Evaluation of PM2.5 exposure and its impact on premature mortality in South and Southeast Asia. *Environmental Research Letters*, *15*(7), 074025. Advance online publication. DOI: 10.1088/1748-9326/ab9375

Zarifhonarvar, A. (2024). Economics of chatgpt: A labor market view on the occupational impact of artificial intelligence. *Journal of Electronic Business & Digital Economics*, *3*(2), 100–116. DOI: 10.1108/JEBDE-10-2023-0021

Zawacki-Richter, O., Marín, V. I., Bond, M., & Gouverneur, F. (2019). Systematic review of research on artificial intelligence applications in higher education – where are the educators? *International Journal of Educational Technology in Higher Education*, *16*(1), 39. DOI: 10.1186/s41239-019-0171-0

Zeng, N., Vignali, G., & Ryding, D. (2023). Understanding the Application of AI-enabled Chatbots in Luxury Fashion Retailing. In *The Garment Economy: Understanding History, Developing Business Models, and Leveraging Digital Technologies* (pp. 369-388): Springer. DOI: 10.1007/978-3-031-33302-6_19

Zhang, Z., Lin, W., Liu, M., & Mahmoud, M. (2020, November). Multimodal deep learning framework for mental disorder recognition. In *2020 15th IEEE International Conference on Automatic Face and Gesture Recognition (FG 2020)* (pp. 344-350). IEEE. DOI: 10.1109/FG47880.2020.00033

Zhang, J., Oh, Y. J., Lange, P., Yu, Z., & Fukuoka, Y. (2020). Artificial intelligence chatbot behavior change model for designing artificial intelligence chatbots to promote physical activity and a healthy diet: Viewpoint. *Journal of Medical Internet Research*, *22*(9), e22845. DOI: 10.2196/22845 PMID: 32996892

Zhang, T., Schoene, A. M., Ji, S., & Ananiadou, S. (2022). Natural language processing applied to mental illness detection: A narrative review. *NPJ Digital Medicine*, *5*(1), 46. DOI: 10.1038/s41746-022-00589-7 PMID: 35396451

Zhao, X., Wu, W., Xu, C., Tao, C., Zhao, D., & Yan, R. (2020). Knowledge-Grounded Dialogue Generation with Pre-trained Language Models. *Proceedings of the 2020 Conference on Empirical Methods in Natural Language Processing (EMNLP)*, 3377–3390. DOI: 10.18653/v1/2020.emnlp-main.272

Zhavoronkov, A. (2022). Rapamycin in the context of Pascal's Wager: Generative pre-trained transformer perspective. *Oncoscience*, *9*, 82–84. DOI: 10.18632/oncoscience.571 PMID: 36589923

Zhou, S., Zhao, J., & Zhang, L. (2022). Application of artificial intelligence on psychological interventions and diagnosis: An overview. *Frontiers in Psychiatry*, *13*, 811665. DOI: 10.3389/fpsyt.2022.811665 PMID: 35370846

Zscaler. (n.d.). What Is the HIPAA Security Rule? Retrieved from https://www.zscaler.com/zpedia/what-is-hipaa-security-rule

About the Contributors

Kadir Uludag, Ph.D., is an accomplished researcher in the field of Applied Psychology, with expertise in areas such as schizophrenia research, drug addiction, machine learning, and educational psychology. He completed his Ph.D. at the Chinese Academy of Sciences and is currently engaged in a postdoctoral research position at Shanghai Jiao Tong University. In addition to his academic pursuits, Kadir is actively involved in knowledge dissemination and community engagement through his website (ifx0.com/), where he facilitates the sharing and discussion of peer-reviewed articles.

Nafees Ahmad obtained CAS-TWAS President's Fellowship Award in 2016 and completed his Ph.D. degree in Physical Chemistry under the supervision of Prof. Huiqiong Zhou from CAS Center for Excellence in Nanoscience, National Center for Nanoscience and Technology, Chinese Academy of Sciences. Then, he worked as a Research Fellow at Tsinghua-Berkeley Shenzhen Institute (TBSI), Tsinghua University. In 2021, he joined the research group of Prof. Liang & Prof. Fan as Postdoctoral Fellow at Shenzhen University and obtained Distinction Certificate in "National Postdoctoral Innovation & Entrepreneurship Competition. https://orcid.org/0000-0003-2120-4750.

* * *

Vishnu Achutha Menon is an independent journalist, writer, researcher, and an Indian percussionist. He is a recipient of the Junior Scholarship the Ministry of Culture awarded. His research interests are film studies, verbal & nonverbal communication, south Asian performances, Natyasastra, media studies, media analysis techniques, Laban Movement Analysis, and Ethnomusicology.

Mirza Jahanzeb Beg is a psychologist and author specialising in Human Behavioural and Mental Health Disorders. He received training in Diplomacy,

International law, and United Nations procedures at the Department of Law, University of New South Wales, Sydney. He has a Bachelor of Science (Hons) degree in Psychology and a Master of Science degree in Clinical Psychology, earning a Gold Medal for his achievements. Currently, he is pursuing a PhD research programme in psychology with a specific emphasis on the use of artificial intelligence in the field of mental health. He contributes to a range of academic journals, magazines, and newspapers. He is also interested in poetry, Sufi music, philosophy and research methods.

Vishvak Chanthar is a distinguished Endocrine and Breast Surgeon renowned for his expertise in comprehensive Breast cancer care as well as Endocrine surgeries. With a solid background in endocrine (thyroid, parathyroid, adrenal, endocrine pancreas) surgery, breast surgery, and clinical research, he brings a wealth of experience to his practice. Specializing in Endocrine and Breast Surgery, Dr. Vishvak Chanthar is highly proficient in thyroid, parathyroid, endocrine pancreas, adrenal surgeries, mastectomy, breast conservation, Oncoplastic breast reconstruction, risk reduction breast surgery, sentinel lymph node biopsy, and microwave ablation of thyroid and breast lesions. His professional journey includes significant roles at Sanjay Gandhi Postgraduate Institute of Medical Sciences, Lucknow, where he served as an assistant professor in the Department of Endocrine and Breast Surgery, focusing on endocrine procedures, mastectomies, Oncoplastic breast conservation techniques, and breast reconstruction. He has further honed his skills through experiences at the breast unit in Guys and St Thomas NHS Foundation Hospital in London, United Kingdom and at the Minimal Invasive Endocrine Division of Police General Hospital in Bangkok, Thailand. Dr. Vishvak's academic achievements are noteworthy, marked by numerous accolades and awards. Actively engaged with esteemed international and national surgical societies, he has contributed significantly to the field's literature. Moreover, he is a seasoned educator, mentoring undergraduates, postgraduates, MCh, and DNB trainees specializing in Endocrine and Breast Surgery. He has served as faculty in various prestigious breast and endocrine surgery conferences, workshops, and masterclasses. Currently, Dr. Vishvak Chanthar serves as a Consultant in Surgical Oncology (Onco Breast Surgery Unit) at the Rajiv Gandhi Cancer Institute and Research Centre, Delhi, where he continues to provide exceptional care and expertise in his field.

Lavleen Kaur is a counselling psychologist at Infiheal, where she applies her extensive knowledge and skills to support individuals in overcoming various mental health challenges. She excels in collaborative healthcare environments that prioritize wellness and values working with other healthcare professionals to deliver comprehensive care. At Infiheal, Lavleen not only provides counselling services but also develops psychometric tests to address mental health issues across diverse populations. Lavleen holds an MA in Psychology from Punjabi University, where she authored three research papers and was honoured with the Young Scientist Award. This recognition underscores her expertise and dedication to advancing mental health practices. Her research experience has equipped her with a profound understanding of evidence-based practices, further enhancing her analytical and critical thinking abilities.

Abhinanda Patra is a Counseling and Research psychologist at Infiheal who believes that empirical and analytical skills are a fundamental part of academic excellence and the building blocks of critical thinking in practicing psychology. In addition to providing counseling services at Infiheal, Abhinanda also creates various psychometric tests to address mental health challenges in diverse populations. Abhinanda holds a M.Sc in Psychology from Banaras Hindu University where she has researched on risk factors of suicidality in the adolescent population. Her professional journey reflects a commitment to research findings to improve mental health outcomes.

Archana Sowbarnika is a psychologist at Infiheal, dedicated to research and constantly upgrading her skills for her practice. She holds dual master's degrees: an M.Sc. in Applied Psychology and a Master of Business Administration. Her research includes a thesis on the "Impact of Mother's Relationship & Parenting Styles on the Development of Self-Concept among Adolescents" (2021) and a study on "Employee Satisfaction and Self-Empowerment" (2017). She has also published on "Addressing Self-Esteem and Perceived Social Support in the Elderly" in the Global Journal for Research Analysis (2015). Her research enhances her analytical and critical thinking abilities. By integrating research findings with practical applications, she also empowers clients to be active participants in their healing process.

Srishti Srivastava is an entrepreneur and health care technologist who founded mental health startup Infiheal. She graduated from IIT Bombay in 2014 with a dual degree (M.Tech and B.Tech) in Chemical Engineering. Thereafter she worked in KPMG as a consultant, and then went on to work in the Government as a public policy consultant. She has done an Executive MBA from Cornell University focused on entrepreneurship (Cornell Maha 60). In 2023, she was invited by World Bank round table on entrepreneurship. Her startup received a mention by the Honourable Prime Minister of India, Mr. Narendra Modi in his 108th National Address.

Sruthi Suresh is a doctoral research scholar in Psychology at CHRIST (Deemed to be University) and an IB Psychology Educator and TOK Coordinator at Knowledgeum Academy, Bengaluru. In 2018, she completed her M.Sc. in

Counseling Psychology and worked as an IB DP Psychology Faculty for the next two years. After joining the Ph.D. program in 2020, she has been an active scholar and engaged with the department as a Research Assistant, Teaching Assistant, Impact Assessment Research Team Lead, and Department Magazine Editor. She writes and presents widely on issues related to child and adolescent mental health, teacher education, and social emotional learning.

Manish Kumar Verma is an esteemed professor of Psychology and serves as the department head at Lovely Professional University, Phagwara, Punjab.

Liangshun Wu received the Ph.D. degree from Wuhan University, in 2021, the first M.S. degree from Wuhan University, Wuhan, China, in 2017, the second M.S. degree in computer information technology from Northern Arizona University, Flagstaff, Arizona, in 2022, the third M.S. degree in communications engineering from Xi'an University of Posts and Telecommunications, Xi'an, China, in 2023, and the B.S. degree from Central South University, Changsha, China, in 2014. He is a Research Assistant and a Postdoctoral Fellow with Shanghai Jiao Tong University, Shanghai, China.

Index

A

C

D

P

R

S

T

www.ingramcontent.com/pod-product-compliance
Lightning Source LLC
LaVergne TN
LVHW080638011026
849160LV00014B/1251
9798337300924